Regenerative Medicine

Editor

SANTOS F. MARTINEZ

PHYSICAL MEDICINE AND REHABILITATION CLINICS OF NORTH AMERICA

www.pmr.theclinics.com

Consulting Editor
SANTOS F. MARTINEZ

November 2016 • Volume 27 • Number 4

ELSEVIER

1600 John F. Kennedy Boulevard • Suite 1800 • Philadelphia, Pennsylvania, 19103-2899

http://www.theclinics.com

PHYSICAL MEDICINE AND REHABILITATION CLINICS OF NORTH AMERICA Volume 27, Number 4
November 2016 ISSN 1047-9651, ISBN 978-0-323-47692-8

Editor: Lauren Boyle
Developmental Editor: Donald Mumford

Reprints. For copies of 100 or more of articles in this publication, please contact the Commercial Reprints Department, Elsevier Inc., 360 Park Avenue South, New York, NY 10010-1710. Tel.: 212-633-3874; Fax: 212-633-3820; E-mail: reprints@elsevier.com.

Physical Medicine and Rehabilitation Clinics of North America (ISSN 1047-9651) is published quarterly by Elsevier Inc., 360 Park Avenue South, New York, NY 10010-1710. Months of issue are February, May, August, and November. Business and Editorial Offices: 1600 John F. Kennedy Blvd., Suite 1800, Philadelphia, PA 19103-2899. Customer Service Office: 3251 Riverport Lane, Maryland Heights, MO 63043. Periodicals postage paid at New York, NY and additional mailing offices. Subscription price per year is $280.00 (US individuals), $538.00 (US institutions), $100.00 (US students), $335.00 (Canadian individuals), $709.00 (Canadian institutions), $210.00 (Canadian students), $415.00 (foreign individuals), $709.00 (foreign institutions), and $210.00 (foreign students). Foreign air speed delivery is included in all *Clinics* subscription prices. All prices are subject to change without notice. **POSTMASTER:** Send address changes to *Physical Medicine and Rehabilitation Clinics of North America*, Customer Service Office: Elsevier Health Sciences Division, Subscription Customer Service, 3251 Riverport Lane, Maryland Heights, MO 63043. **Customer Service: 1-800-654-2452 (US). From outside of the United States, call 314-447-8871. Fax: 314-447-8029. E-mail: JournalsCustomer Service-usa@elsevier.com (for print support); JournalsOnlineSupport-usa@elsevier.com (for online support).**

Physical Medicine and Rehabilitation Clinics of North America is indexed in *Excerpta Medica, MEDLINE/ PubMed (Index Medicus), Cinahl,* and *Cumulative Index to Nursing and Allied Health Literature.*

Contributors

CONSULTING EDITOR

SANTOS F. MARTINEZ, MD, MS
Diplomate of the American Academy of Physical Medicine and Rehabilitation,
Certificate of Added Qualification Sports Medicine, Assistant Professor, Department of
Orthopaedics, Campbell Clinic Orthopaedics, University of Tennessee, Memphis,
Tennessee

EDITOR

SANTOS F. MARTINEZ, MD, MS
Diplomate of the American Academy of Physical Medicine and Rehabilitation,
Certificate of Added Qualification Sports Medicine, Assistant Professor, Department of
Orthopaedics, Campbell Clinic Orthopaedics, University of Tennessee, Memphis,
Tennessee

AUTHORS

ROBERT W. ALEXANDER, MD, DMD, FICS
Clinical Associate Professor, Department of Surgery, University of Washington,
Stevensville, Montana

MATTHEW C. BAYES, MD
Bluetail Medical Group, St Louis, Missouri; Chesterfield, Missouri

KWADWO BOACHIE-ADJEI, BS, CPH
Department of Physiatry, Hospital for Special Surgery, New York, New York

JOANNE BORG-STEIN, MD
Chief of Sports and Musculoskeletal Rehabilitation; Medical Director; Associate
Professor, Department of Physical Medicine and Rehabilitation, Newton-Wellesley
Hospital Spine Center, Spaulding Rehabilitation Hospital, Harvard Medical School,
Wellesley, Massachusetts

MICHAEL N. BROWN, DC, MD
Bellevue, Washington; Monterey, California

CHRISTOPHER J. CENTENO, MD
Centeno Schultz Clinic, Broomfield, Colorado

XAVIER CHEVALIER, MD
Professor, Department of Rheumatology, Hopital Henri Mondor, UPEC Paris XII
University, Creteil, France

HONGSIK CHO, PhD
Associate Professor, Department of Orthopaedic Surgery and Biomedical Engineering, Campbell Clinic/UTHSC, VA Medical Center, Memphis, Tennessee

DAVID M. CRANE, MD
Bluetail Medical Group, St Louis, Missouri; Naples, Florida; Chesterfield, Missouri

JASON M. CUÉLLAR, MD, PhD
Spine Surgeon, Department of Orthopaedic Surgery, Cedars-Sinai Medical Center, Los Angeles, California

VANESSA GABROVSKY CUÉLLAR, MD
Private Practice Hand and Microvascular Surgeon, Beverly Hills, California

ROBERT DIAZ, MD
Resident Physician, Department of Physical Medicine and Rehabilitation, Spaulding Rehabilitation Hospital, Harvard Medical School, Charlestown, Massachusetts

CHRISTOPHER H. EVANS, PhD
Director, Rehabilitation Medicine Research Center, Mayo Clinic, Rochester, Minnesota

MAYO F. FRIEDLIS, MD
Stem Cell Arts, Chevy Chase, Maryland

ALFRED C. GELLHORN, MD
Division of Rehabilitation Medicine, Weill Cornell Medical College, New York-Presbyterian Hospital, New York, New York

JULIAN HARRISON, BS
Department of Physiatry, Hospital for Special Surgery, New York, New York

KAREN A. HASTY, PhD
VA Research Career Scientist, George Thomas Wilhelm Professor, Department of Orthopaedic Surgery and Biomedical Engineering, Campbell Clinic/UTHSC, VA Medical Center, Memphis, Tennessee

PENNY L. HEAD, PT, MS, SCS, ATC, CSCS
Assistant Professor, Department of Physical Therapy, University of Tennessee Health Science Center, Memphis, Tennessee

GREGORY LUTZ, MD
Associate Professor of Clinical Rehabilitation Medicine, Weill Cornell Medical College; Department of Physiatry, Hospital for Special Surgery, New York, New York

ANGELIE MASCARINAS, MD
Department of Physiatry, Hospital for Special Surgery, New York, New York

KRISTIN S. OLIVER, MD, MPH
Bluetail Medical Group, St Louis, Missouri; Columbia, Missouri; Naples, Florida; Chesterfield, Missouri

DAVID P. RABAGO, MD
Associate Professor, Department of Family Medicine and Community Health, University of Wisconsin School of Medicine and Public Health, Madison, Wisconsin

ETHAN RAND, MD
Division of Rehabilitation Medicine, Weill Cornell Medical College, New York-Presbyterian Hospital, New York, New York

KENNETH DEAN REEVES, MD
Private Practice, Roeland Park, Kansas; Clinical Assistant; Associate Professor (1986–2015), Department of Physical Medicine and Rehabilitation, University of Kansas Medical Center, Kansas City, Kansas

DAVID R. RICHARDSON, MD
Department of Orthopaedic Surgery and Biomedical Engineering, University of Tennessee-Campbell Clinic, Memphis, Tennessee

DAVID J. RUTA, MD
St. Luke's Department of Orthopedics and Sports Medicine, Duluth, Minnesota

MICHAEL SCARPONE, DO
Trinity Sports Medicine and Performance Center, Steubenville, Ohio

GAETANO J. SCUDERI, MD
Orthopaedic Spine Surgeon, Jupiter, Florida

BRIAN J. SHIPLE, DO
Glenn Mills, Pennsylvania

REGINA W.S. SIT, MD
Assistant Professor, The Jockey Club School of Public Health and Primary Care, The Chinese University of Hong Kong, Hong Kong

ARTURO D. VILLARREAL, MD
Department of Orthopaedic Surgery and Biomedical Engineering, University of Tennessee-Campbell Clinic, Memphis, Tennessee

PETER WEHLING, MD, PhD
CEO, Orthogen AG, Düsseldorf, Germany

PETER I-KUNG WU, MD, PhD
Resident Physician, Department of Physical Medicine and Rehabilitation, Spaulding Rehabilitation Hospital, Harvard Medical School, Charlestown, Massachusetts

Contents

> Healing is a complex process of orchestrated reactions and interactions with the goal of restoring structure and physical properties to damaged tissues. The musculoskeletal system is composed of different types of connective tissues. When healthy, each has a unique structure, function, and remodeling process. When damaged, they demonstrate unique healing processes. However, similarities in the process exist. Understanding these properties of healing is critical in the development and application of regenerative therapeutics. This article describes the common phases of healing, differences between healing in musculoskeletal tissues, factors that affect healing, and strategies to facilitate and optimize healing.

> Dextrose prolotherapy (DPT) is a treatment for chronic pain involving the injection of hypertonic dextrose at soft tissue attachments or within joint spaces. The mechanism of action of DPT is likely multifactorial. Controlled animal and human trials have reported proliferation of soft tissue and a potential direct neural effect of dextrose injections. Systematic review of clinical trials show that DPT reduces pain and improves function in the long term for knee osteoarthritis; existing studies also suggest that DPT is efficacious for finger/hand osteoarthritis and Osgood Schlatter disease, and may be efficacious for rotator cuff tendinopathy, lateral epicondylosis, and sacroiliac pain.

> Platelet-rich plasma (PRP) is a growing and robust therapeutic option in musculoskeletal medicine. PRP is a preparation of autologous plasma enriched with a platelet concentration above that normally contained in whole blood. The rationale for use and therapeutic potential of a high concentration of platelets is based on their capacity to supply supraphysiologic amounts of essential growth factors to provide a regenerative stimulus that promotes repair in tissues with low healing potential. This article reviews the latest basic science on PRP, clinical evidence for its use in musculoskeletal medicine, limitations in current knowledge, and critical areas for future research.

Although there is ample evidence that beneficial results can be obtained from the use of mesenchymal stem cells, several questions regarding their use remain to be answered. For many of these questions, preclinical models will be helpful, but the task of evaluating and implementing these findings for orthopaedic patients falls onto the shoulders of clinical researchers. Evaluation of these questions is daunting, but such a challenge fits the concept of personalized medicine in today's medicine.

"Using your own tissues to heal" represents a major health care paradigm change and is one of the most exciting minimally invasive options currently available. Biocellular regenerative therapies are rapidly improving in documentation and cellular analyses and are gaining good safety and efficacy profiles. Once considered purely experimental, they have entered into an accepted, translational period to clinical providers, backed by improving science supporting the basic hypotheses. It is a well-recognized and reported alternative to many traditional medical/surgical interventions.

Autologous conditioned serum was developed in the mid 1990s as an expeditious, practical, and relatively inexpensive means of generating the interleukin-1 receptor antagonist, a naturally occurring inhibitor of the cytokine interleukin-1. The latter is thought to be an important mediator of inflammation, pain, and tissue destruction in musculoskeletal conditions. ACS has been widely and successfully used in the local treatment of human and equine osteoarthritis and radicular compression; it has also shown promise in treating tendinopathies, muscle injuries, and tunnel widening after reconstruction of the anterior cruciate ligament. Experience suggests that autologous conditioned serum is safe and effective.

α_2-Macroglobulin (A2M) is a plasma glycoprotein best known for its ability to inhibit a broad spectrum of serine, threonine, and metalloproteases as well as inflammatory cytokines by a unique bait-and-trap method. A2M has emerged as a unique potential treatment of cartilage-based pathology and inflammatory arthritides. This article describes the unique method by which A2M not only inhibits the associated inflammatory cascade but also disrupts the catabolic process of cartilage degeneration. Autologous concentrated A2M from plasma is currently in use to successfully treat various painful arthritides. Future directions will focus on recombinant variants that enhance its anti-inflammatory and disease-modifying potential.

Bone marrow aspiration (BMA) is increasingly being used to harvest stem cells for use in regenerative medicine. The focus of BMA in interventional orthopedics is to maximize the yield of mesenchymal stem cells. The authors present an improved method for BMA that involves fluoroscope or ultrasound guidance combined with anesthesia; in the authors' experience, it produces the highest possible stem cell yield and is well tolerated by patients. The authors provide a step-by-step guide to the process, along with a discussion of technical and other considerations and quick reference guides for ultrasound- and fluoroscope-guided BMA.

Tendon and ligament injuries and degenerative conditions of these soft tissues have poor healing potential and healing is often incomplete. Biocellular and orthobiologic approaches including PRP and stem cell therapies are reviewed. A review of some of the regenerative medicine science and difficulties facing physicians exploring these methods is presented. A series of cases are reviewed demonstrating the application of these principles. Clinical experience with many of these biocellular interventions is outpacing validation in basic science studies. Clinical experience dictates the need for repeated clinical and imaging evaluation and the need for repeated intervention or change in strategies when needed.

This article reviews the current options in orthobiologics for the clinical treatment of knee osteoarthritis (OA). We describe a new model of knee OA that fills the gap in our understanding of it as a purely traumatic and/or inflammation-induced cartilage degenerative condition, to a current model of multinodal pathophysiology. We discuss graft choice and patient selection in the current state of understanding of the treatment of knee OA in a tissue engineering model with orthobiologics. We present a sample treatment algorithm and decision nest for deciding how to proceed with patient care.

A literature review of clinical and translational studies was performed to provide an overview of current concepts on regenerative treatments for

The limited natural capacity for articular cartilage to regenerate has led to a continuously broadening array of surgical interventions. Typically employed once patients' symptoms are no longer relieved by nonoperative management, these methods share the goals of joint preservation and restoration. Techniques include bone marrow stimulation, whole-tissue transplantation, and cell-based strategies, each with its own variations. Many of these interventions are performed arthroscopically or with extended-portal techniques. Indications, operative techniques, unique benefits, and limitations are presented.

Rehabilitation and regenerative medicine therapies has shown improved outcomes for tissue regeneration. Regenerative rehabilitation guides protocols regarding when to start therapy, types of stimuli administered, and graded exercise programs, taking into account biological factors and technologies designed to optimize healing potential. Although there are currently no evidence-based guidelines for rehabilitation, fundamental physical therapy principles likely apply. Immobilization tends to have deleterious effects on musculoskeletal tissues; mechanical loading promotes tissue healing and regeneration. Common physical therapy interventions may provide beneficial effects after the application of regenerative therapies. Research is needed to determine optimal rehabilitation protocols to enhance tissue healing and regeneration.

PHYSICAL MEDICINE AND REHABILITATION CLINICS OF NORTH AMERICA

VISIT THE CLINICS ONLINE!
Access your subscription at:
www.theclinics.com

Preface

Maybe There Is an Alternative Treatment Option

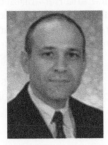

Santos F. Martinez, MD, MS
Editor

The growth in regenerative medical efforts to enhance one's natural reserves to facilitate healing and resolution of musculoskeletal conditions is appealing and thought provoking. Our prior issue focused on outpatient ultrasound-guided procedures, further expanding the field of the neuromusculoskeletal or orthopedic Interventionalist. This regenerative issue certainly further pushes the envelope into an area that is certainly sure to challenge some practitioners' comfort levels, but it is possibly a glimpse of what may be a paradigm shift. Preliminary studies, clinical experience, and patient anecdotal reports on the positive effects of regenerative treatments make it difficult to discount these modalities. Frequently, the only other options open for these patients through our traditional treatment algorithms were surgery. As with many technological advances, theories and claims frequently outpace literature. The lack of high-quality studies, especially in the human model, makes it difficult to establish a sound standard of care in this ever-expanding field. Many questions remain unanswered regarding efficacy, appropriate patient candidacy, optimal graft sources and harvesting techniques, quantification of mesenchymal cells, use of growth factor facilitators, nutritional support, and various other novel techniques to downregulate nociceptors and enhance autonomic contributors to healing.

This issue of *Physical Medicine and Rehabilitation Clinics of North America* in some ways may seem premature because the data certainly are in their infancy, but at the same time, it is hoped, may serve as a catalyst. The issue of safety is certainly of concern as regulatory agencies struggle to balance the scale between encouraging innovation while safeguarding patient safety. Fortunately, a concerted effort is evolving to more definitively answer many of these questions. The clinician must temper enthusiasm for meeting the demand of an ever-expanding patient market with techniques based on sound scientific reasoning while remaining within governmental guidelines.

The editor is extremely grateful to the authors and their willingness to share their diverse approaches and expertise. They take us from basic science and physiology

Phys Med Rehabil Clin N Am 27 (2016) xiii–xiv
http://dx.doi.org/10.1016/j.pmr.2016.09.001
1047-9651/16/© 2016 Published by Elsevier Inc.

pmr.theclinics.com

to didactic-oriented clinical techniques treating a variety of musculoskeletal conditions. The frontier for the minimally invasive musculoskeletal and regenerative practitioner is encouraging, challenging a complacency of what currently is for a vision of what can be. I hope the reader will enjoy the journey.

Santos F. Martinez, MD, MS
American Academy of Physical Medicine and Rehabilitation
Campbell Clinic Orthopaedics
Department of Orthopaedics
University of Tennessee
Memphis, TN, USA

E-mail address:
smartinez@campbellclinic.com

The Healing Cascade
Facilitating and Optimizing the System

Ethan Rand, MD, Alfred C. Gellhorn, MD*

KEYWORDS

- Regenerative medicine • Healing • Repair • Regeneration • Inflammation
- Proliferation • Remodeling

KEY POINTS

- When healthy, each type of musculoskeletal tissue has a unique structure, function, and remodeling process.
- When damaged, each type of musculoskeletal tissue demonstrates a unique process in healing.
- Understanding the unique properties of healing is critical in regenerative medicine, and in the development and application of regenerative therapeutics.
- There are many intrinsic and extrinsic factors that affect healing. An understanding of these factors can facilitate and optimize healing.

INTRODUCTION

Healing is a complex process of orchestrated reactions and interactions with the goal of restoring structure and physical properties to damaged tissues. The musculoskeletal system is composed of different types of connective tissues, including muscle, tendon, ligament, cartilage, and bone. When healthy, each type of tissue has a unique structure, function, and remodeling process. When damaged these tissues also demonstrate unique processes in healing. Despite unique features of repair in each tissue type, overarching similarities in the repair process also exist. Understanding these properties of healing is critical in regenerative medicine, and in the development and application of regenerative therapeutics. This article describes the common phases of healing, differences between healing in musculoskeletal tissues, factors that affect healing, and strategies to facilitate and optimize healing.

PHASES OF HEALING

Although each tissue type has unique aspects to healing, traditionally, healing has been divided into 3 common phases: inflammation, proliferation, and maturation.

Division of Rehabilitation Medicine, Weill Cornell Medical College, New York-Presbyterian Hospital, 525 East 68th Street, New York, NY 10065, USA
* Corresponding author.
E-mail address: alg9109@med.cornell.edu

Phys Med Rehabil Clin N Am 27 (2016) 765–781
http://dx.doi.org/10.1016/j.pmr.2016.07.001
1047-9651/16/© 2016 Elsevier Inc. All rights reserved.

Inflammation (from Injury Through Days 4 to 6)

Hemostasis

Hemostasis and inflammation begin immediately after injury and initiate healing. The body begins by controlling bleeding: injured blood vessels vasoconstrict and the coagulation cascade is activated. Platelets aggregate to form a clot made of collagen, thrombin, and fibronectin. The clot serves as a scaffold for invading cells and stimulates the release of cytokines and growth factors from the platelets, initiating the inflammatory pathway. Cytokines target hematopoietic cells to control immune response, and include chemokines, lymphokines, monokines, interleukins (ILs), colony-stimulating factors, and interferons. Growth factors act on nonhematopoietic cells to modulate healing, and include transforming growth factor (TGF), platelet-derived growth factor (PDGF), vascular endothelial growth factor (VEGF), epidermal growth factor, fibroblast growth factor (FGF), connective tissue growth factor, and insulin-like growth factor, among others. Overall, this phase results in vasodilatation and increased vascular permeability and migration of cells.

Inflammation

Inflammatory mediators modulate this phase of healing. Eicosanoids, a family of arachidonic acid (ArA) metabolites, including prostaglandins and leukotrienes, accumulate, drawing neutrophils into the injured area by IL-1, tumor necrosis factor (TNF)-α, platelet factor (PF)-4, and TGF-β. Neutrophils begin clearing cellular debris using proteolytic enzymes, including serine proteases and metalloproteinases, which digest collagen and break down the existing extracellular matrix (ECM) at the site of injury. Uninjured tissue is protected from these enzymes by protease inhibitors but may be overwhelmed by a robust inflammatory response.[1]

Phagocytosis

Monocytes are attracted to the area by TGF-β, PDGF, PF4, IL-1, and leukotriene B4. Monocytes transform into macrophages around 48 to 96 hours after injury. The macrophages phagocytize the neutrophils and are stimulated by TNF and IL-1 to generate nitric oxide (NO), and additional matrix metalloproteinases (MMPs), clearing and allowing for cell migration into the ECM. Activated macrophages are critical in recruiting fibroblasts to the injured site, transitioning to the proliferative stage of healing. As the number of neutrophils and platelets increase, a cessation of the inflammatory phase of healing is triggered by lipoxins.[2]

Proliferation (Day 4 Through 14)

Angiogenesis

The proliferative stage of healing is led by fibroblasts and epithelial cells. VEGF attracts endothelial cells to the injured area and initiates angiogenesis with the formation of new capillaries. The endothelial cells produce NO via endothelial NO synthase in response to hypoxia, causing vasodilation and increased blood flow to the site of injury.

Fibroplasia

Additional fibroblasts migrate to the injured site and are stimulated primarily by PDGF and TNF-α–derived from platelets and macrophages to begin synthesizing collagen, and a provisional matrix composed of type III collagen, glycosaminoglycans, and fibronectin.[3] TGF-β further directs ECM production and a decrease in its degradation, stimulating fibroblasts to increase production of collagen.

Maturation and Remodeling (Day 8 to 1 Year)

The main feature of the maturation and remodeling phase is strengthening of the ECM and production of collagen in an organized network. Disruption of this stage may affect the strength and appearance of the repaired tissue. The preliminary ECM, composed of fibrin and fibronectin, glycosaminoglycans, proteoglycans, and other proteins, is replaced by an organized matrix made of stronger collagen fibrils. Over time, collagen deposition thickens and is organized along lines of stress. Even after maturation, the collagen in the repaired tissue will never become as organized or strong as the collagen found in uninjured tissues.[4]

MUSCULOSKELETAL TISSUE TYPES: DIFFERENCES IN HEALING

To understand how each tissue type in the musculoskeletal system responds to injury, the basic structures and functions of each respective tissue must first be explored.

Muscle

Structure and function

Muscle is capable of contraction, which generates loads that are transmitted across joints to facilitate motion and provide stability. Myofibrils contain actin and myosin filaments, forming sarcomeres, the fundamental unit of muscle contraction. Myofibrils aggregate within the muscle cell to form fibers and are surrounded by endomysium. Fibers aggregate to form fascicles, encased by perimysium. Finally, fascicles aggregate and are surrounded by epimysium.

Healing

Repair of muscle tissue proceeds through the phases of inflammation, proliferation, and remodeling.[5,6] When muscle tissue is injured, myofibers rupture along with local capillaries, a flux of calcium is released, and clot formation begins. Inflammatory cells migrate to the injured site, leading to phagocytosis of damaged tissues, and activation of fibroblast and satellite cells, which are myogenic stem cells.[7-9] During the proliferative phase, satellite cells differentiate into myoblasts, fusing with the injured myofibers. In the remodeling phase, the new myofibers grow and differentiate into fully mature muscle fibers.[8]

Tendon

Structure and function

Tendon is a mechanosensitive tissue that connects muscle to bone and transmits force to produce motion. Tendon attaches to muscle through the myotendinous junction and to bone through the fibrocartilaginous enthesis, rich in type II cartilage.[10] Tendon has a hierarchical fibrillar structure. Triple-helical type I collagen molecules assemble densely into fibrils within an ECM, parallel to the muscle tendon axis, and along lines of stress. The ECM is composed of collagens, elastin, proteoglycans, and glycoproteins. Fibrils are then assembled into fibers, which are assembled into fascicles, surrounded by endotenon. Ultimately fascicles are bundled and surrounded by epitenon, forming the tendon unit.

Healing

Acute and chronic tendon injury may disrupt the highly organized structure of collagen in tendon. Most commonly, tendon injury results in tendinopathy but may also result in tendon tear. The pathophysiology of tendinopathy is not completely understood and is thought to result in part from impaired healing, with increased noncollagenous ECM, hypercellularity, and neovascularization.[11] Additionally, the role of inflammation is not clearly established and is a point of controversy.[12]

Tendon healing follows the phases of inflammation, proliferation, and remodeling.[13,14] These tissues may heal at a slower rate than other connective tissues due to their dense and hypocellular nature.[15] During the phases of tendon healing, tendon fibroblasts, or tenocytes, are the primary cell regulating homeostasis and respond to chemical and mechanical changes in the environment.[16] These cells are responsible for collagen and other ECM matrix proteins during the proliferative stage of healing. Initially, these proteins are highly disorganized, primarily composed of type III collagen, and subsequently undergo remodeling during the final phase of healing, resulting in replacement with type I collagen, decreased cellularity and vascularity, and improved structure and strength.[17,18] However, as with other connective tissues, healed tendon does not have the same mechanical properties of uninjured tissue.[19]

Ligament

Structure and function
Ligament has a similar hierarchical structure to tendons, linking bone with bone, stabilizing joints, and generally operating under a reduced load compared with tendon. Predominantly, type I collagen is organized into parallel, crosslinked fibers along lines of stress. Ligaments function to provide passive joint stability through normal range of motion and to provide joint proprioception.[20]

Healing
Ligaments are most often injured in traumatic joint injuries, resulting in either partial or complete discontinuity. Ligament healing proceeds through the 3 phases of inflammation, proliferation, and remodeling. Ligament healing depends on the size of the initial injury and whether contact exists between torn segments. During the first phase, retraction of the disrupted segments of ligament leads to gap formation that is filled with clot, which is subsequently resorbed and replaced with cellular infiltrate. Of note, several intra-articular ligaments, such as the anterior cruciate ligament, have limited clot formation at the site of injury, perhaps due to circulating levels of plasmin within the synovial fluid, which may prematurely dissolve the fibrin clot.[21,22]

In the next phase, fibroblast proliferation increases production of collagen and ECM, bridging the torn ends of the ligament. Initially, this disorganized tissue is primarily composed of type III collagen. As healing proceeds into the remodeling phase, the healed tissue becomes more organized and collagen is arranged longitudinal to the multiple planes of force transmitted. Several changes persist after the conclusion of the healing cascade, including limited collagen crosslinking,[23] increased cellularity, smaller collagen fibril size,[24] increased vascularity,[25] and abnormal innervation. Functionally, healed ligamentous tissue is less elastic than healthy tissue.[26]

Bone

Structure and function
Bone provides structure and support for attaching soft tissues. Functionally, bone also serves as a home for hematopoiesis and calcium metabolism. Bone is a composite structure, including cells, ECM, and lipids. The fundamental unit of cortical bone is the osteon, a cylindrical structure, surrounded by several layers of lamellae, containing ECM and osteocytes. Lamellae are densely packed together and surrounded by a highly vascularized periosteum.

Healing

Bone also proceeds through the typical phases of inflammation, proliferation, and remodeling. The inflammatory phase of bone healing begins with bleeding from the periosteal vessels and clot formation at the site of fracture. Cytokines and growth factors are released and responsible for the migration and proliferation of chondroblasts and osteoblasts. The fracture gap is initially filled with granulation tissue and a primitive callus develops, providing some degree of stability at the fracture site.[27,28]

During proliferation, the formation of callus continues, with the differentiation of chondrogenic stem cells into chondrocytes, producing cartilage to initially form of a soft callus.[29,30] Osteoblasts gradually replace the cartilage in the soft callus with immature woven bone via endochondral bone formation, further stabilizing the injured site and forming a hard callus.[31] The hard callus is further reinforced during the remodeling phase, where irregular woven bone is converted into lamellar bone, along lines of force, restoring strength and stability to the repaired bone.[27] Remodeling may occur over months to years.[29]

Cartilage

Structure and function

Articular, or hyaline cartilage lines the end of bones within joints. It can withstand tremendous forces generated through joints and allows for smooth gliding motion without significant friction. Articular cartilage is a highly organized, smooth, translucent tissue, which is hypocellular, aneural, avascular, alymphatic, and composed primarily of type II collagen, ground substance composed of proteoglycans, and elastin. The ECM of cartilage is hyperhydrated with water accounting for over 80% of the total weight.[32] Chondrocytes are located within the ECM of the cartilage and are responsible for synthesis and maintenance of the ECM.

Anatomically, there are 4 main zones within articular cartilage that facilitate its attachment to subchondral bone. The superficial zone is the thinnest, with type II collagen oriented parallel to the articulating surface and with flattened chondrocytes. There is a random organization of type II collagen and spherical chondrocytes within the intermediate zone. The deep zone has type II collagen oriented perpendicular to the joint surface, with spherical chondrocytes. A tidemark then separates this basal layer from the final calcified cartilage zone that participated in endochondral ossification during growth.[33]

Healing

The intrinsic capability of articular cartilage to repair is limited by the lack of vascularity and density of the ECM.[33] The absence of blood supply inhibits the normal healing response that is present in the other connective tissues (see previous discussion). Chondrocytes are present in cartilage but trapped in lacunae and cannot easily migrate to damaged sites. Partial-thickness chondral defects may not show any healing response.[34] On the other hand, a defect that penetrates the subchondral plate has a greater capacity to heal because it may facilitate clot formation and cell migration.[35] However the resulting repair typically resembles fibrocartilage, rather than hyaline cartilage, with less stiffness and resilience.[33,36]

FACTORS THAT AFFECT HEALING

With an understanding of the phases of healing and the unique characteristics of each tissue type, one can appreciate the multiple factors that may alter the complex orchestrated process of repair and work toward optimizing the healing.

Local Factors

Oxygen

Healing requires energy in the form of adenosine triphosphate (ATP). Initially, anaerobic conditions produce ATP via glycolysis.[37] As healing progresses, there is an increased need for energy and ATP is produced via oxidative phosphorylation and requires a rich blood supply. Limitation in oxygen available to the healing site may slow or halt healing.[38] Fibroblasts are resistant to hypoxia and still proliferate in low oxygen environments. However, there is a marked decrease in collagen production in the presence of hypoxia. Hypoxia is also a powerful stimulus for angiogenesis and may explain the abnormal neovascularization seen in some forms of tendinopathy.[39]

Hyperbaric oxygen therapy (HBOT) has been advocated as a treatment option for chronic wounds for many years, with the rationale that this may increase available oxygen at the site of wound healing. HBOT is not widely available and its use remains controversial. A systematic review has shown that HBOT decreases the rate of amputations in patients with diabetic foot ulcers but there does not seem to be a similar beneficial effect for other types of wounds, such as those due to venous stasis, arterial deficiency, or pressure.[40] In musculoskeletal tissues specifically, HBOT does not affect recovery from delayed onset muscle soreness,[41] and no clinical studies in humans have evaluated HBOT effects on tendon, ligament, and bone healing.

Pressure

Edema or elevated tissue pressures can prolong the inflammatory stage and delay the healing response. Mast cells produce numerous cytokines, histamines, and NO associated with increased inflammatory reaction, edema, and possible ischemia-reperfusion injury.[42] A rise in internal or external pressure can increase capillary closure, thereby causing hypoxia and associated ischemic sequelae.

Mechanical

Normal development and remodeling of musculoskeletal connective tissues occurs with repetitive healthy loading. Mechanical loading is also essential in tissue response and repair to injury, particularly in the proliferation and remodeling phases because loads drive the anabolic response and reorganization of collagen and the ECM, as well as fluid exchange. Mechanical stimuli lead to a signaling response, involving growth and transcription factors; however, the precise involvement of these factors in development and repair is not completely understood. For instance, in tendon, tensile loads stretch tenocytes and activate protein kinases and an anabolic response, promoted by TGF-β, FGF, and transcription factors, including scleraxis, which is critical to tendon formation, differentiation, and modulating collagen synthesis.[43–47]

Loading, rather than immobilization, may facilitate healing in tendon tissue. For example, loading stimulates repair of the Achilles tendon, which is impaired with immobilization.[48] Immobilization in this case has been associated with decreased levels of ECM expression, loss of normal ECM structure, and altered tenocyte morphology, resulting in impaired function.[16] Eccentric exercise therapy, with activation of the muscle and tendon while lengthening, has become a primary treatment for tendinopathy.[49–51] These exercises improve symptoms and tendon structure.[52] Optimal load, speed, number of cycles, and duration require further investigation for each tissue type. For instance, in the case of tendon healing, a 4% strain produced tenogenic differentiation, whereas an 8% strain initiated more adipogenic, chondrogenic, and osteogenic differentiation of tendon-derived stem cells.[46] These different cellular responses to loading during healing may explain some features of failed healing in which tendons exhibit bone, fat, and cartilage tissue in areas of chronic injury. Tendon response to load is best understood in the context of a generalized stress-strain curve as shown in **Fig. 1**. Using the correlation between tensile load and tendon deformation, it can be seen that various inflection points along the curve are areas for potential intervention. That is, an exercise program that could reliably produce 4% strain in a tendon would have potentially far-reaching clinical applications. However, in vivo measurement of tendon strain remains technically challenging. Newer imaging techniques, such as shear wave elastography, may offer guidance in these types of measurements in the future.

Bone healing is also affected by mechanical loading. Dynamic and cyclical, rather than static loading, stimulates proliferation of bone. Low-magnitude, high-frequency loads with periods of rest between loading periods have the greatest effect on healing.[53–56] Additionally, compressive loading, rather than shear or tensile loading, produces increased mineralization and strength of callus formation.[57–60] These observations form the basis for the use of low intensity ultrasound in bone healing. Ultrasound activates cell surface mechanoreceptors on osteoblasts, upregulating the production of growth factors and other proteins important in the healing response.

Systemic

Systemic conditions that affect healing have been studied in surgical patients to predict complications in reconstructive surgery.[61] Though these factors have been described primarily in injuries to cutaneous and subcutaneous tissues, the same principles impact healing musculoskeletal injuries. These conditions may affect wound healing for a multitude of reasons. For instance, diabetes mellitus (DM) affects healing via vascular, metabolic, and neuropathic pathways. Conditions that significantly alter the immune system, resulting in increased immune response, inflammation, or immunosuppression can affect the healing. Additionally, age is associated with impaired

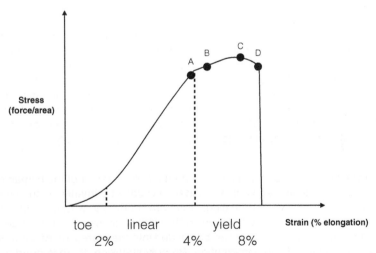

Fig. 1. Generalized stress-strain curve. Point A is the elastic limit. Tissue will have plastic deformation with further stress. B is the yield point. Relatively little stress produces large strain. Point C is the ultimate material strength. Point D is rupture. In the toe region, relatively little stress is required to uncrimp the tendon fibers. In the linear region, fibers are aligned and more stress is required to produce additional elongation. Near the end of this region, additional stress will begin to separate the collagen fibers, resulting in microinjury, corresponding to breaking crosslinks between fibrils. Macrofailure occurs at 8% to 10%.

healing; however, it is difficult to distinguish age alone from those of diseases commonly associated with increased age.[37]

Perfusion

Decreased perfusion can be local (see previous discussion) or systemic due to cardiac dysfunction, peripheral vascular disease, or decreased circulatory volumes. Conditions that reduce systemic perfusion or decrease systemic oxygen concentrations will impair healing. Likewise, cardiovascular exercise can enhance perfusion and thus have a positive impact on healing.

Systemic diseases

Systemic diseases that alter immune function, protein metabolism, or collagen formation can impact tissue repair. Several examples include connective tissue disorders (CTDs), DM, hypothyroidism, malignancy, and organ failure. CTDs, such as Ehlers-Danlos syndrome or osteogenesis imperfecta, result in alterations in tissue strength, elasticity, integrity, and healing. Increased serum glucose levels in DM have significant deleterious effects on healing. The pathophysiology of impaired healing in DM was traditionally thought of as a microvascular occlusive process, though evidence supports additional mechanisms that impair healing, including increased levels of sorbitol, a toxic byproduct of glucose metabolism that may accumulate in tissues.[62] Hypothyroidism is associated with decreased fibroblast function and collagen production, as well as systemic complications. Improved control of these conditions may result in improved healing response.

Malignancies can detrimentally affect healing for a multitude of reasons, including poor nutrition, organ compromise, immunosuppression, and hematologic effects; or as a result of therapeutics, such as antimetabolic, cytotoxic and steroidal agents, immunotherapy, and radiation. Chemotherapy results in bone marrow suppression and inhibits an appropriate inflammatory response and fibroblast collagen formation,[63] whereas radiation increases free radical production, reduces tissue oxygenation, fibroblast proliferation, and inflammatory response.[37]

Organ failure, whether gastrointestinal, renal, hepatic, or cardiopulmonary interferes with tissue repair. Gastrointestinal failure leads to disruption in absorption of critical nutrients and energy. Renal failure increases uremic toxins and a metabolic acidosis can affect healing by altering the immune system. Additionally, there are decreased neutrophil and lymphocyte responses in the setting of dialysis.[37] Hepatic failure decreases clotting factors, protein production, and alters glucose regulation. Finally, failure of the cardiopulmonary system results in reduced perfusion or gas exchange and leads to hypoxemia and resultant tissue hypoxia at the site of injury.

Nutrition

Literature specifically evaluating the role of nutrition in the repair of the human musculoskeletal tissues is limited and current evidence is based primarily on animal models and research in surgical wound healing. Nutritional compounds play a critical role in protein synthesis and immune function, both integral to the healing process. The impact of nutrition on tissue repair can be divided into the correction of nutritional deficiencies and nutritional supplementation. Broadly speaking, there is good scientific support for correcting any nutritional deficiencies in the setting of healing but supra-normal doses of micronutrients and vitamins do not seem to accelerate or improve a healing response.

Deficiencies of energy, macronutrients, and micronutrients can all impair healing.[64] When metabolic requirements of healing exceed caloric intake, body fat and protein are consumed, particularly skeletal muscle. Insufficient nutrition can also elevate endogenous steroid levels, which is associated with muscle catabolism. Careful attention to energy intake is also needed. Following musculoskeletal injury, mobilization and activity levels are often reduced. Thus, one may conclude that energy requirements will decrease significantly following injury; however, this is not necessarily the case. Though prior activity levels will be reduced, tissue repair is an energy intensive process, with an increase of 15% to 50% depending on the type and severity of injury.[65] Additionally, altered mobility may require increased energy expenditure. For example, ambulating with crutches may require 2 to 3 times the energy of normal ambulation.[66]

Healing is heavily reliant on protein synthesis and the formation of collagen. Insufficient protein and amino acid intake will impair healing and increase inflammation.[67] Arginine and methionine are important in collagen and matrix deposition, cellular proliferation, and angiogenesis.[68] Supplementation with arginine has been shown to accelerate healing of pressure ulcers.[69] Glutamine enhances the action of lymphocytes, macrophages, and neutrophils, whereas glycine plays a role in inhibiting leukocytes and is important in reducing inflammation-related tissue injury. High-quality or complete proteins found in animal products, meat, and soy contain all essential amino acids.

Oxandrolone, a synthetic analog of testosterone, has been studied in the setting of critical illness and burns, in which there is an increase in catabolism and decrease in protein reserve. In burn patients, the use of oxandrolone results in decreased nitrogen loss, lower loss of lean body mass, and shorter healing time for the donor site for skin grafts. Because musculoskeletal injury does not typically result in similar catabolic states, it is unclear if significant beneficial effects would be expected from similar treatments. The use of oxandrolone has not been formally evaluated in the healing of musculoskeletal Injuries.

Omega-3 fatty acids have anti-inflammatory and immunomodulatory properties.[70] Supplementation may be beneficial for inflammatory conditions or with excessive or prolonged inflammation.[70] However, inflammation is a key phase of healing and careful consideration and use of anti-inflammatory nutrients is necessary because there is some evidence of impaired healing with supplementation of omega-3 fatty acids.[71–73] Dietary fatty acids also play an important role in enhancing bone formation and suppressing bone resorption.[74]

Micronutrients, including vitamins and minerals, are critical in immune function and healing (**Table 1**). Trace metals are cofactors in collagen production.[68] Deficiency is associated with impaired healing but there is no clear evidence to support supranormal intake during tissue repair.[67] Vitamin C influences collagen modification, neutrophil function, acts as an antioxidant, and is the main vitamin associated with impaired healing. Supplementation with vitamin C has been shown to accelerate healing of pressure ulcers.[75] It has also been shown to accelerate fracture healing in animal models.[76] Vitamin A increases collagen synthesis, crosslinking, and inflammatory response. Importantly, vitamin A has been shown to reverse corticosteroid-induced inhibition of wound healing.[77,78] High intake, however, may be linked to increased incidence of hip fractures and poor bone quality.[79] Vitamin D is involved in controlling blood calcium levels, and appropriate levels of both substances are required for bone health and healing.[80] Low vitamin D levels are also associated with delayed healing and reduced strength of rotator cuff tendons in animal models.[81]

Of many trace elements, zinc, copper, and iron have the closest relationship with healing. Zinc is an essential trace element and functions as a cofactor in several enzymatic reactions involved in healing. It influences collagen deposition and lymphocyte activity. Zinc also increases alkaline phosphatase activity and may have a role in

Table 1
Nutrients and micronutrients important for musculoskeletal tissue healing

Nutrient	Normal Range[a]	Function in Healing
Vitamin D	Deficiency <20 ng/mL Insufficiency 20–29 ng/mL Optimum 30–80 ng/mL Toxicity >150 ng/mL	Control of blood calcium levels.
Vitamin A	0.3–1.20 mg/L	Epithelial and bone formation, cellular differentiation
Vitamin C	23–114 μmol/L	Collagen and proteoglycan formation, tissue antioxidant, neutrophil migration
Vitamin E	5.5–18.0 mg/L	Lipid soluble antioxidant in the skin; if levels are too high, inhibition of collagen synthesis
Folate	5.9–24.8 ng/mL	Bone marrow production of red blood cells
Transferrin	0.16–0.36 g/dL	Binds iron, marker of overall nutritional status
Zinc	60–120 μg/dL	DNA synthesis, cell division, protein synthesis
Copper	70–140 μg/dL	Angiogenesis, synthesis, and stabilization of ECM proteins
Magnesium	—	Collagen synthesis
Albumin	3.5–5.5 g/dL	Protein synthesis, wound remodeling; arginine and glutamine are particularly important
Prealbumin	16.0–35.0 mg/dL	Marker of protein-calorie malnutrition

[a] Normal ranges are for laboratory screening for nutritional deficiency.

fracture healing.[80] Magnesium, copper, and iron function as a cofactors in collagen synthesis.[82] Additional nutritional substances, such as curcumin, a diarylheptanoid found in turmeric, are currently being studied to possibly modulate the healing response, and for use as anti-inflammatory agents.[83,84] Given the positive effect of nutrition on fostering healing, one may consider checking laboratory values, such as vitamin D, vitamin C, vitamin A, folate, zinc, copper, magnesium, albumin, prealbumin, and iron levels. Supplementation with a multivitamin and other nutrients to address any deficiencies should be considered.

Age

With increasing age, individuals heal more slowly.[85] The effect of age is likely due to physiologic changes that occur, including a decrease in protein production, differences in the production of growth factors, collagen and elastin production,[37,86] as well as the increased comorbidities, including cardiovascular disease and diabetes, associated with age.

Although increased sarcopenia in muscle tissue and osteoporosis in bone are clearly associated with increased age, the effects of age on tendon are less conclusive,[86] and may be related to increased MMP activity and a decrease in number of viable tenocytes.[87] Likewise, with aging, chondrocytes decline in number, further impairing the ability for damaged cartilage to heal.[88]

Smoking and alcohol

Smoking and alcohol use both impair tissue repair. The impact of smoking on healing is multifactorial, with nicotine causing vasoconstriction, decreasing erythrocyte, macrophage and fibroblast proliferation, carbon monoxide decreasing oxygen-carrying capacity, and hydrogen cyanide inhibiting oxidative metabolism enzymes. Additionally, smoking increases blood viscosity, platelet aggregation, and decreases collagen deposition.[89] Certain levels of acute and chronic alcohol ingestion impair muscle protein synthesis, wound healing, and increases muscle loss during immobilization.[90–93]

Nonsteroidal anti-inflammatory drugs and corticosteroids

Nonsteroidal anti-inflammatory drugs (NSAIDs) are routinely used in the treatment of musculoskeletal injuries to reduce pain and inflammation. NSAIDs inhibit cyclooxygenase (COX) enzymes in the ArA pathway. By disrupting the ArA pathway, prostaglandin production is decreased and thereby mitigates inflammation. Prostaglandins play a role in many other functions, including renal, gastrointestinal, coagulation, vascular tone, and pregnancy.[94] NSAIDs can selectively inhibit COX-2 activity (eg, celecoxib), or nonselectively inhibit both COX-1 and COX-2 enzymes (eg, ibuprofen). The effect of NSAIDs on healing of musculoskeletal tissues has been studied in animal models and literature is limited regarding the implications on human healing. Overall, the use of nonselective NSAIDs and selective COX-2 inhibitors may impair musculoskeletal connective tissue healing; however, there are conflicting and varied results.[95] For example, early NSAID administration led to a reduction in tensile strength in a rat model of Achilles tendinopathy. Furthermore, NSAIDs lead to decreased presence of prostaglandin but increased levels of leukotriene B4, which leads to increased neutrophil infiltration and leukocyte activation. The type of NSAID, dose, duration, and timing of treatment all likely affect healing.[96,97]

There are several clinical instances when NSAID use may have a greater impact on tissue repair. Animal studies have demonstrated a negative effect on bone healing, particularly in the first week of fracture.[98,99] This effect seems to be caused by inhibition of COX-2 because COX-1 knockout mice had normal bone healing.[100] A retrospective study of NSAID and radiation use for the prevention of heterotopic ossification after hip fracture demonstrated a significant increase in fracture nonunions among the indomethacin group.[101] In the same study, NSAIDs were successfully used in the prevention of heterotopic ossification, which develops through endochondral ossification, the same process seen in bone healing.[102] With this in mind, NSAID use may be useful in the case of deep muscle contusion to prevent heterotopic ossification.[95,98]

When clinicians consider regenerative treatments, such as platelet rich plasma injection, there is often consideration of stopping NSAIDs before and after treatment. Following PRP injection in vivo, the platelets are activated through several different pathways, including exposure to ArA, collagen, adenosine diphosphate, or thrombin receptor activating peptide-6. When PRP is prepared in the setting of NSAID use, there is decreased platelet activation through the ArA pathway in an in vitro experimental setting but no difference in activation through other pathways.[103] Because platelet activation in vivo is likely achieved through multiple pathways, it is unlikely that NSAID administration before use will result in a significant decrease in actual activation. However, given the theoretic concerns, additional research is needed to delineate whether NSAIDs should be stopped before PRP administration and to elucidate the ideal time course for cessation.

Corticosteroids similarly reduce prostaglandin production but have a greater impact on the immune response and healing because they inhibit phospholipase and, thereby, mitigate production of ArA and all products of the ArA pathway. These medications, therefore, reduce neutrophil and macrophage activity, and production of growth factors, leading to a diminished inflammatory response and inhibition of cell growth and production.[78,104] Animal models of tendinopathy show in vivo increased collagen disorganization and necrosis, as well as decreased mechanical properties, following steroid administration. Also, there is emerging clinical evidence in humans to support avoidance of steroids: complete recovery rates are lower in patients with lateral epicondylitis who receive steroid injections compared with placebo.[105] Specific conditions, such as trigger finger and de Quervain tenosynovitis, still show definite therapeutic benefit with steroid injection, so there remains a place for judicious use of steroids in the setting of musculoskeletal tissue injury and healing.

SUMMARY: STRATEGIES TO FACILITATE AND OPTIMIZE HEALING

Novel treatment options have been developed using knowledge of the unique healing characteristics of each musculoskeletal tissue type, as well as an understanding of the factors that can impair or improve healing. Some of these treatments include platelet-rich plasma, autologous conditioned serum, adipose and bone marrow derived stem cells, gene therapy, prolotherapy, exercise programs, and tissue manipulation techniques, such as tenotomy. The application of these agents must be considered in the context of the healing cascade both temporally and spatially, and combined with optimizing local and systemic factors, including control of systemic disease, nutrition, and exercise to promote healing.

REFERENCES

1. Yager DR, Nwomeh BC. The proteolytic environment of chronic wounds. Wound Repair Regen 1999;7(6):433–41.
2. Nathan C. Points of control in inflammation. Nature 2002;420(6917):846–52.
3. Pierce GF, Mustoe TA, Altrock BW, et al. Therapeutic application of growth factors. J Cell Biochem 1991;45(4):319–65.
4. Liu SH, Yang RS, al-Shaikh R, et al. Collagen in tendon, ligament, and bone healing. A current review. Clin Orthop Relat Res 1995;(318):265–78.
5. Tidball JG, Villalta SA. Regulatory interactions between muscle and the immune system during muscle regeneration. Am J Physiol Regul Integr Comp Physiol 2010;298(5):R1173–87.
6. Shin EH, Caterson EJ, Jackson WM, et al. Quality of healing: defining, quantifying, and enhancing skeletal muscle healing. Wound Repair Regen 2014; 22(Suppl 1):18–24.
7. Baoge L, Van Den Steen E, Rimbaut S, et al. Treatment of skeletal muscle injury: a review. ISRN Orthop 2012;2012:689012.
8. Tidball JG. Mechanisms of muscle injury, repair, and regeneration. Compr Physiol 2011;1(4):2029–62.
9. Järvinen TAH, Järvinen TLN, Kääriäinen M, et al. Muscle injuries: biology and treatment. Am J Sports Med 2005;33(5):745–64.
10. Zelzer E, Blitz E, Killian ML, et al. Tendon-to-bone attachment: from development to maturity. Birth Defects Res C Embryo Today 2014;102(1):101–12.
11. Magnusson SP, Langberg H, Kjaer M. The pathogenesis of tendinopathy: balancing the response to loading. Nat Rev Rheumatol 2010;6(5):262–8.
12. Rees JD, Stride M, Scott A. Tendons–time to revisit inflammation. Br J Sports Med 2014;48(21):1553–7.
13. Voleti PB, Buckley MR, Soslowsky LJ. Tendon healing: repair and regeneration. Annu Rev Biomed Eng 2012;14:47–71.
14. Sandrey MA. Acute and chronic tendon injuries: factors affecting the healing response and treatment. J Sport Rehabil 2003;12(1):70–91.
15. Tozer S, Duprez D. Tendon and ligament: development, repair and disease. Birth Defects Res C Embryo Today 2005;75(3):226–36.

16. Wang JH-C. Mechanobiology of tendon. J Biomech 2006;39(9):1563–82.
17. Juneja SC, Schwarz EM, O'Keefe RJ, et al. Cellular and molecular factors in flexor tendon repair and adhesions: a histological and gene expression analysis. Connect Tissue Res 2013;54(3):218–26.
18. Sharma P, Maffulli N. Tendon injury and tendinopathy: healing and repair. J Bone Joint Surg Am 2005;87(1):187–202.
19. Galloway MT, Lalley AL, Shearn JT. The role of mechanical loading in tendon development, maintenance, injury, and repair. J Bone Joint Surg Am 2013; 95(17):1620–8.
20. Frank CB. Ligament structure, physiology and function. J Musculoskelet Neuronal Interact 2004;4(2):199–201.
21. Rość D, Powierza W, Zastawna E, et al. Post-traumatic plasminogenesis in intra-articular exudate in the knee joint. Med Sci Monit 2002;8(5):CR371–8.
22. Brommer EJ, Dooijewaard G, Dijkmans BA, et al. Depression of tissue-type plasminogen activator and enhancement of urokinase-type plasminogen activator as an expression of local inflammation. Thromb Haemost 1992;68(2):180–4.
23. Frank C, McDonald D, Wilson J, et al. Rabbit medial collateral ligament scar weakness is associated with decreased collagen pyridinoline crosslink density. J Orthop Res 1995;13(2):157–65.
24. Frank C, McDonald D, Bray D, et al. Collagen fibril diameters in the healing adult rabbit medial collateral ligament. Connect Tissue Res 1992;27(4):251–63.
25. Bray RC, Rangayyan RM, Frank CB. Normal and healing ligament vascularity: a quantitative histological assessment in the adult rabbit medial collateral ligament. J Anat 1996;188(Pt 1):87–95.
26. Thornton GM, Leask GP, Shrive NG, et al. Early medial collateral ligament scars have inferior creep behaviour. J Orthop Res 2000;18(2):238–46.
27. Schindeler A, McDonald MM, Bokko P, et al. Bone remodeling during fracture repair: The cellular picture. Semin Cell Dev Biol 2008;19(5):459–66.
28. Oryan A, Monazzah S, Bigham-Sadegh A. Bone injury and fracture healing biology. Biomed Environ Sci 2015;28(1):57–71.
29. Pilitsis JG, Lucas DR, Rengachary SS. Bone healing and spinal fusion. Neurosurg Focus 2002;13(6):e1.
30. Geris L, Gerisch A, Sloten JV, et al. Angiogenesis in bone fracture healing: a bioregulatory model. J Theor Biol 2008;251(1):137–58.
31. Goldhahn J, Féron J-M, Kanis J, et al. Implications for fracture healing of current and new osteoporosis treatments: an ESCEO consensus paper. Calcif Tissue Int 2012;90(5):343–53.
32. Bora FW, Miller G. Joint physiology, cartilage metabolism, and the etiology of osteoarthritis. Hand Clin 1987;3(3):325–36.
33. Mobasheri A, Kalamegam G, Musumeci G, et al. Chondrocyte and mesenchymal stem cell-based therapies for cartilage repair in osteoarthritis and related orthopaedic conditions. Maturitas 2014;78(3):188–98.
34. Gelse K, von der Mark K, Schneider H. Cartilage regeneration by gene therapy. Curr Gene Ther 2003;3(4):305–17.
35. Goldberg VM, Caplan AI. Biologic restoration of articular surfaces. Instr Course Lect 1999;48:623–7.
36. Nehrer S, Spector M, Minas T. Histologic analysis of tissue after failed cartilage repair procedures. Clin Orthop Relat Res 1999;365:149–62.
37. Broughton G, Janis JE, Attinger CE. Wound healing: an overview. Plast Reconstr Surg 2006;117(7 Suppl):1e-S–32e-S.

38. Kivisaari J, Vihersaari T, Renvall S, et al. Energy metabolism of experimental wounds at various oxygen environments. Ann Surg 1975;181(6):823–8.
39. Steinbrech DS, Longaker MT, Mehrara BJ, et al. Fibroblast response to hypoxia: the relationship between angiogenesis and matrix regulation. J Surg Res 1999; 84(2):127–33.
40. Roeckl Wiedmann I, Bennett M, Kranke P. Systematic review of hyperbaric oxygen in the management of chronic wounds. Br J Surg 2005;92(1):24–32.
41. Mekjavic IB, Exner JA, Tesch PA, et al. Hyperbaric oxygen therapy does not affect recovery from delayed onset muscle soreness. Med Sci Sports Exerc 2000;32(3):558–63.
42. Allen DB, Maguire JJ, Mahdavian M, et al. Wound hypoxia and acidosis limit neutrophil bacterial killing mechanisms. Arch Surg 1997;132(9):991–6.
43. Murchison ND, Price BA, Conner DA, et al. Regulation of tendon differentiation by scleraxis distinguishes force-transmitting tendons from muscle-anchoring tendons. Development 2007;134(14):2697–708.
44. Scott A, Danielson P, Abraham T, et al. Mechanical force modulates scleraxis expression in bioartificial tendons. J Musculoskelet Neuronal Interact 2011; 11(2):124–32.
45. Mendias CL, Gumucio JP, Bakhurin KI, et al. Physiological loading of tendons induces scleraxis expression in epitenon fibroblasts. J Orthop Res 2012; 30(4):606–12.
46. Zhang J, Wang JH-C. Mechanobiological response of tendon stem cells: implications of tendon homeostasis and pathogenesis of tendinopathy. J Orthop Res 2010;28(5):639–43.
47. Zhang J, Wang JH-C. The effects of mechanical loading on tendons–an in vivo and in vitro model study. PLoS One 2013;8(8):e71740.
48. Killian ML, Cavinatto L, Galatz LM, et al. The role of mechanobiology in tendon healing. J Shoulder Elbow Surg 2012;21(2):228–37.
49. Arampatzis A, Peper A, Bierbaum S, et al. Plasticity of human Achilles tendon mechanical and morphological properties in response to cyclic strain. J Biomech 2010;43(16):3073–9.
50. Rees JD. Current concepts in the management of tendon disorders. Rheumatology 2006;45(5):508–21.
51. Alfredson H, Pietilä T, Jonsson P, et al. Heavy-load eccentric calf muscle training for the treatment of chronic Achilles tendinosis. Am J Sports Med 1998;26(3): 360–6.
52. Ohberg L, Lorentzon R, Alfredson H. Eccentric training in patients with chronic Achilles tendinosis: normalised tendon structure and decreased thickness at follow up. Br J Sports Med 2004;38(1):8–11 [discussion: 11].
53. Rubin C, Turner AS, Bain S, et al. Low mechanical signals strengthen long bones. Nature 2001;412(6847):603–4.
54. Gilsanz V, Wren TAL, Sanchez M, et al. Low-level, high-frequency mechanical signals enhance musculoskeletal development of young women with low BMD. J Bone Miner Res 2006;21(9):1464–74.
55. Robling AG, Hinant FM, Burr DB, et al. Improved bone structure and strength after long-term mechanical loading is greatest if loading is separated into short bouts. J Bone Miner Res 2002;17(8):1545–54.
56. Srinivasan S, Weimer DA, Agans SC, et al. Low-magnitude mechanical loading becomes osteogenic when rest is inserted between each load cycle. J Bone Miner Res 2002;17(9):1613–20.

57. Schell H, Epari DR, Kassi JP, et al. The course of bone healing is influenced by the initial shear fixation stability. J Orthop Res 2005;23(5):1022–8.
58. Augat P, Merk J, Wolf S, et al. Mechanical stimulation by external application of cyclic tensile strains does not effectively enhance bone healing. J Orthop Trauma 2001;15(1):54–60.
59. Augat P, Burger J, Schorlemmer S, et al. Shear movement at the fracture site delays healing in a diaphyseal fracture model. J Orthop Res 2003;21(6):1011–7.
60. Klein P, Schell H, Streitparth F, et al. The initial phase of fracture healing is specifically sensitive to mechanical conditions. J Orthop Res 2003;21(4):662–9.
61. Lingen MW. Role of leukocytes and endothelial cells in the development of angiogenesis in inflammation and wound healing. Arch Pathol Lab Med 2001; 125(1):67–71.
62. He Z, King GL. Microvascular complications of diabetes. Endocrinol Metab Clin North Am 2004;33(1):215–38, xi–xii.
63. de Waard JW, de Man BM, Wobbes T, et al. Inhibition of fibroblast collagen synthesis and proliferation by levamisole and 5-fluorouracil. Eur J Cancer 1998; 34(1):162–7. Available at: http://www.ncbi.nlm.nih.gov/pubmed/9624252. Accessed February 27, 2016.
64. Tipton KD. Nutritional Support for Exercise-Induced Injuries. Sports Med 2015; 45(Suppl 1):93–104.
65. Frankenfield D. Energy expenditure and protein requirements after traumatic injury. Nutr Clin Pract 2006;21(5):430–7.
66. Waters RL, Campbell J, Perry J. Energy cost of three-point crutch ambulation in fracture patients. J Orthop Trauma 1987;1(2):170–3.
67. Arnold M, Barbul A. Nutrition and wound healing. Plast Reconstr Surg 2006; 117(7 Suppl):42S–58S.
68. Ruberg RL. Role of nutrition in wound healing. Surg Clin North Am 1984;64(4): 705–14.
69. Leigh B, Desneves K, Rafferty J, et al. The effect of different doses of an arginine-containing supplement on the healing of pressure ulcers. J Wound Care 2012;21(3):150–6.
70. Calder PC. n-3 fatty acids, inflammation and immunity: new mechanisms to explain old actions. Proc Nutr Soc 2013;72(3):326–36.
71. Albina JE, Gladden P, Walsh WR. Detrimental effects of an omega-3 fatty acid-enriched diet on wound healing. JPEN J Parenter Enteral Nutr 1993;17(6): 519–21.
72. Lopez HL. Nutritional interventions to prevent and treat osteoarthritis. Part I: focus on fatty acids and macronutrients. PM R 2012;4(5 Suppl):S145–54.
73. Otranto M, Do Nascimento AP, Monte-Alto-Costa A. Effects of supplementation with different edible oils on cutaneous wound healing. Wound Repair Regen 2010;18(6):629–36.
74. Watkins BA, Li Y, Seifert MF. Dietary ratio of n-6/n-3 PUFAs and docosahexaenoic acid: actions on bone mineral and serum biomarkers in ovariectomized rats. J Nutr Biochem 2006;17(4):282–9.
75. Taylor TV, Rimmer S, Day B, et al. Ascorbic acid supplementation in the treatment of pressure-sores. Lancet 1974;2(7880):544–6.
76. Sarisözen B, Durak K, Dinçer G, et al. The effects of vitamins E and C on fracture healing in rats. J Int Med Res 2002;30(3):309–13.
77. Hunt TK, Ehrlich HP, Garcia JA, et al. Effect of vitamin A on reversing the inhibitory effect of cortisone on healing of open wounds in animals and man. Ann Surg 1969;170(4):633–41.

78. Anstead GM. Steroids, retinoids, and wound healing. Adv Wound Care 1998; 11(6):277–85.
79. Binkley N, Krueger D. Hypervitaminosis A and bone. Nutr Rev 2000;58(5): 138–44.
80. Giganti MG, Tresoldi I, Masuelli L, et al. Fracture healing: from basic science to role of nutrition. Front Biosci (Landmark Ed) 2014;19:1162–75.
81. Angeline ME, Ma R, Pascual-Garrido C, et al. Effect of diet-induced vitamin D deficiency on rotator cuff healing in a rat model. Am J Sports Med 2014; 42(1):27–34.
82. Chow O, Barbul A. Immunonutrition: role in wound healing and tissue regeneration. Adv Wound Care 2014;3(1):46–53.
83. Aggarwal BB, Gupta SC, Sung B. Curcumin: an orally bioavailable blocker of TNF and other pro-inflammatory biomarkers. Br J Pharmacol 2013;169(8): 1672–92.
84. Buhrmann C, Mobasheri A, Busch F, et al. Curcumin modulates nuclear factor κB (NF-κB)-mediated Inflammation in human tenocytes in vitro. J Biol Chem 2011;286(32):28556–66.
85. Van de Kerkhof PC, Van Bergen B, Spruijt K, et al. Age-related changes in wound healing. Clin Exp Dermatol 1994;19(5):369–74.
86. Dressler MR, Butler DL, Boivin GP. Age-related changes in the biomechanics of healing patellar tendon. J Biomech 2006;39(12):2205–12.
87. Yu T-Y, Pang J-HS, Wu KP-H, et al. Aging is associated with increased activities of matrix metalloproteinase-2 and -9 in tenocytes. BMC Musculoskelet Disord 2013;14:2.
88. Goggs R, Carter SD, Schulze-Tanzil G, et al. Apoptosis and the loss of chondrocyte survival signals contribute to articular cartilage degradation in osteoarthritis. Vet J 2003;166(2):140–58.
89. Broughton G, Janis JE, Attinger CE. The basic science of wound healing. Plast Reconstr Surg 2006;117(7 Suppl):12S–34S.
90. Lang CH, Frost RA, Kumar V, et al. Impaired protein synthesis induced by acute alcohol intoxication is associated with changes in eIF4E in muscle and eIF2B in liver. Alcohol Clin Exp Res 2000;24(3):322–31.
91. Parr EB, Camera DM, Areta JL, et al. Alcohol ingestion impairs maximal post-exercise rates of myofibrillar protein synthesis following a single bout of concurrent training. PLoS One 2014;9(2):e88384.
92. Jung MK, Callaci JJ, Lauing KL, et al. Alcohol exposure and mechanisms of tissue injury and repair. Alcohol Clin Exp Res 2011;35(3):392–9.
93. Vargas R, Lang CH. Alcohol accelerates loss of muscle and impairs recovery of muscle mass resulting from disuse atrophy. Alcohol Clin Exp Res 2008;32(1): 128–37.
94. Su B, O'Connor JP. NSAID therapy effects on healing of bone, tendon, and the enthesis. J Appl Physiol 2013;115(6):892–9.
95. Radi ZA, Khan NK. Effects of cyclooxygenase inhibition on bone, tendon, and ligament healing. Inflamm Res 2005;54(9):358–66.
96. Dimmen S, Engebretsen L, Nordsletten L, et al. Negative effects of parecoxib and indomethacin on tendon healing: an experimental study in rats. Knee Surg Sports Traumatol Arthrosc 2009;17(7):835–9.
97. Virchenko O, Skoglund B, Aspenberg P. Parecoxib impairs early tendon repair but improves later remodeling. Am J Sports Med 2004;32(7):1743–7.
98. Ziltener J-L, Leal S, Fournier P-E. Non-steroidal anti-inflammatory drugs for athletes: an update. Ann Phys Rehabil Med 2010;53(4):278–82, 282–8.

99. Cottrell J, O'Connor JP. Effect of non-steroidal anti-inflammatory drugs on bone healing. Pharmaceuticals 2010;3(5):1668–93.

100. Simon AM, Manigrasso MB, O'Connor JP. Cyclo-oxygenase 2 function is essential for bone fracture healing. J Bone Miner Res 2002;17(6):963–76.

101. Burd TA, Lowry KJ, Anglen JO. Indomethacin compared with localized irradiation for the prevention of heterotopic ossification following surgical treatment of acetabular fractures. J Bone Joint Surg Am 2001;83-A(12):1783–8.

102. Saudan M, Saudan P, Perneger T, et al. Celecoxib versus ibuprofen in the prevention of heterotopic ossification following total hip replacement: a prospective randomised trial. J Bone Joint Surg Br 2007;89(2):155–9.

103. Schippinger G, Prüller F, Divjak M, et al. Autologous platelet-rich plasma preparations: influence of nonsteroidal anti-inflammatory drugs on platelet function. Orthop J Sports Med 2015;3(6). 2325967115588896.

104. Petratos PB, Felsen D, Trierweiler G, et al. Transforming growth factor-beta2 (TGF-beta2) reverses the inhibitory effects of fibrin sealant on cutaneous wound repair in the pig. Wound Repair Regen 2002;10(4):252–8.

105. Coombes BK, Bisset L, Brooks P, et al. Effect of corticosteroid injection, physiotherapy, or both on clinical outcomes in patients with unilateral lateral epicondylalgia: a randomized controlled trial. JAMA 2013;309(5):461–9.

Dextrose Prolotherapy
A Narrative Review of Basic Science, Clinical Research, and Best Treatment Recommendations

 CrossMark

Kenneth Dean Reeves, MD[a,b,*], Regina W.S. Sit, MD[c],
David P. Rabago, MD[d]

KEYWORDS

- Prolotherapy • Dextrose • Regenerative medicine • Osteoarthritis, Knee
- Tendinopathy

KEY POINTS

- Animal models suggest specific tissue responses to hypertonic dextrose, including proliferation.
- Clinical benefit in human studies is not explained by proliferation alone; the mechanism of dextrose prolotherapy (DPT) is likely multifactorial.
- DPT is efficacious for knee osteoarthritis and likely efficacious for finger osteoarthritis and Osgood-Schlatter disease.
- Moderate-quality randomized clinical trial (RCT) evidence supports use of DPT in rotator cuff tendinopathy, lateral epicondylosis, plantar fasciopathy and nonsurgical sacroiliac pain.

INTRODUCTION

Prolotherapy is an injection-based treatment of chronic musculoskeletal pain. A general surgeon in the United States, George Hackett, formalized injection protocols in the 1950s, based on 30 years of clinical experience.[1] Prolotherapy has been identified as a regenerative injection therapy[2] but is differentiated from other regenerative injection therapies, such as platelet-rich plasma (PRP) and stem cell injection by the absence of a biologic agent.

[a] Private Practice, 4740 El Monte Roeland Park, KS 66205, USA; [b] Department of Physical Medicine and Rehabilitation, University of Kansas Medical Center, 3901 Rainbow Blvd, Kansas City, KS 66160, USA; [c] The Jockey Club School of Public Health and Primary Care, The Chinese University of Hong Kong, 30-32 Ngan Shing Street, School of Public Health Building, Prince of Wales Hospital, Shatin, New Territory, Hong Kong; [d] Department of Family Medicine and Community Health, University of Wisconsin School of Medicine and Public Health, 1100 Delaplaine Ct, Madison, WI 53715, USA
* Corresponding author. 4740 El Monte, Roeland Park, KS, 66205-1348.
E-mail address: DeanReevesMD@gmail.com

Phys Med Rehabil Clin N Am 27 (2016) 783–823
http://dx.doi.org/10.1016/j.pmr.2016.06.001
1047-9651/16/© 2016 Elsevier Inc. All rights reserved.

pmr.theclinics.com

Prolotherapy is increasingly popular in the United States and internationally. The current number of practitioners of prolotherapy in the United States is estimated as several thousand based on conference attendance and physician listings on relevant Web sites, including both independent physicians and members of multispecialty groups. Currently, Prolotherapy Regenerative Medicine is one of the 23 specialty colleges of the American Osteopathic Association (http://www.prolotherapycollege.org). Training of doctors of medicine and doctors of osteopathy is primarily outside medical schools, for example, through postgraduate-level conferences and service learning projects through universities, professional organizations, and foundations (www.fammed.wisc.edu/prolotherapy, www.aaomed.org, and www.hacketthemwallpatterson.org).

Hypertonic dextrose is the most commonly used prolotherapy solution, with favorable outcomes shown in multiple clinical trials.[3] It is inexpensive, readily available, and reported to be safe. This review focuses on the basic science and clinical evidence of prolotherapy using hypertonic dextrose solutions. The term *dextrose* is interchangeable with *glucose* because dextrose is the dexter (right-handed) form of glucose found in animals and humans. For this discussion, the term dextrose is preferred.

METHODS

A search of electronic databases was performed by the University of Kansas library staff, including Medline, Web of Science, and ClinicalTrials.gov, from 1980 to 2016, without language restrictions. Search specifics included (1) prolotherapy; (2) (regenerative OR tendon OR tendinopathy OR ligament OR osteoarthritis) AND (dextrose OR glucose); and (3) dextrose injection from 1980 to 2016. Basic science studies were included in this review if they featured blinded histologic, histochemical, or radiographic outcome assessment. Clinical studies were included if randomized assignment was used and a dextrose arm was included. The strength of each RCT was assessed by 2 reviewers (K.D.R. and R.W.S.S.) using the Cochrane risk of bias tool.[4] Disagreements were resolved by consensus and presented in descriptive and tabled form.

RESULTS

Of 469 studies identified, 48 met inclusion criteria and were grouped into the following 2 areas: basic science (n = 33) and clinical research (n = 15).

Basic Science Findings

In vitro effects of dextrose on cytokine levels

Transport of dextrose into human cells uses a family of transport proteins, GLUTs 1–4, that interact with cytokines in a crucial way to signal either cell growth or repair.[5] DNA expression changes favoring production of multiple cytokines have been measured within 20 minutes of exposure to in vitro elevation of pericellular dextrose levels to as little as 30 mM (0.54%)[6] in a variety of animal and human cells, including fibroblasts,[6–10] chondrocytes,[11,12] and nerve cells.[13,14]

Proliferative tissue changes in diabetic patients who have frequent elevations of pericellular dextrose in the 30-mM range are prominent, such as with diabetic proliferative retinopathy.[15] Such effects are of unclear significance, however, given that elevated glucose levels in cases of diabetes seem to trigger interrelated complex pathophysiologic mechanisms,[15] which may vary greatly from the effect of brief and isolated dextrose elevation on injection in either nondiabetics or diabetics. For example, the duration of glucose elevation is important to production of favorable[16] or unfavorable cytokines.[17]

Animal studies on cartilage and other soft tissue proliferation
Animal studies on femoral cartilage equivalent Kim and colleagues[18] reported chondrocytic tissue filling of 2-mm punch lesions in adult rabbit femoral cartilage on blinded histologic evaluation 6 weeks after injection of 10% dextrose or platelet-poor plasma but not in controls (noninjected). Histologic images were limited in this Korean language study. Park and colleagues[19] demonstrated a protective effect of injector-blinded weekly 10% dextrose injection versus saline injection in a rabbit osteoarthritis model (anterior cruciate ligament [ACL] transection) on masked Mankin[20] grading analysis at 19 weeks. The dextrose injection solution, however, contained amino acids and ascorbic acid as well, so the chondroprotective effect cannot be ascribed to dextrose alone.

Animal studies on Achilles tendon A transient reduction in tensile strength of the healthy rat Achilles tendon was not demonstrable at 0 days, 5 days, or 10 days by Martins and colleagues[21] after masked injection of 12.5% dextrose compared with normal saline injection or no injection. Injured rat Achilles tendon (transected and sutured) injected with 20% dextrose by Ahn and colleagues[22] showed significantly more fibroblasts on blinded histologic review at 4 weeks compared with injured but noninjected control tendons. Kim and colleagues[23] reported that single injection of either 5% dextrose (D5W) or 20% dextrose made hypertonic with saline (1100 mOsm) into noninjured rat Achilles tendon resulted in a significant increase in tendon diameter and fibroblast counts per high-power field (hpf) compared with equimolar (1100-mOsm) saline, suggesting a nonosmolar mechanism of dextrose-induced proliferation. In another study Kim and colleagues[24] showed that oral nonsteroidal anti-inflammatory drug (NSAID) (celecoxib) administration did not limit the increase in Achilles diameter or fibroblast count per hpf at 6 weeks, suggesting a noninflammatory mechanism of proliferation.

Animal studies on medial collateral ligament equivalent Jensen and colleagues[25] demonstrated an inflammatory response to needling alone or needling with either saline or 15% dextrose in noninjured rat MCL. One measurable difference in the inflammatory responses was that, at 24 hours postdextrose injection, ED2$^+$ macrophages and CD43$^+$ leukocytes increased compared with saline-injection and needle-stick controls ($P<.05$). Another study by Jensen and colleagues[26] using MCL ligaments with a standardized subfailure stretch injury[27] showed no significant differences in MCL strength or fibroblast number 3 weeks after injection with 15% dextrose or saline, although the cross-sectional area was significantly increased in the dextrose-injected MCLs ($P<.05$). This time frame was short compared with other animal model studies, perhaps too short to evaluate the effect of dextrose.[21]

Animal studies on transverse carpal ligament equivalent (subsynovial connective tissue) A study by Oh and colleagues[28] demonstrated noninflammatory (no neutrophil invasion at 1 week, 2 weeks, 4 weeks, or 8 weeks) collagen bundle thickening at 8 weeks in the transverse carpal ligament rabbit equivalent after a single injection of 0.05 mL of 10% dextrose into the carpal tunnel equivalent (subsynovial space) through a small incision with a 30-gauge needle. This initial study was followed by 3 randomized, masked, 2-arm studies that compared 10% dextrose versus normal saline. One[29], two[30] or four[31] injections, given at weekly intervals, were evaluated in successive studies with findings measured at 12 weeks, 12 weeks, and 16 weeks, respectively, after the first dextrose injection. Energy absorption and load to failure of the subsynovial connective tissue (SSCT) were measured using a standardized approach.[32] The 3 studies demonstrated consistent and significant increases in tensile load to rupture (**Fig. 1**), total energy

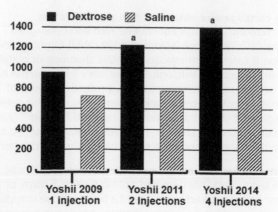

Fig. 1. Tensile load to rupture of the SSCT, comparing forepaws of each rabbit, with randomized injection of either 0.1 mL of 10% dextrose or 0.1 mL of NS on 1, 2, or 4 occasions. [a] $P<.05$.

absorption to rupture (**Fig. 2**), and thickening of the SSCT, presented in **Fig. 3** graphically and by a representative biopsy in **Fig. 4**.

Median nerve flattening was noted in the 2-weekly and 4-weekly injection studies[30,31] along with a relative increase in latency of the median motor conduction ($P = .08$), edema in the median nerve bundles, a thinner myelin sheath and observation of poorly myelinated nerve fibers, and evidence of wallerian degeneration.[31] The author's hypothesis that noninflammatory progressive transverse carpal ligament (or equivalent in animal) proliferative thickening (fibrosis) leads to eventual median neuropathy, is supported by these studies.

Human studies on cartilage and other soft tissue proliferation
Human studies on cartilage proliferation Rabago and colleagues[33] reported no changes in cartilage volume on blinded pretreatment and post-treatment MRI knee scans obtained at 1 year between dextrose-injected participants with symptomatic

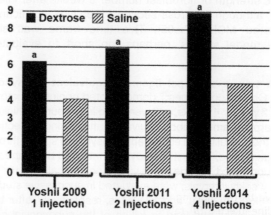

Fig. 2. Total energy absorption to rupture of the SSCT, comparing forepaws of each rabbit with randomized injection of either 0.1 mL of 10% dextrose or 0.1 mL of NS on 1, 2, or 4 occasions. [a] $P<.05$.

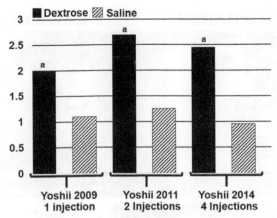

Fig. 3. Thickness of the SSCT in millimeters, comparing forepaws of each rabbit with randomized injection of either 0.1 mL of 10% dextrose or 0.1 mL of NS on 1, 2, or 4 occasions. [a] $P<.05$.

knee osteoarthritis and those who received saline injections or exercise prescription. Direct arthroscopic visualization of the joint surface, however, is superior to MRI evaluation,[34] and a recent study by Topol and colleagues[35] used pretreatment and post-treatment video-arthroscopy documentation, to compare pre and post treament denuded femoral cortex surfaces for evidence of cartilage growth. This was by methylene blue stain for chondrocyte growth, with biopsy of new areas of methylene blue uptake after treatment to evaluate for cartilage type (I = fibrocartilage and II = hyaline-like cartilage) by quantitative polarized light microscopy (QPLM) and immunohistologic straining with photographic documentaton of the biopsy defect area. Biopsies were obtained from areas of new uptake of methylene blue with photographic

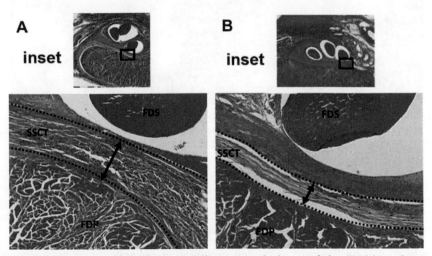

Fig. 4. Representative biopsy showing difference in thickness of the SSCT in a dextrose-injected (*A*) and saline-injected (*B*) rabbit forepaw after 4 weekly injections. The main map for A and B includes an outlined area shown below as a magnified inset map. FDP, flexor digitorum profoundus; FDS, flexor digitorium superficialis. The *arrow* depicts the thickness of the subsynovial connective tissue (SSCT).

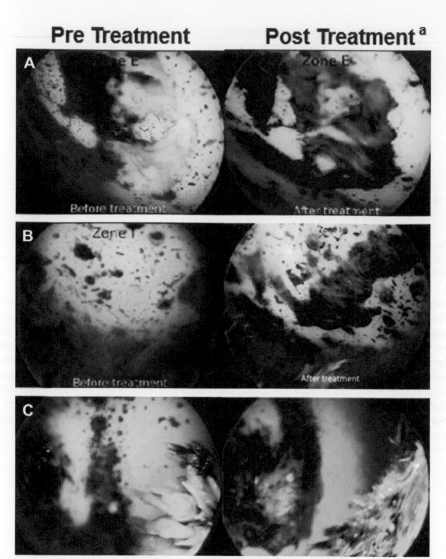

Fig. 5. Prearthroscopy and postarthroscopy showing areas of new methylene blue uptake in representative participants (A–C). [a] Area of new uptake is a combination of fibrocartilage and hyaline-like cartilage, as confirmed by QPLM and immunohistologic straining.

documentation of the biopsy defect area (**Fig. 5**); QPLM and immunohistologic stains showed a mixture of fibrocartilage and hyaline-like cartilage in the biopsies. Although the study was limited by the small sample size of participants and the lack of a control group, it suggests that dextrose may stimulate or mediate chondrogenesis.

Human studies on ligament or tendon proliferation Several studies have followed clinical and radiographic changes in parallel. Rabago and colleagues[36] demonstrated clinical benefit from dextrose injection in lateral epicondylosis in the absence of demonstrable MRI changes at 16 weeks. Bertrand and colleagues[37] used a systematic ultrasound rotator cuff tendinopathy grading method[38] to evaluate pretreatment and post-treatment images and showed no significant differences at 9 months despite significant postprolotherapy clinical improvement. Two other second-look ultrasound studies have also indicated improvement in tendinosis, but these studies were not controlled, and standardization of ultrasound imaging is always challenging for clinical studies.[39,40]

Human studies on a potential sensorineural mechanism

A direct sensorineural effect of dextrose injection has been proposed based on the observation that analgesia results from subcutaneous perineural injection of dextrose along tender peripheral nerves in some chronic pain patients.[41] Hypothesizing a potential analgesic effect of D5W, Maniquis-Smigel and colleagues[42] conducted a double-blind randomized controlled trial of the effect of epidural injection of D5W versus normal saline in 35 participants with chronic nonsurgical low back pain and buttock or leg pain. A significant analgesic effect was seen in those who received D5W in comparison to those who received normal saline from 15 minutes to 48 hours ($P<.05$). The speed of analgesia onset after epidural[42] or subcutaneous[41] injection of dextrose suggests a potential direct effect of dextrose on peripheral nerves.[41]

The transient receptor potential cation channel subfamily V member 1 (TRPV-1), formerly called the capsaicin receptor, is known to produce nociceptive pain with up-regulation.[43] Bertrand and colleagues[44] stimulated the TRPV-1 receptor using a capsaicin cream model to produce pain. Mannitol-containing cream or a control (vehicle) cream was then applied to the painful area in a double-blind manner. Mannitol is a 6-carbon sugar alcohol chemically related to dextrose. Pain resolution was reported faster with mannitol (**Fig. 6**). Researchers hypothesized that the TRPV-1 receptors were down-regulated or that other related ion channels or receptors were directly affected.[44,45]

Summary of basic science–related literature

Key findings from basic science studies are summarized in **Box 1**. Basic science studies suggest that dextrose has independent effects that may promote local healing of chronically injured extra-articular and intra-articular tissue through

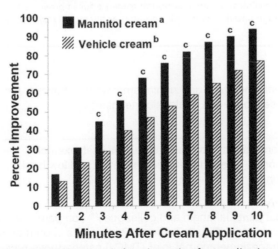

Fig. 6. Minute-by-minute improvement in burning pain after application of mannitol cream or vehicle cream to opposite sides of a lip made to burn by application of capsaicin. [a] Mannitol is similar in structure to dextrose and similar in observed analgesic effect on perineural injection but has minimal sweetness, which is easily masked in cream. [b] Natural degradation occurs in the burning pain on lips after capsaicin application. [c] $P<.05$.

Box 1
Summary of basic science findings from animal or human trials (along with primary/example reference)

1. Dextrose elevation to as little as 0.6% around fibroblasts and chondrocytes results in a rise in the level of complex proteins (cytokines) responsible to signal growth or breakdown of human tissue in vitro.

2. The duration of dextrose elevation in vitro influences the balance of cytokines toward repair or disrepair.

3. Dextrose injection (noninflammatory; 10%) may stimulate repair of rabbit femoral cartilage punch lesions.

4. Dextrose injection (10%) may slow the development of osteoarthritis in a rabbit ACL-transection model.

5. Healthy Achilles tendon in rats shows no temporary weakening after direct intratendinous injection.

6. Healthy Achilles tendon in rats shows an increase in tendon diameter and an increase in fibroblast counts by DPT, which is not imitated by equimolar (hypertonic) saline injection and is not altered by administration of an NSAID, suggesting a mechanism of action not based primarily on hyperosmolarity or inflammation.

7. Multiple randomized and saline injection–controlled injections under the transverse carpal ligament equivalent in rabbits demonstrate a consistent and significant thickening of the ligament and an increase in both tensile load to rupture and energy absorption to rupture.

8. An increase in volume of cartilage in the human osteoarthritic knee has not been demonstrated after DPT.

9. A chondrogenic effect of intraarticular dextrose in humans has been demonstrated in a small proof of concept study using second-look arthroscopy with cartilage cell staining and biopsy for immunohistologic evaluation of cartilage type showing a mixture of fibro and hyaline-like cartilage.

10. Clinical studies on lateral epicondylosis with interval MRI testing and rotator cuff tendinopathy with internal ultrasonography have not shown a significant proliferation effect to explain clinical benefits, although evidence for improvement in tendinosis has been suggested in patellar tendinosis and plantar fasciopathy by interval ultrasound examination.

---

stimulating both inflammatory and noninflammatory pathways; recent studies also suggest a direct sensorineural analgesic mechanism.

Clinical Research

The most important aspects of several studies that exemplify the effects of DPT in discrete conditions—osteoarthritis, tendinopathy, and low back pain—are summarized in this section.

Hand osteoarthritis

Trapeziometacarpal joint Jahangiri and colleagues[46] compared DPT to steroid injection in a 2-arm blinded trial (**Fig. 7, Table 1**). Participants in both groups with chronic thumb pain and trapeziometacarpal joint (TMCJ) osteoarthritis received 1-mL intra-articular and 1-mL extra-articular injection through the anatomic snuff box at 0 months, 1 month, and 2 months. Effects were assessed at 6 months by a 0 to 10 Visual Analog Scale (VAS) for pain, a Health Assessment Questionnaire Disability Index (HAQ-DI), and lateral pinch strength in pounds by a hydraulic pinch gauge.

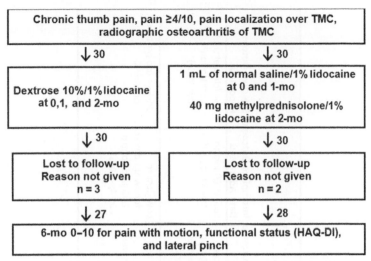

Fig. 7. Flow diagram for Jahangiri et al. (*Data from* Jahangiri A, Moghaddam FR, Najafi S. Hypertonic dextrose versus corticosteroid local injection for the treatment of osteoarthritis in the first carpometacarpal joint: a double-blind randomized clinical trial. J Orthop Sci 2014;19:737–43.)

Participants had statistically similar baseline characteristics. At 6 months the DPT group improved more in pain on movement (3.8 points ± 0.9 points [76%] vs 2.1 points ± 1.0 points [46%]; P = .02) and hand function (HAQ-DI) function score (3.0 points ± 2.2 points [65%] vs 1.77 points ± 1.0 points [41%]; P = .01) than the steroid group (**Fig. 8**).

Trapeziometacarpal joint, proximal interphalangeal joint, or distal interphalangeal joint of fingers 2–4 Reeves and Hassanein[47] compared DPT to blinded lidocaine injections in a 2-arm blinded trial (**Fig. 9**, see **Table 1**). Participants with chronic thumb or finger pain and radiographic hand osteoarthritis received treatment at 0 months, 2 months, and 4 months, with optional open-label dextrose injection after 6 months. All symptomatic joints were treated and participants were analyzed based on the average change across all joints treated, with effects assessed at 6 months (blinded) and 12 months (open label) using a 0 to 10 numeric rating scale (NRS) pain score and flexion range of motion.

Participants were similar statistically at baseline. The DPT group improved more in pain on movement (1.9 points ± 1.5 points [42%] vs 0.6 points ± 1.0 points [14%]; P = .027) and flexion range of motion (+8.0 ± 3.6° vs −8.8 ± 2.9°; P = <.01) than the lidocaine group at 6 months (**Figs. 10** and **11**). DPT administration to the lidocaine group after 6 months resulted in a similar pattern of improvement as the original dextrose group.

Summary of hand osteoarthritis Both HOA studies were double-blind trials but lacked a robust study design (see **Table 1**); whereas DPT is likely to be efficacious in HOA, higher-quality evidence is needed to confirm the role of DPT.

Intraarticular dextrose versus intraarticular lidocaine Reeves and Hassanein[48] compared DPT to blinded lidocaine injections in a 2-arm blinded trial using an intraarticular-only injection protocol (**Fig. 12**, **Table 2**) Participants with chronic knee

Table 1
Hand osteoarthritis risk of bias table

Source	Sequence Generation	Allocation Concealment	Blinding of Participants and Researchers	Blinding of Outcome Assessment	Incomplete Outcome Data Addressed	Selective Outcome Reporting
Jahangiri et al,[46] 2014	Low (A computer-generated randomization)	Low (sequentially numbered sealed envelopes used for assignment)	Unclear (information was not reported)	Unclear (clinician masked to group but who assessed outcome is not stated)	Low (5/60 lost to follow-up; <10%)	Low (clinical trial registration available)
Reeves & Hassanein,[47] 2000	Low (a random number table was utilized)	Unclear (clinicians and research coordinator masked. Assignments not made off-site)	Low (the solutions were identical in color and viscosity)	Low (assessor and database coordinator were masked)	Low (lost to follow-up dextrose 2/13 and control 0/14; <10%)	Unclear (no protocol provided)

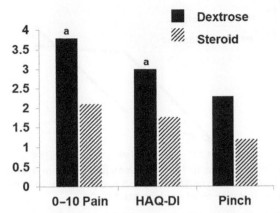

Fig. 8. Numeric improvement at 6-month follow-up on 0 to 10 VAS for pain with movement, 0 to 9 function scale (HAQ-DI hand portion), and lateral grip pinch in pounds comparing DPT and steroid injection. [a] $P<.05$.

pain and Kellgren-Lawrence (KL) stages II–IV radiographic knee osteoarthritis received injections at 0 months, 2 months, and 4 months, with optional open-label dextrose injection after 6 months. Primary measures were 0 to 10 NRS for walking pain and goniometrically measured knee range of motion.

Participants had statistically similar baseline characteristics. Range-of-motion gains favored the DPT group at 6 months ($13.2 \pm 2.1°$ vs $7.7 \pm 2.2°$; $P = .015$). The 2 groups did not have a statistically significant difference in walking pain (**Fig. 13**).The DPT

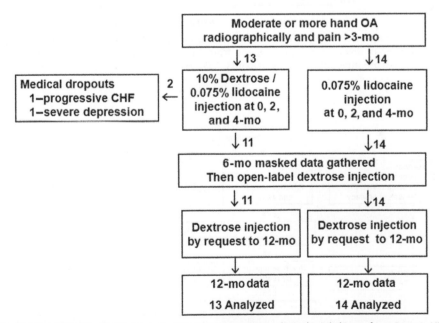

Fig. 9. Flow diagram for Reeves et al hand osteoarthritis clinical trial. (*Data from* Reeves KD, Hassanein K. Randomized prospective placebo-controlled double-blind study of dextrose prolotherapy for osteoarthritic thumbs and fingers [DIP, PIP and trapeziometacarpal Joints]: evidence of clinical efficacy. J Altern Complement Med 2000;6:311–20.)

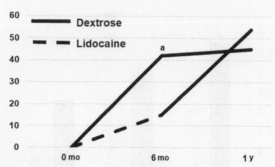

Fig. 10. Percentage improvement in finger movement pain from 0 to 6 months (masked period) after injection of dextrose or lidocaine, and from 6 months to 12 months (open label) after offering dextrose injection to all participants. [a] $P<.05$.

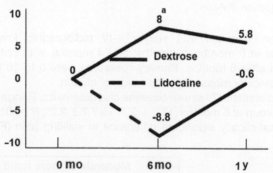

Fig. 11. Improvement in finger flexion range in degrees from 0 to 6 months (masked period) after injection of dextrose or lidocaine, and from 6 months to 12 months (open-label) after offering dextrose injection to all participants. [a] $P<.05$.

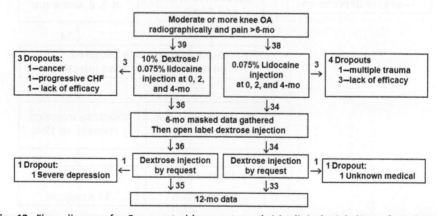

Fig. 12. Flow diagram for Reeves et al knee osteoarthritis clinical trial. (*Data from* Reeves KD, Hassanein K. Randomized prospective double-blind placebo-controlled study of dextrose prolotherapy for knee osteoarthritis with or without ACL laxity. J Altern Complement Med 2000;6:68–80.)

Table 2
Knee osteoarthritis risk of bias table

Source	Sequence Generation	Allocation Concealment	Blinding of Participants and Researchers	Blinding of Outcome Assessment	Incomplete Outcome Data Addressed	Selective Outcome Reporting
Reeves & Hassanein,[48] 2000	Low (a random number table was used)	Unclear (relevant information was not reported)	Low (identical control solution was used)	Low (assessor and database coordinator masked)	High (9/77 [11.7%]; >10%).	Unclear (no protocol provided)
Hashemi et al,[49] 2015	Unclear (randomization method was not mentioned)	Unclear (relevant information was not reported)	Unclear (relevant information was not reported)	Unclear (relevant information was not reported)	Unclear (relevant information was not reported)	Unclear (no protocol provided)
Dumais et al,[50] 2012	Unclear (random sequencing method not described)	Low (opaque sealed envelopes were used)	High (open-label trial)	Low (outcome assessors masked to group)	High (>10% lost to follow-up from each group)	Unclear (no protocol provided)
Rabago et al,[52] 2013	Low (random sequence generated by computer)	Low (off-site assignment and opaque sealed envelopes)	Low (both active and control solutions looked similar)	Low (outcome assessor masked to group allocation)	Low (no lost to follow-up cases)	Unclear (no protocol provided)

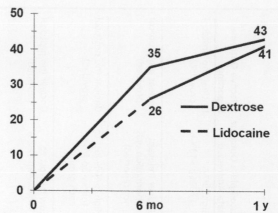

Fig. 13. Percentage improvement in knee pain with walking from 0 months to 6 months (masked period) after injection of dextrose or lidocaine, and from 6 months to 12 months (open label) after offering dextrose injection to all participants.

group, however, showed continuing improvement at 12 months and the lidocaine group, after unblinding, received DPT and also showed continuing improvement to 12 months (see **Fig. 13**).

Intraarticular dextrose versus intraarticular ozone Hashemi and colleagues[49] compared DPT to ozone injection in a 2-arm randomized open-label trial (**Fig. 14**; see **Table 2**). Participants with KL I–II knee osteoarthritis of undocumented duration received 3 treatments at 7-day to 10-day intervals of intra-articular dextrose or intra-articular ozone. Effects were assessed at 3 months using 0 to 10 VAS pain levels and Western Ontario and McMaster Universities Arthritis Index (WOMAC), 0–100 points.

Participants had statistically similar baseline characteristics. At 3-month follow-up, the DPT group and the ozone group did not differ with respect to VAS pain level improvement (4.8 points vs 5.1 points) or WOMAC composite score improvement (25.3 vs 25.2) (**Fig. 15**).This is a comparison, however, of 2 active treatment groups, both of which demonstrated significant improvement in pain and WOMAC scores compared with the pretreatment baseline.

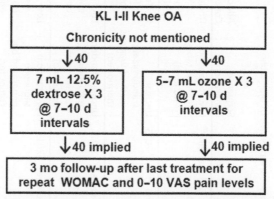

Fig. 14. Flow diagram for Hashemi et al. (*Data from* Hashemi M, Jalili P, Mennati S, et al. The effects of prolotherapy with hypertonic dextrose versus prolozone [intraarticular ozone] in patients with knee osteoarthritis. Anesth Pain Med 2015;5:e27584.)

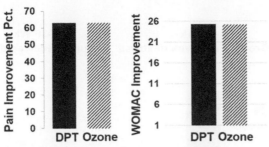

Fig. 15. Percentage improvement in 0 to 10 knee pain intensity 3 months after 3 intra-articular injections of dextrose or ozone.

Exercise plus intraarticular and collateral ligament dextrose injection versus exercise alone Dumais and colleagues[50] compared DPT plus a home-based physical therapy program to home-based physical therapy alone in a randomized crossover trial (**Fig. 16**; see **Table 2**). Participants with chronic knee pain and any KL grading received injections at 0 weeks, 4 weeks, 8 weeks, and 12 weeks of 20% dextrose intra-articularly and 15% dextrose in collateral ligaments versus therapy only. Assessments were performed at week 16. After that, the 2 arms crossed over with a second assess-ment at week 36.

Participants had statistically similar baseline characteristics, and 86% were KL III or IV. Improvement in composite WOMAC score was significantly more in the group receiving DPT for period 1 (21.8 ± 12.5 vs 6.1 ± 13.9; $P<.05$) and period 2 (9.3 ± 11.4 vs 1.2 ± 10.7; $P<.05$) with an overall significance of $P<.001$ using a stan-dard statistical method of crossover design analysis[51] (**Fig. 17**).

Intraarticular and multiple extraarticular dextrose or saline injection versus exercise alone Rabago and colleagues[52] conducted a 3-arm RCT comparing DPT to normal saline injection and a home-based exercise group (**Fig. 18**; see **Table 2**). Participants with chronic knee pain and any radiological evidence of osteoarthritis by KL grading were randomized to receive injection at 1 weeks, 5 weeks, and 9 weeks with optional treatments at 13 and 17 weeks consistent with a published protocol.[53] Effects were

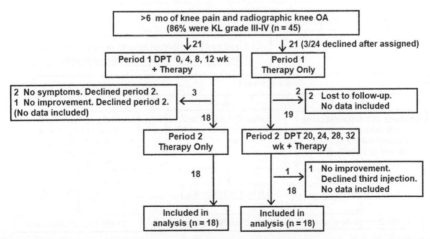

Fig. 16. Flow diagram for Dumais et al. (*Data from* Dumais R, Benoit C, Dumais A, et al. Ef-fect of regenerative injection therapy on function and pain in patients with knee osteoar-thritis: a randomized crossover study. Pain Med 2012;13:990–9.)

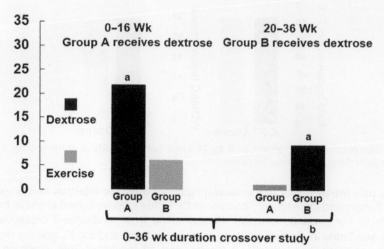

Fig. 17. Ordinal improvement in WOMAC Score during period 1 (0–16 weeks) and period 2 (20–36 weeks) of Dumais and colleagues' crossover trial of knee osteoarthritis treatment.[50] [a] Change in DPT group greater than change in group receiving exercise alone (P<.05). [b] Change in DPT group greater than change in group receiving exercise along during the entire 0 to 36-week period (P<.001).

assessed using the WOMAC questionnaire at 0 weeks, 5 weeks, 9 weeks, 12 weeks, 26 weeks, and 52 weeks.

Participants had statistically similar baseline characteristics and 63% were rated KL III–IV. By 9 weeks, participants receiving DPT reported substantial improvement in the WOMAC composite score (13.91 ± 3.2 points) compared with both control therapies (**Fig. 19**). Maximum benefits were recorded by 24 weeks and persisted through 52 weeks. At 52 weeks, the DPT group improved more than either the saline injection or exercise groups in WOMAC composite score (15.3 ± 3.3 vs 7.6 ± 3.4 vs 8.2 ± 3.3, respectively; P<.05) (see **Fig. 19**).

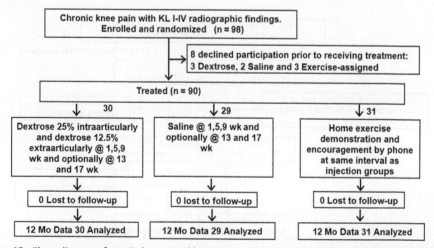

Fig. 18. Flow diagram from Rabago et al knee osteoarthritis clinical trial. (*Data from* Rabago D, Patterson JJ, Mundt M, et al. Dextrose prolotherapy for knee osteoarthritis: a randomized controlled trial. Ann Fam Med 2013;11:229–37.)

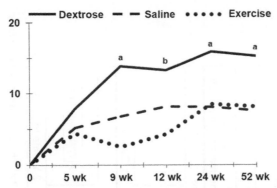

Fig. 19. Improvement in WOMAC score comparing dextrose injection, saline injection and home-based exercise in knee OA. [a] Change in DPT group greater than change in either saline or exercise group. (P<.05). [b] Change in DPT group greater than change in exercise group (P<.05). Change in DPT group not significantly greater than in the saline group.

Summary of knee osteoarthritis The role of DPT in knee osteoarthritis is supported by level I evidence in the form of a systemic review and meta-analysis published in 2016.[54] A standardized mean difference was used to evaluate the effect size. Four RCTs were included in the review.[33,48,50,52] Analysis of pooled data indicated that peri-articular and intra-articular hypertonic dextrose knee injections in 3 to 5 sessions have a statistically significant and clinically relevant effect in the improvement of WOMAC composite score (0.81; 95% CI, 0.18–1.45, $P = .012$; $I_2 = 53.6\%$); functional subscale (0.78; 95% CI, 0.25–1.30; $P = .001$; $I_2 = 34.5\%$); and pain subscale (0.62; 95% CI, 0.04–1.20; $P = .035$; $I_2 = 46.2\%$) at 12 to 16 weeks compared with formal at-home exercise. Benefits, generally higher than the minimal clinically important difference (MCID), were sustained to 1 year.

Low back pain or sacroiliac pain
Low back pain Yelland and colleagues[55] compared DPT to normal saline injection in addition to either exercise or usual care in a factorial design (**Fig. 20, Table 3**). Participants with chronic back pain and failure of conservative treatment received 6 treatments at 2-week intervals and then as needed at 4 months, 6 months, 12 months, and 24 months, consistent with a published protocol.[56] Participants were masked to solution type for the 24-month period of the study. Effects were assessed using the Roland-Morris (R-M) disability score and a 0 to 100 VAS for pain. Data were collected at 12 months and 24 months.

Participants had statistically similar baseline characteristics. At 12 months, no statistical difference was found between exercise and normal activity. DPT and not significant (NS) groups also did not differ in terms of the change in R-M disability score (5.5 ± 0.9; 36% vs 4.5 ± 0.8; 26%; $P = .60$) or pain intensity measured by a VAS (18.6 ± 3.2 points; 36% vs 18.4 ± 4.0 points; 33%; $P = .93$). However, 12-month improvements exceeded the minimally important change for the R-M disability score (30% or 5.0)[57] in the dextrose group and the 0 to 100 VAS pain score (20% or 15 points)[57] in both groups (**Fig. 21**). Greater than 50% pain reduction was observed in 46% and 36% of dextrose and saline groups respectively at 12 months. Improvements were durable to 24 months.

Sacroiliac pain Kim and colleagues[58] compared DPT to steroid injection in a 2-arm blinded trial (**Fig. 22, see Table 3**). Participants with pain more than 3 months localized below the posterior superior iliac spine with positive Patrick or Gaeslen test, and pain

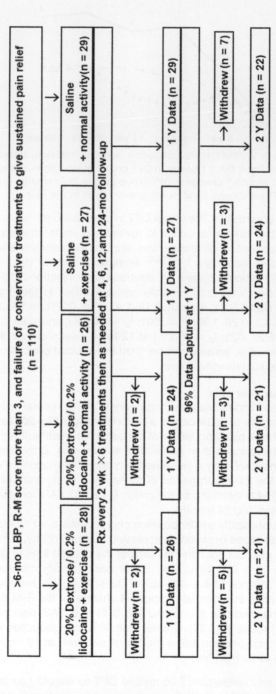

Fig. 20. Flow diagram for Yelland et al low back pain study. (*Data from* Yelland MJ, Glasziou PP, Bogduk N, et al. Prolotherapy injections, saline injections, and exercises for chronic low-back pain: a randomized trial. Spine 2004;29:9–16.)

Table 3
Low back pain and sacroiliac pain risk of bias table

Source	Sequence Generation	Allocation Concealment	Blinding of Participants and Researchers	Blinding of Outcome Assessment	Incomplete Outcome Data Addressed	Selective Outcome Reporting
Yelland et al,[55] 2004	Low (computer-generated random number system)	Low (off-site randomization)	Low (off-site solution preparation)	Low (assessors masked)	Low 4% loss of data to 1 y (Intention to treat utilized)	Unclear (no protocol was provided)
Kim et al,[58] 2010	Low (computer-generated random table)	Unclear (relevant information was not reported)	Low (researcher and patient masked. Injector not masked but no other interaction with participant)	Low (outcome assessor was blinded)	Low (only 2/48 lost to follow-up)	Unclear (no protocol was provided)

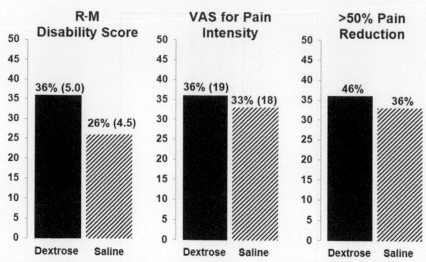

Fig. 21. Percentage improvement in R-M disability score, percentage improvement in VAS for pain intensity at 12 months, and percentage of participants with more than 50% pain reduction.

reduction more than 50% with fluoroscopic injection of 0.25% levobupivacaine, were recruited in this study. Injections were performed at 0 weeks, 2 weeks, and 4 weeks or until pain improvement more than 90% was reached. The primary measure was a 0 to 10 NRS pain scale and data were collected pretreatment and 2 weeks, 6 months, 10 months, and 15 months after the last injection.

Participants had statistically similar baseline characteristics. The dextrose group received more injections than the steroid group (2.7 ± 1.1 vs 1.5 ± 0.8) to achieve an initial 90% improvement. **Fig. 23** reinforces the diagnostic specificity for SI joint pain source, with greater than or equal to 50% pain reduction achieved by all participants at 2 weeks post-treatment. By 6 months, significantly more participants in the dextrose group than steroid group remained more than 50% improved. At 9 months

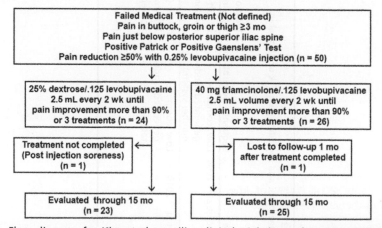

Fig. 22. Flow diagram for Kim et al sacroiliac clinical trial. (*Data from* Kim WM, Lee HG, Jeong CW, et al. A randomized controlled trial of intra-articular prolotherapy versus steroid injection for sacroiliac joint pain. J Altern Complement Med 2010;16:1285–90.)

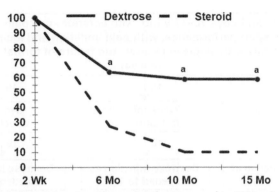

Fig. 23. Percentage of participants with greater than or equal to 50% pain reduction at 2, 6, 10, and 15 months after treatment completion for sacroiliac pain. [a] Change in DPT group greater than change in steroid group ($P<.01$).

the between group difference was maximal, ($58.7 \pm 20.8\%$ vs $10.2 \pm 16.9\%$; $P<.01$) and was sustained to follow-up at 15 months (**Fig. 23**).

Summary of low back pain and sacroiliac pain A Cochrane review by Dagenais and colleagues[59] in 2007 evaluated the role of prolotherapy in low back pain. The review included 5 eligible studies[55,60–63] and concluded that prolotherapy alone is not effective for chronic low back pain; however, 4 of the 5 studies[60–63] used a mixture of prolotherapy solutions containing dextrose, glycerine, and phenol, which may not allow full evaluation of DPT alone in low back pain. More high-quality RCTs using DPT alone are needed to confirm or refute DPT efficacy in lumbosacral pain. However, intrarticular injection of dextrose into symptomatic SI joints appears to result in significant and sustained benefit in comparison injection of steroid.[58]

Osgood-Schlatter disease
Topol and colleagues[64] conducted a 3-arm RCT comparing usual-care with double-blind injection of 1% lidocaine solution with or without 12.5% dextrose (**Fig. 24**, **Table 4**). Preteens and teens with chronic anterior knee pain localized to the tibial tuberosity with a single leg squat received treatment at 0 months, 1 months, and 2 months, and all groups were offered dextrose injection after 3 months by request. The primary measure for assessment was the 0 to 7 Nirschl Pain Phase Scale (NPPS),[65,66] chosen because a score of 0 indicates both no pain and no stiffness, consistent with full symptom resolution. A 0 to 10 NRS pain score was the secondary measure. Data were collected at 3 months (blinded) and 1 year (open-label).

Participants had statistically similar baseline characteristics. DPT resulted in more improvement of the NPPS score at 3 months than either lidocaine injection or usual care (3.9 ± 0.3 points vs 2.4 ± 0.3 points vs $1.2 \pm .4$ points, respectively; $P<.05$) and lidocaine injection was superior to usual care ($P<.05$) (**Fig. 25**). At 1 year, 32/38 (84%) of knees treated with DPT were asymptomatic (NPPS = 0) compared with 6/13 (46%) or 2/14 (14%) of knees receiving lidocaine injection or usual care throughout the year (see **Fig. 25**).

Temporomandibular subluxation with pain
Multiple needling with either dextrose plus mepivicaine or mepivicaine alone-Study 1 Refai and colleagues[67] compared DPT with mepivacaine to mepivacaine-

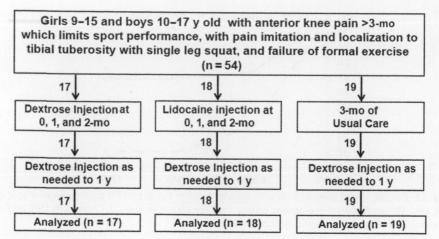

Fig. 24. Flow diagram for Topol et al. (*Data from* Topol GA, Podesta LA, Reeves KD, et al. Hyperosmolar dextrose injection for recalcitrant Osgood-Schlatter disease. Pediatrics 2011;128:e1121–8.)

only injection in a 2-arm blinded trial (**Fig. 26**, **Table 5**) Participants with symptoms of temporomandibular joint (TMJ) locking and facial pain, with CT confirmation of an anteriorly positioned condyle with wide mouth opening received treatment at 0 weeks, 6 weeks, 12 weeks, and 18 weeks, which involved needle insertion into superior and inferior capsular attachments, superficial to the TMJ capsule and joint capsule, and into the superior joint space. Effects were assessed by maximal interincisal opening in millimeters, 0 to 10 VAS for pain with palpation, and in the number of locking episodes per month. Data collection was 3 months after the last injection.

Participants had similar baseline characteristics. Three months after the last treatment, the dextrose group significantly improved in laxity, as reflected in a reduction of excess interincisal opening (dextrose 7 mm [8.6%] vs mepivacaine 0 mm [0%]; $P = .039$). At 3 months, 5/6 (83%) of participants in each group no longer had any pain with palpation of the TMJ, and locking episodes were no longer reported in 6/6 dextrose and 5/6 mepivacaine recipients, with no statistically significant difference between groups (**Fig. 27**).

Multiple needling with either dextrose plus mepivicaine or mepivicaine alone-Study 2 Kilic and Güngörmüş[68] also compared DPT with mepivacaine to mepivacaine-only injection in a 2-arm blinded trial (**Fig. 28**, see **Table 5**). Participants with symptoms of TMJ locking, facial pain, and CT confirmation of an anteriorly positioned condyle with wide mouth opening received injection at 0 weeks, 4 weeks, and 8 weeks into the superior and inferior capsular attachments, posterior disk attachment, stylomandibular ligament, and superior joint space. Effects were assessed by maximal interincisal opening in millimeters and 0 to 10 VAS for participant self-reported pain (not pain with examiner's palpation). The number of subluxations was not monitored. Data were collected at 0 and 12 months.

Participants had statistically similar baseline characteristics. At 1-year follow-up, excess mouth opening was improved significantly but equally in both dextrose and mepivacaine groups (−2.9 mm vs −2.7 mm; $P > .05$). Jaw pain substantially improved in each group (dextrose 79% and mepivacaine 68%) with no significant difference between the 2 groups (**Fig. 29**).

Table 4
Osgood-Schlatter disease risk of bias table

Source	Sequence Generation	Allocation Concealment	Blinding of Participants and Researchers	Blinding of Outcome Assessment	Incomplete Outcome Data Addressed	Selective Outcome Reporting
Topol et al,[64] 2011	Low (a random numbers table was used for assignment)	Unclear (relevant information was not reported)	Low (identical control solution prepared in manner that blinded the subjects and treating/evaluating physicians)	Low (outcome assessor blinded)	Low (no loss to follow-up)	Unclear (no protocol was provided)

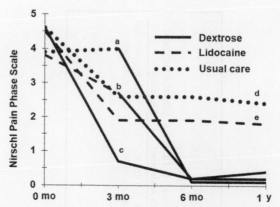

Fig. 25. Improvement in NPPS from 0 to 3 months (masked period) after injection of dextrose, injection of lidocaine, or usual care and improvement pattern from 3 months to 12 months after offering dextrose injection to all participants with Osgood-Schlatter disease. [a] Conversion of a dotted line to a solid line represents the mean NPPS score pattern of participants who received usual care for 3 months and then chose to receive dextrose injection beginning at 3 months. [b] Conversion of a dashed line to a solid line represents the mean NPPS score pattern of participants who received lidocaine injection for 3 months and then chose to receive dextrose injection beginning at 3 months. [c] NPPS change in DPT group from 0 to 3 months was greater than the NPPS change with lidocaine injection ($P<.01$) or usual care ($P<.001$). The DPT group more likely to be symptom free with sport (NPPS = 0) at 3 months than with lidocaine ($P<.01$) or usual care ($P<.001$). NPPS change in lidocaine group greater than change with usual care ($P = .024$). [d] Dextrose-treated knees more frequently asymptomatic with sport 1 year than knees treated with exercise only ($P<.001$). [e] Dextrose-treated knees more frequently asymptomatic with sport 1 year than knees treated with lidocaine only ($P = .024$).

Summary of temporomandibular dysfunction The studies discussed previously suggest that DPT does not perform better than mepivacaine injection alone in improving TMJ pain and laxity, although pain relief was substantial and laxity reduction measurable in both injection groups in each study, suggesting a potential therapeutic effect of

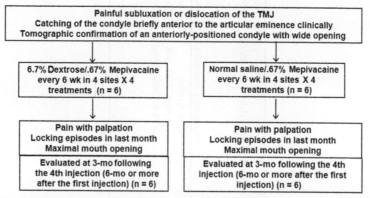

Fig. 26. Flow diagram for Refai et al. (*Data from* Refai H, Altahhan O, Elsharkawy R. The efficacy of dextrose prolotherapy for temporomandibular joint hypermobility: a preliminary prospective, randomized, double-blind, placebo-controlled clinical trial. J Oral Maxilofac Surg 2011;69:2962–70.)

Table 5
Temporomandibular dysfunction painful subluxation risk of bias table

Source	Sequence Generation	Allocation Concealment	Blinding of Participants and Researchers	Blinding of Outcome Assessment	Incomplete Outcome Data Addressed	Selective Outcome Reporting
Rafai et al,[67] 2011	Unclear (random sequence mentioned but method was not described)	Unclear (relevant information was not reported)	Low (the solutions were identical in color)	Low (outcome assessor blinded)	Unclear (relevant information was not reported)	Unclear (no protocol was provided)
Kilic & Güngörmüş,[68] 2016	Unclear (random sequence mentioned but method was not described)	Unclear (relevant information was not reported)	Unclear (relevant information was not reported)	Unclear (relevant information was not reported)	High (4/30 [13.3%] lost to follow-up and intention to treat not used)	Unclear (no protocol was provided)

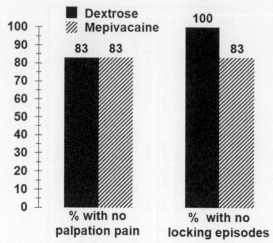

Fig. 27. Percentage of participants with no palpation pain and with no locking episodes 3 months after treatment completion in participants with TMD hypermobility and locking.

injection alone. Both studies had a high risk of bias (see **Table 5**). Larger double-blinded RCTs with more robust methods should be conducted to confirm the efficacy of DPT in the TMJ and preferably include those with other types of TMD, because those with painful hyperlaxity are a subset of the those with TMD. One such larger RCT has recently reported favorable preliminary results.[69]

Tendinopathy

Achilles tendinosis Yelland and colleagues[70] compared DPT to eccentric loading exercises (ELEs) and to combined DPT and ELEs in a 3-arm randomized trial (**Fig. 30**, **Table 6**). ELE is a standard-of-care treatment of Achilles tendinosis with a high success rate.[71,72] Participants had 6 weeks or more of midsubstance Achilles tendinopathy, and clinical severity on the Victorian Institute of Sport Assessment-Achilles

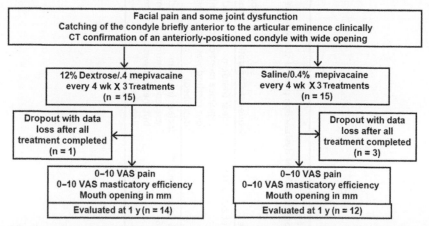

Fig. 28. Flow diagram for Kilic et al. (*Data from* Kilic SC, Güngörmüş M. Is dextrose prolotherapy superior to placebo for the treatment of temporomandibular joint hypermobility? A randomized clinical trial. Int J Oral Maxillofac Surg 2016;45(7):813–9.)

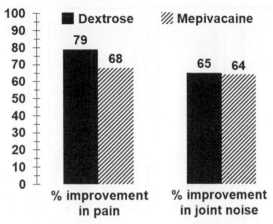

Fig. 29. Percentage improvement in a 0 to 10 VAS for jaw pain and a 0 to 10 VAS for joint noise 1 year after treatment completion in participants with TMD hypermobility and locking.

(VISA-A) score of less than 80 for athletes and less than 70 for nonathletes (higher scores are better). The primary effect measure was the 0 to 100 point VISA-A, measured to 12 months. Injection-treated participants received 9.5 ± 2.8 weekly peritendinous subcutaneous injections according to a published protocol[73]; ELE participants performed eccentric training for 12 weeks according to a published protocol,[74] and combined treatment participants received 8.7 ± 2.9 DPT injections with ELE.

Participants had statistically similar baseline characteristics. By 12 months the improvement in VISA-A scores was more in the combined treatment than ELE-only group (41.1 ± 11.8 vs 23.7 ± 8.1; *P* = .007) (**Fig. 31**) with intermediate results for the DPT-only group (27.5 ± 14.7). One partial Achilles tear occurred in the ELE group.

Lateral epicondylosis Rabago and colleagues[36] compared DPT versus injection of dextrose plus sodium morrhuate versus delayed treatment in a 3-arm trial with

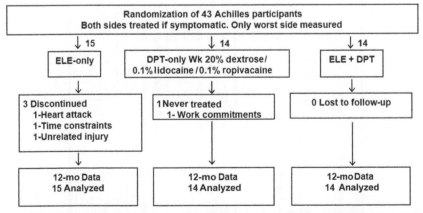

Fig. 30. Flow diagram for Yelland et al Achilles tendinosis clinical trial. (*Data from* Yelland MJ, Sweeting KR, Lyftogt JA, et al. Prolotherapy injections and eccentric loading exercises for painful Achilles tendinosis: a randomised trial. Br J Sports Med 2011;45:421–8.)

Table 6
Tendinopathy risk of bias table

Source	Sequence Generation	Allocation Concealment	Blinding of Participants and Researchers	Blinding of Outcome Assessment	Incomplete Outcome Data Addressed	Selective Outcome Reporting
Yelland et al,[70] 2011	Low (computer-generated random table)	Low (randomization generated and administered by a separate statistics center)	High (open-label trial)	Low (outcome assessor blinded)	Low (4/43 [<10%] dropped out, but intention to treat used)	Unclear (no protocol was provided)
Rabago et al,[36] 2013	Low (computer-generated randomization)	Low (randomization generated and administered by a separate statistical center)	Unclear (relevant information was not reported)	Low (outcome assessor blinded, identical solution)	Low (no lost to follow-up)	Measures agree with (clinical trial registration)
Kim & Lee,[76] 2014	High (randomization by odd and even sequence number)	High (predictable allocation sequence)	High (PRP and dextrose were 2 different modalities)	Unclear (relevant information was not reported)	Low (0/11 dextrose and 1/10 PRP lost to follow-up)	Unclear (no protocol provided)
Bertrand et al,[37] 2016	Low (randomization by blocks of 3)	Low (allocation by off-site pharmacists)	Low (the solutions were identical, participants and injectors blinded)	Low (outcome assessor blinded)	Low (loss to follow-up: 5/77 [6.5%] Intention to treat used)	Low (measures agree with clinical trial registration)

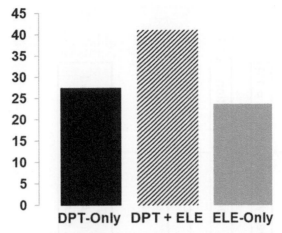

Fig. 31. Improvement in VISA-A score at 12 months comparing DPT versus combination DPT + ELE versus ELE-only in participants with Achilles tendinopathy.

masked injection arms (**Fig. 32**, see **Table 6**). Participants received treatment at 1 week, 4 weeks, and 8 weeks with data collection at 16 weeks, at which time those in the wait-and-see group were offered DPT as their incentive for participation. The prolotherapy groups were then followed to 32 weeks. Effects were assessed using the composite Patient Rated Tennis Elbow Evaluation (PRTEE) score, which has pain (5-item) and function (10-item) subscales[75] and dynamometer-measured grip strength in pounds.

At 16 weeks, the dextrose-morrhuate group improved significantly more than the wait-and-see group on the composite PRTEE (17.5 [54%] vs 9.3 [18%]; $P<.05$) (**Fig. 33**), and the dextrose group outperformed the wait-and-see group on the function subscale of the PRTEE (7.3 vs 5.4; $P<.05$), and further improvement was noted at 32 weeks. Grip strength improvement at 16 weeks in the dextrose group was significantly greater than either the dextrose-morrhuate or wait-and-see groups (65.0 pounds vs 0.9 pounds vs 18.7 pounds, respectively; $P<.05$) (**Fig. 34**). At 32 weeks, the difference between the 2 injection groups was no longer significant for grip strength improvement (69.5 pounds [dextrose] vs 38.6 pounds [dextrose-morrhuate]; $P>.05$) (see **Fig. 34**).

Plantar fasciosis Kim and colleagues compared DPT to injection of autologous PRP in a 2-arm blinded trial (**Fig. 35**, see **Table 6**). Participants with chronic medial arch pain imitated with palpation over the plantar fascia origin and failure of conservative treatments, such as NSAIDs, stretching PT, night split, arch supports, or steroid injection received injection at 0 and 2 weeks. Effects were assessed using the Foot Function Index (FFI).[77,78] Data were collected before the first injection, and 2 weeks, 10 weeks, and 28 weeks after the last injection.

The 2 groups were statistically similar at baseline. The between-group difference in improvement on the FFI did not reach statistical significance at any point in time (**Fig. 36**).This is a comparison, however, of 2 active treatment groups, both of which resulted in clinically significant improvement at more than twice the minimal perceptible change of 11.9 for the FFI[79] in these participants with a mean pain duration of 2.9 years.

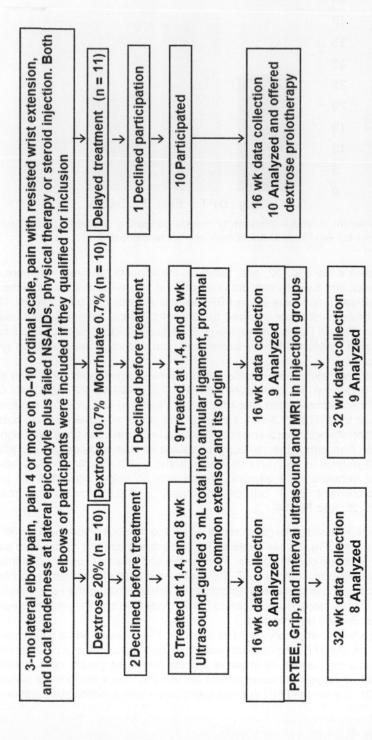

Fig. 32. Flow diagram for Rabago et al lateral epicondylosis clinical trial. (*Data from* Rabago D, Lee KS, Ryan M, et al. Hypertonic dextrose and morrhuate sodium injections [prolotherapy] for lateral epicondylosis [tennis elbow]: results of a single-blind, pilot-level, randomized controlled trial. Am J Phys Med Rehabil 2013;92:587–96.)

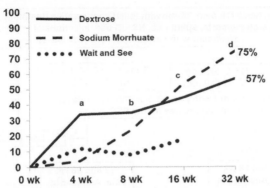

Fig. 33. Percentage improvement in composite PRTEE over time in treatment of lateral epicondylosis. [a] Change in DPT group greater than change in dextrose-morrhuate injection group and wait-and-see group ($P<.05$). [b] Change in DPT group greater than change in the wait-and-see group ($P<.05$) but not greater than change in the dextrose-morrhuate group. [c] Change in the dextrose morrhuate group greater than change in the wait-and-see group ($P<.05$). Change in the DPT group greater than wait-and-see group on functional component of PRTEE. No significant difference between DPT and dextrose-morrhuate. Change in DPT group significantly greater than baseline ($P<.05$). [d] No significant difference between DPT and dextrose-morrhuate. Change in DPT and dextrose-morrhuate group significantly greater than baseline ($P<.05$).

Rotator cuff tendinopathy Bertrand and colleagues[37] conducted a 3-arm blinded RCT comparing DPT (group 1) to lidocaine alone on painful entheses (group 2) to lidocaine alone with superficial injections over painful entheses without touching the entheses (group 3) (**Fig. 37**, see **Table 6**). Participants with chronic shoulder pain and confirmation of rotator cuff tendinopathy by clinical examination and ultrasound

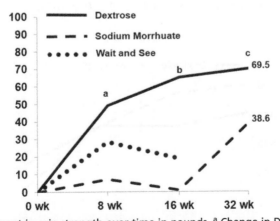

Fig. 34. Improvement in grip strength over time in pounds. [a] Change in DPT group greater than change in dextrose-morrhuate injection group and wait-and-see group ($P<.05$). [b] Change in DPT group greater than change in dextrose-morrhuate injection group and wait-and-see group ($P<.05$). Change in DPT group significantly greater than baseline ($P<.05$). [c] No significant difference between DPT and dextrose-morrhuate. Change in DPT group significantly greater than baseline ($P<.05$).

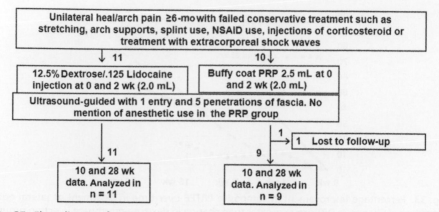

Fig. 35. Flow diagram for Kim et al plantar fasciosis clinical trial. (*Data from* Kim E, Lee JH. Autologous platelet-rich plasma versus dextrose prolotherapy for the treatment of chronic recalcitrant plantar fasciitis. PM R 2014;6:152–8.)

confirmation received injections at 0 months, 1 months, and 2 months, and all received physical therapy during the period of injection. The primary outcome measure was achieving an improvement in maximal current shoulder pain greater than or equal to 2.8 points on a 0 to 10 VAS score, which is twice the MCID for shoulder pain improvement in rotator cuff tendinopathy.[80] Data were collected at 0 and 9 months for pain improvement and for 0 to 10 participant satisfaction (10 = completely satisfied.)

Participants had statistically similar baseline characteristics. A post-treatment questionnaire indicated that blinding of participants was effective. The percentage of participants reaching shoulder pain improvement greater than or equal to 2.8 points on the 0 to 10 VAS at 9 months favored DPT over the superficial lidocaine injection control (59% vs 27%; $P = .017$) (**Fig. 38**) but not the lidocaine enthesis injection group (59% vs 37%; $P = .088$). Patient satisfaction was greater in the DPT group than with superficial lidocaine injection (6.7 ± 3.2 vs 3.9 ± 3.1; $P = .003$) but not compared with lidocaine enthesis injection (6.7 ± 3.2 vs 4.7 ± 4.1; $P = .079$).

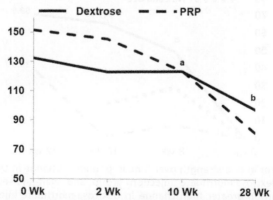

Fig. 36. Change in FFI from 0 to 28 weeks. [a] Change in PRP group significantly better than baseline ($P<.05$). No significant difference between PRP and DPT. [b] Change in PRP and DPT group significantly better than baseline ($P<.05$). No significant difference between PRP and DPT.

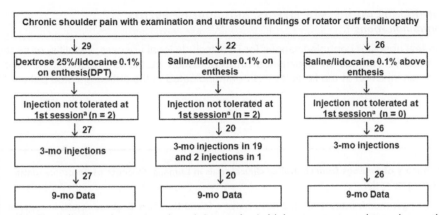

Fig. 37. Flow diagram for Bertrand et al. [a] Anesthetic blebs were not used to enhance the ability to blind between superficial and deep injection groups. Several patients could not tolerate injection. (*Data from* Bertrand H, Reeves KD, Bennett CJ, et al. Dextrose prolotherapy versus control injections in painful rotator cuff tendinopathy. Arch Phys Med Rehabil 2016;97:17–25.)

Summary of tendinopathy Studies show that prolotherapy is effective in both reducing pain and improving function for lower limb tendinopathy and fasciopathy, with no study reporting a mean negative or non significant outcome after prolotherapy injection; DPT injections provides equal or superior short-term, intermediate-term, and long-term results to alternative treatment modalities, including ELEs for Achilles tendinopathy, plantar fasciopathy treatment with PRP, and usual care or lignocaine injections for Osgood-Schlatter disease. The use of DPT on rotator cuff tendinopathy needs more study to confirm its role.

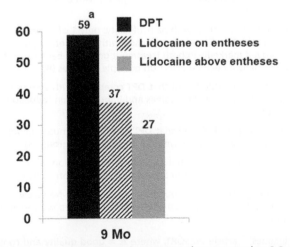

Fig. 38. Percentage of participants improving greater than or equal to 2.8 points on the 0 to 10 VAS at 9 months. [a] Percentage of DPT participants favored DPT over the superficial lidocaine injection control (*P* = 017) but not the lidocaine enthesis injection group (*P* = .088).

CONTRAINDICATIONS, SIDE EFFECTS, AND ADVERSE EVENTS
Contraindications

The few absolute contraindications for DPT include local abscess, cellulitis, or septic arthritis. Knowledge of a patient's anticoagulation status is important, however, because injection at the facet level is contraindicated in the anticoagulated patient.[81]

Box 2
Summary of findings from controlled clinical trials in humans (Strength of Recommendation Taxonomy scale)

1. Finger/thumb osteoarthritis: 2 RCT results; 1 found that 10% dextrose results in superior pain reduction and functional improvement compared with corticosteroid injection in trapeziometacarpal (TMC) OA, and the second found that DPT improves pain and joint flexibility significantly more than anesthetic injection in symptomatic TMC thumb and 2nd through 5th finger proximal interphalangeal (PIP) and distal interphalangeal (DIP) osteoarthritis (B).

2. Knee osteoarthritis: 3 RCT results; 1 study found that DPT improves knee range of motion in advanced knee osteoarthritis, 1 that DPT plus exercise improves pain, function, and stiffness significantly more than exercise alone, and 1 that DPT improves function and pain levels significantly in comparison with both injection control and exercise. A recently published meta-analysis concluded that the effects of DPT are both positive and significantly beneficial in symptomatic knee osteoarthritis (A).

3. Low back pain: 1 study found that DPT is not superior to injection of multiple entheses with saline, although treatment in both groups resulted in significant and sustainable functional gains to 1 year (B).

4. Sacroiliac pain: 1 study found that intraarticular injection of dextrose compared with steroid injection resulted in superior long-term pain reduction in those with a diagnostic-injection–confirmed sacroiliac pain source (B).

5. Osgood-Schlatter disease: 1 study found that DPT significantly improves the frequency of unrestricted sport and asymptomatic sport compared with usual-care exercise and lidocaine injection. (A)

6. Temporomandibular dysfunction with painful laxity: only 1 of 2 studies showed that DPT reduced laxity in painful lax TMJs in comparison with anesthetic injection. Jaw pain and subluxation improved markedly in both treatment groups in each study, for reasons unclear, but potentially a needlng effect on multiple entheses (B).

7. Achilles tendinopathy: 1 study found that DPT combined with standard-of-care therapy (ELEs) results in better functional outcomes and improved pain reduction at 12 months than ELEs alone (B).

8. Lateral epicondylosis: 1 study found that DPT and DPT/morrhuate improve function and pain levels in comparison with a delayed treatment control group (B).

9. Plantar fasciosis: 1 study found that DPT and PRP injection both result in clinically significant functional improvement in a treatment comparison study (B).

10. Rotator cuff tendinopathy: 1 study found that, in patients who receive physical therapy, DPT results in improved pain reduction at 9 months compared with superficial anesthetic control injection (B).

Per Ebell and colleagues'[85] article on SORT, where A = good quality and consistent patient-oriented evidence, B = limited quality of inconsistent patient-oriented evidence, and C = usual practice, consensus, disease-oriented evidence, opinion, or case series evidence.

Common Side Effects

Pain with injection is common, although this may be minimized considerably with use of anesthetic blebs, coupled with tumescent type anesthetic injection through such blebs. Mild bleeding also occurs with injection. Postinjection soreness is common, typically waning by the second day,[53] and mild or limited analgesic use may be helpful for some patients.[52] A self-limited pain flare may occur, typically managed with acetaminophen. NSAIDs are not routinely used postprocedure, due to theoretic interference with 1 or more DPT mechanisms, although histologic evidence does not support that theory.[24]

Adverse Events

Dagenais and colleagues[82] reported the largest survey to date of adverse events associated with prolotherapy to the spine. They sought responses from 308 practicing prolotherapists, with a response rate of 50%. Of the 472 adverse events reported, 174 were spinal headaches, with 123 pneumothoraces, 73 systemic reactions, 54 nerve damage events, 27 hemorrhages, 9 nonsevere spinal cord insults to spinal cord and 2 disk injuries. Their conclusion was that adverse effects are similar to other needling procedures about the spine.

No adverse effects were noted in the randomized trials reviewed in this article. The authors' review for other reports in peer-reviewed literature of DPT-related complications revealed 1 case report of isolated partial R arm numbness related to improper technique in a cervical injection[83] and 1 case report of epidural abscess time-related to perispinal proliferant injection.[84] Despite the rarity of such events, complications after DPT directly relate to the training of the injector and consistency in use of customary antiseptic precautions.[85] As prolotherapy progressively moves toward

---

Box 3
Best practice recommendations with strength of recommendation per Strength of Recommendation Taxonomy scale

1. TMC/finger osteoarthritis: in chronic TMC osteoarthritis DPT is preferable to steroid injection, and in symptomatic PIP and DIP arthritis DPT may reduce pain and stiffness (B).

2. Knee osteoarthritis: DPT should be considered, because its effects are both positive and significantly beneficial in symptomatic knee osteoarthritis (A).

3. Low back pain: no definite recommendations came be made based on literature available.

4. Sacroiliac pain: DPT is preferable to steroid injection in those with sacroiliac pain confirmed by diagnostic injection.

5. Osgood-Schlatter disease: consider DPT for adolescents with Osgood-Schlatter disease who have persistent pain or limitation of sport despite physical therapy.

6. Temporomandibular dysfunction with painful laxity: no definite recommendations can be made based on literature available.

7. Achilles tendinopathy: the combination of DPT and ELEs may be utilized as potentially superior to either treatment alone.

8. Lateral epicondylosis: DPT may improve pain and function in those who have failed NSAIDs, standard physical therapy or steroid injection.

9. Plantar fasciosis: DPT may improve functional status in plantar fasciosis.

10. Rotator cuff tendinopathy: consider DPT administration in combination with physical therapy, or with insufficient or nonsustained response to physical therapy.

routine incorporation in university training programs, systemization of methods is expected to further reduce adverse events.

SUMMARY OF CURRENT LITERATURE STATUS, STRENGTH OF RECOMMENDATION EVIDENCE, AND BEST TREATMENT RECOMMENDATIONS

Box 2 is a summary of clinical findings from the RCTs published at the time of this writing along with their Strength of Recommendation Taxonomy (SORT).[86] **Box 3** lists the current best practice recommendations for use of DPT for osteoarthritis, low back pain and sacroiliac pain, Osgood-Schlatter disease, TMD, and various enthesopathies (Achilles, lateral epicondylosis, and rotator cuff).

INCORPORATING PROLOTHERAPY INTO PRACTICE

DPT is a treatment method with broad applications and this article cannot address methods in any detail. Methods of prolotherapy are described in several textbooks.[1,87,88] Training in DPT is not typically available in medical school and residency programs. More commonly, post graduate training is available through conference settings including the University of Wisconsin Prolotherapy Education and Research Lab (UW-PEARL; http://www.fammed.wisc.edu/prolotherapy/research) in concert with the Hackett Hemwall Foundation (www.hacketthemwall.org/WELCOME.html), the American Association of Orthopaedic Medicine (www.aaomed.org), and the American Osteopathic Association of Prolotherapy Regenerative Medicine (www.prolotherapycollege.org)

REFERENCES

1. Hackett GS, Hemwall GA, Montgomery GA. Ligament and tendon relaxation treated by prolotherapy. Oak Park (IL): Gustav A. Hemwall; 1993.
2. DeChellis DM, Cortazzo MH. Regenerative medicine in the field of pain medicine: prolotherapy, platelet-rich plasma, and stem cell therapy-theory and evidence. Tech Reg Anesth Pain Manag 2011;15:74–80.
3. Rabago D, Slattengren A, Zgierska A. Prolotherapy in primary care practice. Prim Care 2010;37:65–80.
4. Higgins JP, Altman DG, Gøtzsche PC, et al. The Cochrane Collaboration's tool for assessing risk of bias in randomised trials. BMJ 2011;18:d5928.
5. Thorens B, Mueckler M. Glucose transporters in the 21st Century. Am J Physiol Endocrinol Metab 2010;298:E141–5.
6. Murphy M, Godson C, Cannon S, et al. Suppression subtractive hybridization identifies high glucose levels as a stimulus for expression of connective tissue growth factor and other genes in human mesangial cells. J Biol Chem 1999; 274:5830–4.
7. Pugliese G, Pricci F, Locuratolo N, et al. Increased activity of the insulin-like growth factor system in mesangial cells cultured in high glucose conditions. Relation to glucose-enhanced extracellular matrix production. Diabetologia 1996;39: 775–84.
8. Di Paolo S, Gesualdo L, Ranieri E, et al. High glucose concentration induces the overexpression of transforming growth factor-beta through the activation of a platelet-derived growth factor loop in human mesangial cells. Am J Pathol 1996;149:2095–106.
9. Fukuda K, Kawata S, Inui Y, et al. High concentration of glucose increases mitogenic responsiveness to heparin-binding epidermal growth factor-like growth

factor in rat vascular smooth muscle cells. Arterioscler Thromb Vasc Biol 1997;17: 1962–8.

10. Ohgi S, Johnson PW. Glucose modulates growth of gingival fibroblasts and periodontal ligament cells: correlation with expression of basic fibroblast growth factor. J Periodontal Res 1996;31:579–88.

11. Mobasheri A. Glucose: an energy currency and structural precursor in articular cartilage and bone with emerging roles as an extracellular signaling molecule and metabolic regulator. Front Endocrinol 2012;3:153.

12. Cigan AD, Nims RJ, Albro MB, et al. Insulin, ascorbate, and glucose have a much greater influence than transferrin and selenous acid on the in vitro growth of engineered cartilage in chondrogenic media. Tissue Eng Part A 2013;19:1941–8.

13. Russell JW, Golovoy D, Vincent AM, et al. High glucose-induced oxidative stress and mitochondrial dysfunction in neurons. FASEB J 2002;16:1738–48.

14. Stecker MM, Stevenson M. Effect of glucose concentration on peripheral nerve and its response to anoxia. Muscle Nerve 2014;49:370–7.

15. Wong TY, Cheung CM, Larsen M, et al. Diabetic retinopathy. Nat Rev Dis Primers 2016;2:16012.

16. D'Lima DD. Glucose concentration increases IGF expression from human synovial membrane, Technical Report, August 17, 2009. Available at: http://www.aaomed.org/Scripps-Report-Glucose-effect-on-Synovial-tissue-IGF-expression. Accessed August 6, 2016.

17. Laiguillon MC, Courties A, Houard X, et al. Characterization of diabetic osteoarthritic cartilage and role of high glucose environment on chondrocyte activation: toward pathophysiological delineation of diabetes mellitus-related osteoarthritis. Osteoarthritis Cartilage 2015;23:1513–22.

18. Kim SA, Kim EH, Kim SY, et al. The effects of hyperosmolar dextrose and autologous serum injection in the experimental articular defect of rabbit. J Korean Acad Rehabil Med 2006;30:173–8.

19. Park YS, Lim SW, Lee IH, et al. Intra-articular injection of a nutritive mixture solution protects articular cartilage from osteoarthritic progression induced by anterior cruciate ligament transection in mature rabbits: a randomized controlled trial. Arthritis Res Ther 2007;9:R8.

20. Pearson RG, Kurien T, Shu KS, et al. Histopathology grading systems for characterisation of human knee osteoarthritis–reproducibility, variability, reliability, correlation, and validity. Osteoarthritis Cartilage 2011;19:324–31.

21. Martins CA, Bertuzzi RT, Tisot RA, et al. Dextrose prolotherapy and corticosteroid injection into rat Achilles tendon. Knee Surg Sports Traumatol Arthrosc 2012;20: 1895–900.

22. Ahn KH, Kim HS, Lee WK, et al. The effect of the prolotherapy on the injured Achilles tendon in a rat model. J Korean Acad Rehabil Med 2002;26:332–6.

23. Kim HJ, Jeong TS, Kim WS, et al. Comparison of histological changes in accordance with the level of dextrose-concentration in experimental prolotherapy model. J Korean Acad Rehabil Med 2003;27:935–40.

24. Kim HJ, Kim SH, Yun DH, et al. The effects of anti-inflammatory drugs on histologic findings of the experimental prolotherapy model. J Korean Acad Rehab Med 2006;30:378–84.

25. Jensen KT, Rabago DP, Best TM, et al. Early inflammatory response of knee ligaments to prolotherapy in a rat model. J Orthop Res 2008;26:816–23.

26. Jensen KT, Rabago D, Best TM, et al. Longer term response of knee ligaments to prolotherapy in a rat injury model. Am J Sports Med 2008;36:1347–57.

27. Provenzano PP, Hayashi K, Kunz DN, et al. Healing of subfailure ligament injury: comparison between immature and mature ligaments in a rat model. J Orthop Res;20:975–983.

28. Oh S, Ettema AM, Zhao C, et al. Dextrose-induced subsynovial connective tissue fibrosis in the rabbit carpal tunnel: a potential model to study carpal tunnel syndrome? Hand 2008;3:34–40.

29. Yoshii Y, Zhao C, Schmelzer JD, et al. The effects of hypertonic dextrose injection on connective tissue and nerve conduction through the rabbit carpal tunnel. Arch Phys Med Rehabil 2009;90:333–9.

30. Yoshii Y, Zhao C, Schmelzer JD, et al. Effects of hypertonic dextrose injections in the rabbit carpal tunnel. J Orthop Res 2011;29:1022–7.

31. Yoshii Y, Zhao C, Schmelzer JD, et al. Effects of multiple injections of hypertonic dextrose in the rabbit carpal tunnel: a potential model of carpal tunnel syndrome development. Hand (N Y) 2014;9:52–7.

32. Yamaguchi T, Osamura N, Zhao C, et al. The mechanical properties of the rabbit carpal tunnel subsynovial connective tissue. J Biomech 2008;41:3519–22.

33. Rabago D, Kijowski R, Woods M, et al. Association between disease-specific quality-of-life and magnetic resonance imaging outcomes in a clinical trial of prolotherapy for knee osteoarthritis. Arch Phys Med Rehabil 2013;94:2075–82.

34. Munk B, Madsen F, Lundorf E, et al. Clinical magnetic resonance imaging and arthroscopic findings in knees: a comparative prospective study of meniscus anterior cruciate ligament and cartilage lesions. Arthroscopy 1998;14:171–5.

35. Topol GA, Podesta LA, Reeves KD, et al. The chondrogenic effect of intra-articular hypertonic-dextrose (prolotherapy) in severe knee osteoarthritis. PM&R 2016. http://dx.doi.org/10.1016/j.pmrj.2016.03.008.

36. Rabago D, Lee KS, Ryan M, et al. Hypertonic dextrose and morrhuate sodium injections (prolotherapy) for lateral epicondylosis (tennis elbow): results of a single-blind, pilot-level, randomized controlled trial. Am J Phys Med Rehabil 2013;92: 587–96.

37. Bertrand H, Reeves KD, Bennett CJ, et al. Dextrose Prolotherapy Versus Control Injections in Painful Rotator Cuff Tendinopathy. Arch Phys Med Rehabil 2016;97: 17–25.

38. Brose SW, Boninger ML, Fullerton BD, et al. Shoulder ultrasound abnormalities, physical examination findings, and pain in manual wheelchair users with spinal cord injury. Arch Phys Med Rehabil 2008;89:2086–93.

39. Ryan M, Wong A, Rabago D, et al. Ultrasound-guided injections of hyperosmolar dextrose for overuse patellar tendinopathy: a pilot study. Br J Sports Med 2011; 45:972–7.

40. Ryan M, Wong A, Taunton J. Favorable outcomes after sonographically guided intratendinous injection of hyperosmolar dextrose for chronic insertional and mid-portion Achilles tendinosis. Am J Roentgenol 2010;194:1047–53.

41. Lyftogt J. Pain conundrums: which hypothesis? Central nervous system sensitization versus peripheral nervous system autonomy. Australas Musculoskel Med 2008;13:72–4.

42. Maniquis-Smigel L, Reeves KD, Lyftogt J, et al. Analgesic effect of caudal 5% dextrose in water in chronic low back pain (Abs). Arch Phys Med Rehabil 2015;96:e103.

43. Watabiki T, Kiso T, Kuramochi T, et al. Amelioration of neuropathic pain by novel transient receptor potential vanilloid 1 antagonist AS1928370 in rats without hyperthermic effect. J Pharmacol Exp Ther 2011;336:743–50.

44. Bertrand H, Kyriazis M, Reeves KD, et al. Topical Mannitol Reduces Capsaicin-induced Pain: Results of a Pilot Level, Double-Blind Randomized Controlled Trial. PM&R 2015;7:1111–7.
45. Szallasi A, Cortright DN, Blum CA, et al. The vanilloid receptor TRPV1: 10 years from channel cloning to antagonist proof-of-concept. Nat Rev Drug Discov 2007; 6:357–72.
46. Jahangiri A, Moghaddam FR, Najafi S. Hypertonic dextrose versus corticosteroid local injection for the treatment of osteoarthritis in the first carpometacarpal joint: a double-blind randomized clinical trial. J Orthop Sci 2014;19:737–43.
47. Reeves KD, Hassanein K. Randomized prospective placebo-controlled double-blind study of dextrose prolotherapy for osteoarthritic thumbs and fingers (DIP, PIP and trapeziometacarpal Joints): evidence of clinical efficacy. Jnl Alt Compl Med 2000;6:311–20.
48. Reeves KD, Hassanein K. Randomized prospective double-blind placebo-controlled study of dextrose prolotherapy for knee osteoarthritis with or without ACL laxity. Alt Ther Hlth Med 2000;6:68–80.
49. Hashemi M, Jalili P, Mennati S, et al. The effects of prolotherapy with hypertonic dextrose versus prolozone (intraarticular ozone) in patients with knee osteoarthritis. Anesth Pain Med 2015;5:e27584.
50. Dumais R, Benoit C, Dumais A, et al. Effect of regenerative injection therapy on function and pain in patients with knee osteoarthritis: a randomized crossover study. Pain Med 2012;13:990–9.
51. Jones B, Kenward MG. Design and Analysis of Cross-Over Trials. 2nd edition. New York: Chapman & Hall/CRC; 2003.
52. Rabago D, Patterson JJ, Mundt M, et al. Dextrose prolotherapy for knee osteoarthritis: a randomized controlled trial. Annals of family medicine 2013;11:229–37.
53. Rabago D, Zgierska A, Fortney L, et al. Hypertonic dextrose injections (prolotherapy) for knee osteoarthritis: results of a single-arm uncontrolled study with 1-year follow-up. J Altern Complement Med 2012;18:408–14.
54. Sit RWS, Chung VCH, Reeves KD, et al. Hypertonic dextrose injections (prolotherapy) in the treatment of symptomatic knee osteoarthritis: a systematic review and meta-analysis. Scientific Reports 2016;6:25247.
55. Yelland MJ, Glasziou PP, Bogduk N, et al. Prolotherapy injections, saline injections, and exercises for chronic low-back pain: a randomized trial. Spine 2004; 29:9–16.
56. Dhillon GS. Prolotherapy in lumbo-pelvic pain australas musculoskel. Med 1997; 2:17–9.
57. Ostelo RW, Deyo RA, Stratford P, et al. Interpreting change scores for pain and functional status in low back pain: towards international consensus regarding minimal important change. Spine 2008;33:90–4.
58. Kim WM, Lee HG, Jeong CW, et al. A randomized controlled trial of intra-articular prolotherapy versus steroid injection for sacroiliac joint pain. J Altern Complement Med 2010;16:1285–90.
59. Dagenais S, Mayer J, Haldeman S, et al. Evidence-informed management of chronic low back pain with prolotherapy. Spine J 2008;8:203–12.
60. Mathews JA, Mills SB, Jenkins VM, et al. Back pain and sciatica: controlled trials of manipulation, traction, sclerosant and epidural injections. Br J Rheumatol 1987;26:416–23.
61. Klein RG, Eek BC, DeLong WB, et al. A randomized double-blind trial of dextrose-glycerine-phenol injections for chronic, low back pain. J Spinal Disord 1993;6: 23–33.

62. Ongley MJ, Klein RG, Dorman TA, et al. A new approach to the treatment of chronic low back pain. Lancet 1987;18:143–6.
63. Dechow E, Davies RK, Carr AJ, et al. A randomized, double-blind, placebo-controlled trial of sclerosing injections in patients with chronic low back pain. Rheumaology 1999;38:1255–9.
64. Topol GA, Podesta LA, Reeves KD, et al. Hyperosmolar dextrose injection for recalcitrant Osgood-Schlatter disease. Pediatrics 2011;128:e1121–8.
65. Nirschl RP. Elbow tendinosis/tennis elbow. Clin Sports Med 1992;11:851–70.
66. O'Connor FG, Howard TM, Fieseler CM, et al. Managing overuse injuries: a systematic approach. Phys Sportsmed 1997;25:88–113.
67. Refai H, Altahhan O, Elsharkawy R. The efficacy of dextrose prolotherapy for temporomandibular joint hypermobility: a preliminary prospective, randomized, double-blind, placebo-controlled clinical trial. J Oral Maxilofac Surg 2011;69:2962–70.
68. Kilic SC, Güngörmüş M. Is dextrose prolotherapy superior to placebo for the treatment of temporomandibular joint hypermobility? A randomized clinical trial. Int J Oral Maxillofacial Surg 2016.
69. Louw WF. Treatment of Temporomandibular Dysfunction with dextrose prolotherapy: A randomized controlled trial with long term follow-up (abs) North American Primary Care Research Group, 11400 Tomahawk Creek Parkway, Suite 240, Leawood, KS, 66211. Available at: http://wwwnapcrgorg/Conferences/Past MeetingArchives/2016AnnualMeetingArchives/pending 2016.
70. Yelland MJ, Sweeting KR, Lyftogt JA, et al. Prolotherapy injections and eccentric loading exercises for painful Achilles tendinosis: a randomised trial. Br J Sports Med 2011;45:421–8.
71. Kingma JJ, de Knikker R, Wittnick HM, et al. Eccentric overload training in patients with chronic Achilles tendinopathy: a systematic review. Br J Sports Med 2007;41(6):e3.
72. Stevens M, Tan CW. Eccentric lengthening is supported as first line treatment for Achilles and patellar tendinopathy. J Orthop Sports Phys Ther 2014;44:59–67.
73. Lyftogt J. Subcutaneous prolotherapy for Achilles tendinopathy Australas Musculoskeletal. Med 2007;12:107–9.
74. Alfredson H, Pietilä T, Jonsson P, et al. Heavy-load eccentric calf muscle training for the treatment of chronic Achilles tendinosis. Am J Sports Med 1998;26:360–6.
75. Macdermid J. Update: The Patient-rated Forearm Evaluation Questionnaire is now the Patient-rated Tennis Elbow Evaluation. J Hand Ther;18:407–410.
76. Kim E, Lee JH. Autologous platelet-rich plasma versus dextrose prolotherapy for the treatment of chronic recalcitrant plantar fasciitis. PMR 2014;6:152–8.
77. Agel J, Beskin JL, Brage M, et al. Reliability of the Foot Function Index:: A report of the AOFAS Outcomes Committee. Foot Ankle Int 2005;26:962–7.
78. SooHoo NF, Samimi DB, Vyas RM, et al. Evaluation of the validity of the Foot Function Index in measuring outcomes in patients with foot and ankle disorders. Foot Ankle Int 2006;27:38–42.
79. Landorf KB, Radford JA. Minimal important difference: values for the Foot Health Status Questionnaire, Foot Function Index and Visual Analogue Scale. The Foot 2008;18:15–9.
80. Tashjian RZ, Deloach J, Porucznik CA, et al. Minimal clinically important differences (MCID) and patient acceptable symptomatic state (PASS) for visual analog scales (VAS) measuring pain in patients treated for rotator cuff disease. J Shoulder Elbow Surg 2009;18:927–32.

81. Friedrich JM, Harrast MA. Lumbar epidural steroid injections: indications, contra-indications, risks, and benefits. Curr Sports Med Rep 2010;9:43–9.
82. Dagenais S, Ogunseitan O, Haldeman S, et al. Side effects and adverse events related to intraligamentous injection of sclerosing solutions (prolotherapy) for back and neck pain: a survey of practitioners. Arch Phys Med Rehabil 2006; 87:909–13.
83. Yun HS, Sun HS, Seon HJ, et al. Prolotherapy-induced cervical spinal cord injury-A case report. Ann Rehabil Med 2011;35:570–3.
84. Clifton T, Selby M. Epidural abscess from prolotherapy: a cautionary tale. ANZ J Surg 2015.
85. Foster MA, Grigg C, Hagon J, et al. Notes from the Field: Investigation of Hepatitis C Virus Transmission Associated with Injection Therapy for Chronic Pain - California, 2015. MMWR Morb Mortal Wkly Rep 2016;65:547–9.
86. Ebell MH, Siwek J, Weiss BDW, et al. Strength of recommendation taxonomy (SORT): a patient-centered approach to grading evidence in the medical literature. Am Fam Physician 2004;69:549–56.
87. Ravin TH, Cantieri MS, Pasquarello GJ. Principles of prolotherapy. Friesens, Altona, Manitoba, Canada: American Academy of Musculoskeletal Medicine; 2008.
88. Reeves KD, Lyfogt J. Prolotherapy: regenerative injection therapy. In: Waldman SD, editor. Pain management. 2nd edition. Philadelphia: Saunders (Elsevier); 2011. p. 1027–44.

Platelet-Rich Plasma

Peter I-Kung Wu, MD, PhD[a],*, Robert Diaz, MD[a],
Joanne Borg-Stein, MD[b]

KEYWORDS

- Platelet-rich plasma • Musculoskeletal • Healing • Regenerative • Sports
- Rehabilitation • Injection

KEY POINTS

- PRP is a regenerative therapy that has gained popularity in musculoskeletal medicine for its potential to augment repair of tissues with low healing ability.
- Basic science and preclinical studies have begun to elucidate the therapeutic roles of platelets, leukocytes, and red blood cells, suggesting greater benefit from leukocyte-poor PRP.
- Clinical studies have investigated PRP for tendon, ligament, muscle, and cartilage repair, yielding limited Level I evidence supporting use for lateral epicondylosis and knee osteoarthritis.
- Patient selection and education and postprocedural rehabilitation are essential to maximize the therapeutic effect of PRP.
- Investigations are needed to determine the ideal PRP composition, while large clinical trials with standardized reporting of formulations used are needed to determine PRP efficacy.

INTRODUCTION

The clinical application of platelet-rich plasma (PRP) and other regenerative therapies in sports, spine, and musculoskeletal medicine has soared in the last decade. Over this period, many factors have converged to fuel this development. Advances in scientific understanding of tendinopathy as a degenerative cellular and connective tissue process; lack of long-term efficacy of steroid injection therapies, which has prompted the need for alternative therapies; advances in musculoskeletal ultrasound (US) to facilitate diagnosis and guide interventions; as well as translation of treatment paradigms from colleagues in oral and veterinary surgery have all contributed to the advancement of this regenerative field.

Disclosure: There are no commercial or financial conflicts of interest or any funding sources to disclose.
[a] Department of Physical Medicine & Rehabilitation, Spaulding Rehabilitation Hospital, Harvard Medical School, 300 First Avenue, Charlestown, MA 02129, USA; [b] Department of Physical Medicine & Rehabilitation, Newton-Wellesley Hospital Spine Center, Spaulding Rehabilitation Hospital, Harvard Medical School, 65 Walnut Street, Wellesley, MA 02481, USA
* Corresponding author.
E-mail address: iwu3@partners.org

Phys Med Rehabil Clin N Am 27 (2016) 825–853
http://dx.doi.org/10.1016/j.pmr.2016.06.002
1047-9651/16/© 2016 Elsevier Inc. All rights reserved.

This article provides the latest clinically relevant information on the basic science of PRP and practical considerations for its use, evidence for PRP use in musculoskeletal medicine, recommendations for PRP preparation and patient selection, as well as suggested postprocedure rehabilitation and return to sport protocols. The authors will identify the limitations in current knowledge of this regenerative therapy and recommend critical areas for future research.

BASIC SCIENCE AND RATIONALE
Definition of Platelet-Rich Plasma

PRP is a preparation of autologous plasma enriched with a platelet concentration above that normally contained in whole blood.[1] In clinical musculoskeletal medicine, PRP is classically prepared by centrifuging autologous, anticoagulated whole blood to separate its components and concentrate platelets above baseline levels. Typical protocols include either 1 or 2 centrifugation steps to separate whole blood into 3 layers: a top plasma layer, middle leukocyte layer, and bottom red blood cell (RBC) layer, to collect a concentrate of platelets in plasma.[2] The rationale for use and therapeutic potential of a high concentration of platelets is based on their capacity to supply and release supraphysiologic amounts of essential growth factors and cytokines from their alpha granules to provide a regenerative stimulus that augments healing and promotes repair in tissues with low healing potential.

Early Use of Platelet-Rich Plasma

PRP therapy has gained popularity in regenerative medicine and other specialties since the earliest reports of its clinical use in the 1980s and 1990s, with applications traced to the fields of cardiac, dental, and maxillofacial surgery. In cardiac surgery, PRP was shown to be an effective autologous source for transfusion to address surgical blood loss and hematologic derangements from cardiopulmonary bypass.[3,4] In dentistry, Anitua[5] demonstrated application of PRP to tooth extraction sites facilitated bone regeneration in these sockets with compact mature bone that had normal morphology. In maxillofacial surgery, Marx and colleagues[6] evaluated the effect of PRP on bone maturation rate and bone density in bone graft reconstructions of mandibular continuity defects, demonstrating that addition of PRP to grafts resulted in increased bone formation.

Today in musculoskeletal and sports medicine, PRP therapy has become highly attractive for its potential benefit and influence on repairing injured tissue, treating a wide range of degenerative disorders, and accelerating return to sport, finding its role as an injectable biologic used to augment healing of tendon, ligament, muscle, and cartilage.[7]

Basics of Wound Healing

The utility of PRP in promoting healing is especially significant for tendons, ligaments, and cartilage, the repair processes of which can be particularly slow and poor due to their limited blood supply and slow cell turnover.[8,9] In general, wound healing can be separated into 3 phases: inflammation, proliferation, and remodeling.[10] The initial inflammation phase is characterized by hemostasis, with platelets establishing clot formation, and the release of growth factors that aid in activating and attracting inflammatory cells like neutrophils and macrophages to the site of injury. The proliferation phase is characterized by the construction of an extracellular matrix associated with granulation, contraction, and epithelialization.[7,10] Finally, the remodeling phase is associated with production of collagen and scar tissue. The physiologic progression through these phases of wound healing is orchestrated by growth factors and cytokines, many of which are released and modulated by blood components in PRP.

Components of Platelet-Rich Plasma

Platelets

Although platelets play a key role in hemostasis, they are central to mediating the anabolic effects of PRP by virtue of releasing growth factors stored in their alpha granules. During the initial phases of wound repair, activated platelets attract and foster cell migration into the wound by aggregating and forming a fibrin matrix. This matrix then serves as a tissue scaffold for sustained release of platelet growth factors and cytokines, which stimulate cell recruitment, differentiation, and communication.[11] Although both angiogenic and antiangiogenic factors are stored in platelets, they are released differentially.[11,12] Notable growth factors released from platelets that are involved in the healing process include platelet-derived growth factor (PDGF), transforming growth factor (TGF-β), vascular endothelial growth factor (VEGF), epidermal growth factor (EGF), basic fibroblast growth factor (bFGF), and insulin-like growth factor (IGF-1) (**Table 1**).[8]

Leukocytes

Leukocytes are essential mediators of the inflammatory response, host defense against infectious agents, and wound healing.[8] Neutrophils are involved in the inflammation phase of wound healing. Monocytes and macrophages facilitate tissue repair by debriding and phagocytosing damaged tissue and debris. Similar to platelets, macrophages also secrete growth factors that are important in tissue repair and have been shown to contribute to subchondral bone regeneration.[2,13] Although leukocytes play key roles in tissue repair and provide desirable protection against infectious agents, their proinflammatory and immunologic effects can also induce undesirable local

Table 1
Key regenerative growth factors stored in platelet alpha granules and their functions

Growth Factor	Function
PDGF	Stimulates cell proliferation, chemotaxis, and differentiation Stimulates angiogenesis
TGF-β	Stimulates production of collagen type I and type III, angiogenesis, re-epithelialization, and synthesis of protease inhibitors to inhibit collagen breakdown
VEGF	Stimulates angiogenesis by regulating endothelial cell proliferation and migration
EGF	Influences cell proliferation and cytoprotection Accelerates re-epithelialization Increases tensile strength in wounds Facilitates organization of granulation tissue
bFGF	Stimulates angiogenesis Promotes stem cell differentiation and cell proliferation Promotes collagen production and tissue repair
IGF-1	Regulates cell proliferation and differentiation Influences matrix secretion from osteoblasts and production of proteoglycan, collagen, and other noncollagen proteins

Abbreviations: PDGF, platelet-derived growth factor; TGF-β, transforming growth factor-β; VEGF, vascular endothelial growth factor; EGF, epidermal growth factor; bFGF, basic fibroblast growth factor; IGF-1, insulin-like growth factor.
Data from Refs.[1,2,8,12]

cell and tissue damage that opposes the intended healing effects of PRP therapy. In vitro studies have shown that high concentrations of leukocytes in PRP can produce an inflammatory environment that can be detrimental to the healing response.[14–17] In addition, studies of tendon models by Boswell and colleagues[18] showed that reducing leukocyte concentrations, and thus decreasing the inflammatory response, may be more important than maximizing platelet concentrations to optimize PRP efficacy. A summary of several preclinical studies involving leukocyte concentration in PRP is provided in **Table 2**. Further preclinical studies are needed for each target tissue type to elucidate the optimal concentration of leukocytes that can augment healing without inciting damage.

Red blood cells
RBC content is typically reduced or absent in PRP because of the centrifugation process. Using hemoglobin, RBCs perform their primary function of carrying and delivering oxygen, other metabolic gases, nutrients, and regulatory molecules like nitric oxide. Although nitric oxide is known to stimulate vasodilation, it has also been implicated in mediating insensitivity in diseased cartilage to the anabolic effects of IGF-1.[8] During oxidative stress, iron contained in heme molecules can release cytotoxic oxygen free radicals that induce apoptosis of host cells.[8] This destructive process is thought to occur in human synoviocytes treated with RBC concentrates, leading to significantly greater cell death and cartilage degradation.[15,19–21] Such findings suggest that RBC concentrations should be reduced or eliminated in PRP preparations used for intra-articular applications.

Considerations for Platelet-Rich Plasma Use

Differences among platelet-rich plasma products
To date, there is no general consensus on how best to prepare PRP or the optimal concentrations of blood components to include in the product, with each PRP formulation having its own unique biologic properties and effects, which has contributed to

Table 2
Findings from preclinical studies of leukocyte concentration in platelet-rich plasma

Tissue of Interest	Findings
Human synoviocytes[15]	Treatment with leukocyte-rich PRP and RBC concentrates resulted in significant cell death and proinflammatory mediator production. Consider using leukocyte-poor and RBC-free preparations of PRP for intra-articular therapy
Rabbit patellar tendons[16]	Leukocyte-rich PRP resulted in significantly greater inflammatory response 5 d after intratendinous injection compared with leukocyte-poor PRP. There was no difference in inflammatory response 14 d after injection between leukocyte-rich and leukocyte-poor PRP
Human synoviocytes[14]	Leukocyte-rich PRP is able to maintain long-term upregulation of proinflammatory factors and downregulation of anticatabolic mediators in cartilage compared with leukocyte-poor PRP and platelet-poor plasma
Equine flexor digitorum superficialis tendons[13]	High leukocyte concentrations in PRP can contribute to the expression of inflammatory cytokines in flexor digitorum superficialis tendon explants. Leukocyte-poor PRP may be the preferred preparation to stimulate healing without scar tissue formation

mixed results of PRP's clinical efficacy from human trials. In the literature, investigators have used a variety of PRP preparation protocols, differing by preparation kits, centrifugation systems, number of centrifugation steps, activation methods with or without thrombin and/or calcium, and ultimate concentrations of PRP components (platelets, leukocytes, RBCs).[22,23] The large variability in PRP formulations used creates a challenge to accurately draw conclusions from the literature to guide PRP production and determine indications for use, prompting the development of PRP classification schemes to facilitate reporting of clinical investigations.[24–27]

Activated versus nonactivated platelet-rich plasma

PRP preparations are commonly activated before administration in order to induce release of a highly concentrated bolus of growth factors to the target tissue. Up to 70% of growth factor content from activated PRP can be released over 10 minutes.[6] Roh and colleagues[28] demonstrated that PRP activated with a low-dose mixture of thrombin and calcium significantly increased growth factor release over 7 days compared with nonactivated PRP. Nevertheless, uncertainty exists as to whether rapid, bolus delivery of growth factors is ideal. Studies have shown mixed results supporting PRP activation, with activated preparations resulting in less efficient fibroblast differentiation and wound healing but providing equivalent bony regeneration compared with nonactivated preparations.[11,29] Given limited data, there is no agreement on whether activation is beneficial or deleterious, but it is understood that activation alters the properties of PRP and must be considered when comparing results from clinical studies.

Drug interactions

Application of PRP has generally not been recommended in individuals who take or cannot suspend taking antiplatelet therapy, which may inhibit platelet degranulation and release of growth factors and bioactive molecules, thereby significantly reducing the healing potential of this biologic approach. Such antiplatelet agents come from drug classes with various mechanisms of action that include reversible and irreversible cyclo-oxygenase inhibitors, adenosine diphosphate receptor inhibitors, adenosine reuptake inhibitors, phosphodiesterase inhibitors, and glycoprotein IIB/IIIA inhibitors.[30] Autologous PRP produced from subjects taking nonsteroidal anti-inflammatory drugs (NSAIDs), reversible cyclo-oxygenase inhibitors that are commonly taken for anti-inflammation and pain management, was shown to have significantly impaired platelet aggregation and thus potentially diminished therapeutic effect.[31] Other medications may also inhibit platelet function. Pioglitazone, an anti-hyperglycemic medication, was shown to both directly inhibit platelet release of thromboxane, an inducer of platelet aggregation, and potentiate aspirin inhibition of platelet aggregation and ATP release.[32]

EVIDENCE BASE FOR MUSCULOSKELETAL DISORDERS

PRP therapies are used increasingly for treating musculoskeletal soft tissue injuries, including tendinopathies and tendon tears, and ligament, muscle, and cartilage injuries.[33] Therapies have been used as both principal treatment and augmentative therapy alongside surgical repair. A most recent 2014 *Cochrane Review* of single-center, randomized controlled trials (RCTs) of PRP in the literature reveals that evidence for the primary outcomes of function and pain are of low quality and at high risk of bias. Overall results showed PRP provides no clinically significant improvement in short- and long-term function and only a small reduction in short-term pain compared with control. Adverse effects were associated with concerns about persisting pain. Difficulty in drawing clear conclusions from this collection of studies stems from using heterogeneous PRP preparation methods, application techniques, and outcome measures; treating disparate musculoskeletal disorders; and conducting underpowered studies. The current evidence also comprises a collection of earlier, smaller studies, many with nonrandomized or uncontrolled methodology, that demonstrate variable results for the effectiveness of PRP to treat musculoskeletal injuries. The review presented here emphasizes findings from the most recent RCTs over earlier case reports, cohort or retrospective studies.

Tendon

Lateral epicondyle tendinopathy

Results for PRP treatment of lateral epicondyle tendinopathy (LET) have been promising.[34–37] RCTs have demonstrated the efficacy of PRP for treating chronic LET, with superior 1-year[38] and 2-year[39] improvements in function and pain compared with steroid injection. However, more recent RCTs have demonstrated variable efficacy of PRP compared with saline, steroid, autologous whole blood, and bupivacaine:[40–43]

- PRP was superior at reducing pain at 6 weeks[41] but inferior at improving function by 6 months compared with autologous blood injection.[40]
- PRP was no different than steroid or saline at reducing pain and improving function at 3 months, was inferior to steroid at improving pain and function at 1 month, and was associated with greater postinjection pain.[42]
- PRP was superior to bupivacaine at improving pain at 6 months.[43]

A further RCT comparing the efficacy of PRP with that of autologous whole blood injection showed both methods are comparably effective in treating LET, with no significant difference between groups in pain reduction and functional improvement in 12 months of follow-up.[44] Although results suggest there may be no need to have platelet concentration greater than in whole blood to obtain therapeutic effects, limitations of this study included a relatively small number of cases and the absence of a placebo control group; thus, whether these treatment approaches are superior to natural recovery remains unverified.

Results are pending from a multicenter RCT comparing autologous PRP, autologous whole blood, dry needle tendon fenestration, and physical therapy (PT) alone on pain and quality of life in patients with LET (IMpact of Platelet Rich Plasma Over Alternative Therapies in Patients with Lateral Epicondylitis: IMPROVE Trial).[45]

Achilles tendinopathy

Results for PRP treatment of Achilles tendinopathy have been mixed. Earlier return to sport by 8 weeks has been observed after local application of platelet-rich fibrin at the time of open repair of complete Achilles tendon tear.[9] However, PRP injection did not improve mechanical properties or functional performance of Achilles tendon up to 1 year after surgical repair of an acute rupture compared with no PRP injection.[46]

For chronic Achilles tendinopathy, case series,[47–53] pilot studies,[54] and retrospective studies[55–57] have reported promising results for the efficacy of PRP injection, with lasting improvements in functional outcomes at 4 years.[58] RCTs, however, demonstrated no significant difference in outcomes of clinical function, tendon healing, or return to sport times at either 6 months[59] or 1 year between PRP and saline control,[60] nor did PRP injection provide a significantly different neovascularization response or ultrasonographically assessed change in tendon structure over 6 months than saline injection did for chronic Achilles tendinopathy.[61]

Meta-analyses comparing various injection therapies for lateral epicondylitis[62,63] and noninsertional Achilles tendinosis[64] revealed no strong evidence for selecting one injectable over another and indicated large-scale studies are needed before treatment recommendations can be made.

Patellar tendinopathy

Results from case series[49,51,65–67] and retrospective studies[57] have shown promise for PRP injection to improve function in patients with chronic patellar tendinopathy, with lasting effects in functional outcomes at 4 years.[68]

Although a small comparative study did not find the addition of PRP injection to rehabilitation to provide greater pain reduction at 6 months,[69] studies have demonstrated efficacy of PRP for treating patellar tendinopathy, with superior 1-year outcomes compared with extracorporeal shockwave therapy.[70–72]

In an RCT, US-guided PRP injection administered with dry needling accelerated recovery from patellar tendinopathy relative to dry needling alone, but benefits to pain and function dissipated after 3 months, occurring without any significant improvement in quality of life.[73]

Application of PRP to patellar tendon harvest sites for ACL reconstruction was found in RCTs to provide significant reduction in postoperative pain, greater donor patellar tendon healing at 6 months,[74] and greater function at 12 months.[75]

Rotator cuff tendinopathy

Studies of augmentative PRP use alongside rotator cuff repair have been of variable quality and have shown mixed results:

- Following initial safety studies,[76] early, underpowered studies demonstrated no significant benefit to pain or function of PRP augmentation during arthroscopic rotator cuff repair.[77,78]
- Intraoperative local application of autologous PRP to the arthroscopic repair site of complete rotator cuff tears has been associated with significantly less pain within the first postoperative month and greater strength within the first 3 months compared with standard repair alone, with benefit more pronounced for less extensive tears;[79] however, benefits to pain, function, and healing integrity were not found to endure beyond a year for small, moderate,[80] or complete[81–83] rotator cuff tears.
- PRP improved repair integrity for large tears without an associated greater improvement in function[84] and had lower rates of re-tears for small to large tears at 1 year.[79,80,84,85]
- Other studies have demonstrated not only no significant benefit of PRP, but also possible negative effects on rotator cuff healing.[83,86] Platelet-rich fibrin injection during arthroscopic rotator cuff tendon repair was associated with a greater persistence of rotator cuff tendon defect at 3 months.[83] Similarly, PRP injection with arthroscopic acromioplasty in patients with chronic rotator cuff tendinopathy was associated with reduced cellularity and vascularity and increased levels of apoptosis in tendons at 12-week follow-up.[86]

For principal treatment of chronic rotator cuff tendinopathy, PRP injection was no more effective than autologous whole blood by 1 year, but significantly more effective than dry needling by 6 months, in improving pain, disability, and shoulder range of motion.[87,88]

Ligament

Anterior cruciate ligament reconstruction

Several studies of PRP applied during anterior cruciate ligament (ACL) reconstruction demonstrated no benefit to postoperative functional scores. Intraoperative application of PRP during ACL reconstruction using hamstring tendon grafts improved graft maturation[89,90] and anteroposterior knee stability at 6 months[91] but was ineffective in preventing femoral or tibial bone tunnel enlargement[89,92] and improving postoperative functional scores at 15 months.[93] PRP improved maturation of bone-patellar tendon-bone allografts,[94] but did not improve clinical function or biomechanical properties of these grafts at 24 months.[95] PRP application has been inconsistently shown to accelerate graft-to-bone incorporation, ranging from being ineffective for osteoligamentous integration,[89,96,97] to improving healing,[98] reducing edema, increasing vascularity at the bone-graft interface,[99,100] and reducing time for the graft to achieve a "ligamentous-like" MRI signal by 48%.[101] Significantly less swelling and inflammation have been associated with use of PRP without leukocytes to augment ACL reconstruction.[102]

Medial collateral ligament
Presently, there is no strong evidence to support the efficacy of PRP injections for treating medial collateral ligament (MCL) lesions in humans. A case report described favorable outcomes in managing a high-grade acute MCL lesion using PRP treatment.[103] A small study showed PRP augmentation of arthroscopic meniscal repair did not improve reoperation rates or accelerate return to activity.[104]

Plantar fasciopathy
Early cohort studies have reported the benefit of PRP injection on improving pain,[105] function,[106] and tissue structure[107] for chronic plantar fasciopathy.

RCTs have compared PRP with conventional treatments. A most recent double-blinded RCT showed that PRP was as effective as or more effective than corticosteroid injection when compared with normal saline control to reduce pain over 3 months of follow-up and improve functional scores for chronic plantar fasciopathy.[108]

Multiple prior studies have compared the efficacy of PRP and corticosteroid without a placebo control and showed variable results, ranging from PRP providing greater early pain reduction and functional improvement[109,110] with lasting effects at 1[111] and 2 years of follow-up,[112] to being equally effective at 3 months[113] and at 6 months,[111,114] to being less effective in reducing pain at 3 months.[115]

A single-blinded RCT showed PRP was as effective as prolotherapy at reducing pain and improving function at 6 months for plantar fasciopathy.[116]

Further trials showed PRP was as effective as extracorporeal shockwave therapy at improving pain and functional outcomes beyond conventional therapy for plantar fasciitis.[117]

Ankle sprains
A double-blinded RCT comparing the injection of PRP and saline placebo in addition to standard therapy for severe ankle sprains showed no statistically significant difference in pain and function outcomes between groups over 30 days of follow-up.[118]

A separate study comparing the addition of US-guided PRP injection to rehabilitation to treat anterior inferior tibiofibular ligament tears from high ankle sprains in elite athletes showed PRP accelerated return to sport by nearly 3 weeks, improved joint stability, and reduced residual pain.[119]

Ulnar collateral ligament
A case series described favorable outcomes from PRP treatment of partial ulnar collateral ligament tears of the elbow.[120]

Muscle

Following case reports describing the promise of PRP injection for muscle injuries,[121] a small, randomized, nonblinded study demonstrated US-guided PRP treatment for acute muscle injuries (thigh, shoulder, foot, and ankle) compared with conservative therapy provided greater reduction of early pain, improvement of range of motion, and earlier return to sport.[122]

Hamstring

Acute hamstring injury is one of the most common types of muscle injury affecting athletes, resulting in loss of competition time.[123,124] A single-blinded RCT demonstrated PRP significantly reduced pain intensity over 10 weeks and accelerated return to sport by 16 days for acute hamstring partial tears.[125]

Larger, double-blinded RCTs, however, showed PRP injection provided no significant benefit. A single PRP injection in combination with intensive rehabilitation provided no significantly greater benefit when compared with intensive rehabilitation alone to accelerate return to sport, improve muscle strength, or influence reinjury rates after 2 and 6 months in athletes following an acute hamstring injury.[126]

Similarly, US-guided intramuscular injection of PRP compared with saline, both combined with a rehabilitation program, for acute hamstring injury showed no significant difference between groups in reinjury rate at 2 months or 1 year or return to sport at 6 months[127] or 1 year.[128]

Gastrocnemius and rectus femoris

Injection of autologous PRP in combination with standard conservative care compared with standard care alone for gastrocnemius and rectus femoris muscle tears with hematoma did not significantly improve healing.[129]

Cartilage

Although few studies have been published on use of PRP for management of hip and ankle arthritis, several trials have focused on PRP use for knee arthritis.

Knee

Several trials have suggested the efficacy of PRP to improve functional outcomes for mild knee osteoarthritis (OA).[130–140] Overall findings from RCTs have been unable to consistently demonstrate the superiority of PRP over traditional approaches. Comparative trials have demonstrated that autologous PRP intra-articular injections have greater efficacy than hyaluronic acid injections in reducing pain and recovering articular function,[141–143] especially for younger patients and milder knee OA,[144–146] with one study showing benefit of PRP even for grade 3 knee OA.[147] Others have shown inconsistent superiority of PRP over viscosupplementation.[136] In an RCT with 1-year follow-up, PRP was not superior to viscosupplementation for knee OA, with diminishing benefit beyond 9 months.[148,149]

No difference in outcomes for pain and function came from having a single or a double injection of PRP, but both provided superior outcomes compared with saline control.[150] Another study demonstrated superiority of PRP compared with viscosupplementation only when multiple PRP injections were used.[146]

PRP was shown to be superior to steroid injection for knee OA.[151]

Adverse effects have been minor, with leukocyte-rich PRP associated with increased pain and swelling relative to leukocyte-poor PRP.[23]

Hip

Two case series demonstrated the safety and promise of PRP injection for treating hip OA,[152] but with time-dependent benefit and nonsuperiority over viscosupplementation.[153,154]

Ankle

A small, prospective study comparing the efficacy of PRP injection to viscosupplementation for talar osteochondral lesions proved PRP to be significantly more effective in controlling pain and re-establishing function.[155] PRP injection was shown, similarly, to provide clinical improvement for low-grade ankle OA[156] and as an adjunct to arthroscopic microfracture surgery for treating osteochondral talus lesions.[157]

Meniscus

Few studies have evaluated the use of PRP for meniscal applications. A small retrospective study demonstrated the promise of PRP injection to relieve pain, facilitate return to sport, and halt progression of injury over 6 months for intrasubstance, grade 2, knee meniscal lesions.[158] A clinical trial reported PRP augmentation of open meniscal repair improved outcomes compared with open repair alone.[159]

Future Work

Questions remain as to the proper preparation, dosing, and timing of PRP. There is need for future studies to have better randomization and blinding procedures, larger sample sizes, adequate and consistent descriptions of preparation and injection techniques, radiographic data to provide additional objective data for analysis, standard postinjection rehabilitation protocols, longer-term follow-up of at least 2 years, and standard functional outcome scores. Further studies comparing leukocyte-rich to leukocyte-poor PRP are needed.

PATIENT SELECTION AND PREPROCEDURE COUNSELING
Consultation

During the initial consultation, a thorough history of the current injury should be obtained, including pain onset, duration, and quality. A past medical history and current medication list should also be obtained to identify any contraindications to PRP treatment. It is vital to confirm the clinical diagnosis by physical examination and diagnostic workup. Imaging modalities such as MRI, computed tomography, and/or musculoskeletal US should be performed as needed. If uncertainty remains, a diagnostic injection with a local anesthetic like 1% lidocaine may be performed to determine whether symptoms from a potential pain generator are temporarily alleviated. A response to this diagnostic procedure can suggest a potential positive clinical response to PRP.

Furthermore, it is crucial to review prior treatments to identify standard care options that remain to be explored and offered before, along with, or instead of PRP therapy. Therapeutic options may include activity modification, oral and/or topical analgesics, focused PT, orthoses/bracing, alternative injection-based therapies (eg, corticosteroids, hyaluronic acid), and even surgery in some cases. It is not uncommon to repeat standard therapies tried previously for various reasons. For example, a patient's time constraints, goals, or preferences may warrant a repeat corticosteroid injection or course of PT. In some cases, the severity of the condition may indicate surgical intervention as the best option to pursue.

Selection Criteria

Indications

Different clinics may vary in their preference for and experience in using PRP. In some Sports Medicine practices, PRP therapy may be commonly reserved for second-line treatment of chronic conditions like tendinopathy or refractory OA of large joints that have failed first-line conservative management, which may have included activity modification, PT, analgesics, complementary therapies, and steroid injections. Less frequently, PRP may be administered for acute myotendinous injuries. Indications for consideration of PRP can include the following:[7]

1. Pain duration greater than 3 to 6 months that averages higher than 4 on a 0 to 10 visual analog scale.
2. Physical examination, diagnostic imaging, and diagnostic procedures confirming clinical suspicion of tendinopathy, OA, and/or myotendinous injuries.
3. Symptoms refractory to standard conservative care (activity modification, NSAIDs, PT).
4. Patient goals to prolong or avoid surgical intervention.
5. Anticipated recovery time consistent with patient's timeline to return to activity.
6. Patient is dedicated to commit to a postinjection course of PT of at least 6 weeks.

Contraindications

Medical contraindications that warrant caution or avoidance of PRP therapy may include blood dyscrasias, current infections being treated by antibiotics, use of antiplatelet agents, and use of systemic immunosuppressant medications such as oral glucocorticoids. Non-medical contraindications may include being unable to tolerate injection therapies, commit to a PT program, or afford to undergo a potential series of injections.

Patient Education and Counseling

The patient should be informed that PRP injections for musculoskeletal injuries are currently not covered by the Centers for Medicare and Medicaid Services and most medical insurance companies; therefore, the patient should expect to pay "out of pocket" for PRP therapy. Notification of cost at the initial consultation is important because multiple injections may be needed to obtain a desirable clinical outcome.

Because PRP is not considered the standard of care, it is important to educate the patient on evidence from clinical studies that support its use, the variability of outcomes to expect, as well as the variables that can potentially influence response to PRP treatment, including duration of symptoms, injury severity, medical comorbidities, sports participation, and activity level. Although no significant adverse effects have been reported from PRP, patients should be informed that they may experience temporary local discomfort or pain, lasting up to a week, following an injection.

The procedure of preparing and administering PRP should be thoroughly explained. PRP may not be the most appropriate therapy to pursue for a patient who is "needle phobic" because it involves venous blood draws to collect whole blood and potentially multiple PRP injections.

It is common to recommend courses of PT before and after PRP injection to maximize therapeutic effect; therefore, a patient is considered a better candidate for PRP if they can commit adequate time for PT. Athletes, however, require further counseling on the need for postprocedural activity restrictions and sufficient time off from play to allow for optimal recovery and to avoid reinjury by returning to sport too soon.

Postinjection recommendations entail avoiding the use of NSAIDs for 2 to 6 weeks after the procedure. Although no studies have investigated the effect of taking NSAIDs following PRP injections, the theoretic concern involves the capacity of NSAIDs to alter the inflammatory phase of the healing process.[160] Over-the-counter acetaminophen is recommended as an alternative to NSAIDs for postprocedural analgesia.

APPLICATION OF PLATELET-RICH PLASMA
Specifics and Logistics

Studies have shown the best time for PRP injections is 3 to 6 months after injury, with repeat administrations ranging between 2- and 8-week intervals. The efficacy of multiple injections is under investigation, with some studies showing no significant difference in outcomes between single and double injections for knee OA,[150] and others demonstrating the superiority of multiple injections for knee OA[146] and patellar tendinopathy.[72] By alleviating pain and increasing activity tolerance, PRP allows for earlier return to sport and activity by 2 to 3 weeks, compared with no PRP injection (**Box 1**).[7]

Preparation

The numerous names and preparation methods used in studies for this biologic treatment, such as PRP, autologous conditioned plasma, and platelet lysate, as well as newer methods of production, such as preparation rich in growth factors,[161]

Box 1
Clinical use of platelet-rich plasma injections

Indications for PRP therapy

Tendinopathy: lateral and medial epicondyle tendons, rotator cuff, hip girdle, peroneal tendon

Chronic pain and OA: knee, ankle, foot, shoulder, hip

Chronic ligamentous injury and pain: ankle, knee, hip, sacroiliac joint, plantar fascia

Muscle tears

Consider PRP therapy if the following conditions are met:

History:
- Duration of pain >3 to 6 months and is on average >4 on a 0 to 10 visual analog scale
- Signs and symptoms consistent with tendinopathy or muscle or ligamentous injury
- Pain persists despite standard conservative treatments

Workup:
- MRI or US evidence of tendinopathy or muscle or ligamentous injury
- A diagnostic bupivacaine injection was successful

Patient factors:
- No contraindications
- Patient is pursuing a nonsurgical solution and has time to be out of play for about 4 weeks

Contraindications to PRP therapy

Immunocompromised state

Active infection

Inability to comprehend or comply with postprocedure instructions for activity modification

Coagulopathy or anticoagulation, international normalized ratio greater than 2.5

Patients with prosthetic joints

Prosthetic hardware infection

Severe cases of advanced OA

platelet-rich fibrin matrix,[162] simplified buffy coat method, and platelet-rich fibrin,[163] reflect the complexity and diversity of this therapy and the challenges in translating findings from clinical trials to clinical practice.[2] Ongoing efforts strive to elucidate the influence of PRP preparation methods and formulation characteristics on growth factor release, biologic effect, and therapeutic outcomes.

Validation studies have shown that PRP cellular composition and biomolecular characteristics vary according to the preparation protocol[164,165] and system used.[162,166–171] Preclinical investigations suggest PRP preparation methods additionally affect growth factor release kinetics and efficacy, with significant differences between classic PRP and second-generation preparations like platelet-rich fibrin.[172–179] Furthermore, PRP biologic activity is known to diminish with storage time.[180]

Regarding platelet content, the clinical literature has commonly suggested using platelet concentrations 4 to 6 times greater than that in whole blood for PRP. Concentrations greater than an optimal amount may provide no additional effect or even inhibit healing.[18] In vitro studies have shown that 1.5×10^6 PLT/μL was optimal to promote human umbilical vein endothelial cell proliferation, motility, and morphology, with greater concentrations causing inhibition.[181] A range of 0.5 to 1.5×10^6 PLT/μL was optimal for normal human dermal fibroblast proliferation, motility, and wound healing.[182] Tenocyte function plateaued by a concentration of 2.0×10^6 PLT/μL, beyond which no greater benefit to function was achieved.[183]

The superiority of leukocyte-poor or leukocyte-rich PRP has been investigated given concern over the proinflammatory effects of leukocytes and their inhibitory effect on tissue healing.[184] Although interaction between mononuclear cells and platelets results in greater anabolic growth factor release and cellular effect,[185,186] high leukocyte concentrations (>21,000/μL),[16] especially of neutrophils, result in greater release of proinflammatory and catabolic substances[187,188] that is independent of the ratio of platelets to leukocytes,[17] produce an acute inflammatory response,[16] and increase synoviocyte cell death,[15,16] suggesting leukocyte-poor (<1000/μL) PRP is a better option. The optimal concentration of leukocytes and ratio of leukocytes to platelets to have in PRP, however, remain unknown.

Most preparation methods minimize the RBC content in PRP, with concentrations of less than 1000/μL reported.[16]

The role of activation further contributes to variations in growth factor release[28] and has been shown to lower the platelet concentration required to reach a plateau in

Table 3
PLRA classification system

PLRA Classification	Criteria	
P: Platelet count	___P___ Volume Injected	___M___ Cells/μL
L: Leukocyte content[a]	>1% <1%	+ −
R: Red blood cell content	>1% <1%	+ −
A: Activation[b]	Yes No	+ −

[a] If white blood cells are present (+), the percentage of neutrophils should also be reported.
[b] The method of exogenous activation should be reported.
Adapted from Mautner K, Malanga GA, Smith J, et al. A call for a standard classification system for future biologic research: the rationale for new PRP nomenclature. PM R 2015;7(4 Suppl): S53–9.

Table 4
Post-PRP and BMAC Rehabilitation Protocol – PT Version

Phase	Length of Time Post Injection	Restrictions	Rehabilitation
Phase I GOALS: Protect tissue; allow PRP to absorb	Days 0–7	• Doctor may recommend using crutches or walking boot for lower extremity procedures; braces, slings or splints for upper extremity procedures. • No exercise, with exception of this rehabilitation protocol. • If you had an upper extremity injection, no lifting more than a toothbrush. • Avoid NSAIDS (Ibuprofen, Aleve, Advil, etc.). • You may take Tylenol (up to 2500 mg/day) or prescribed medications (Tramadol, Oxycodone, Percocet or Vicodin) for pain after this procedure. • Avoid ice. • Use heat after injection as needed to help with pain control. • You may take a light shower on the same day after the injection. Avoid a hot tub bath or swimming. • You may have driving restrictions for up to 1 wk after your injection	• Pain is expected after your procedure. • Daily activities as tolerated within your provided device; avoid excess loading or stress to treated area. • Gentle movement of the extremity (active range of motion) out of immobilizing device. • Avoid exercise unless approved by your doctor. *PT protocol:* Gentle AROM. If shoulder was injected, PROM to point of tissue resistance. Gentle submax Isometrics. WB restrictions: Foot/Ankle – boot and WBAT with crutches Knee – immobilizer, WBAT with crutches Hip – WBAT with crutches Shoulder/Elbow – sling Wrist –splint May initiate use of modalities for pain management and symptom control: non-thermal ultrasound, cold laser, E-stim.

Phase II GOALS: Protect tissue; start early movement; wean off immobilizing device PT protocol: Facilitate collagen deposition; avoid disruption of collagen crosslink	**Days 8–14**	• Progress to full weight bearing without protective device. • Gradually progress active range of motion without feeling stretching sensation. • No overstressing of the tendon through exercise or impact activity. • If you had an upper extremity injection, no lifting more than a coffee cup. • Avoid NSAIDS and ice.	• Continue Phase I Rehabilitation recommendations. • Consult your physical therapist regarding cross-training and return to exercise options (initiating exercise to upper body if you had a lower body injection or exercise to lower body if you had an upper body injection). *PT protocol:* Continue Phase I exercises. Gradually progress AROM to point of initial tissue resistance. No concentric exercises to affected tissue outside ADLs and ambulation. May continue to utilize modalities for symptom control: non-thermal US, cold laser, Russian E-stim. Initiate appropriate cross training exercises.
Phase III GOALS: Protect tissue; continue gentle movement; minimize deconditioning PT protocol: Facilitate collagen deposition; avoid disruption of collagen crosslink	**Days 15–21**	• Gradually progress active range of motion without feeling stretching sensation. • No overstressing of the tendon through exercise or impact activity. • If you had an upper extremity injection, no lifting more than a dinner plate. • Avoid eccentric exercises (this is the part of exercise when the weight is being lowered). • Avoid NSAIDS and ice.	• Pain with daily activities should be improving. • Consult your physical therapist regarding initiating low resistance exercises. *PT protocol:* Progress AROM to point of initial tissue resistance. Avoid tissue strain with ADLs and exercises. Avoid repetitive use of stairs if lower extremity was injected. Initiate low resistance, high repetition, concentric, open chain exercise (pain should not increase more than 2 points on 11 point VAS). No eccentric exercises to affected tissue. Gentle soft tissue mobilization along the line of the fibers of injected tissue. May continue to utilize modalities for tissue proliferation: non-thermal US, cold laser, Russian E-stim.

(continued on next page)

Table 4
(continued)

Phase	Length of Time Post Injection	Restrictions	Rehabilitation
Phase IV GOALS: Restore normal tissue integrity; improve range of motion PT Protocol: Reparative phase: tissue proliferation; stimulate collagen lay-down in organized fashion	Weeks 3–6	• Progress as tolerated. • Avoid NSAIDs and ice.	• Consult your physical therapist regarding initiation of eccentric exercise, proprioceptive training, preparation for plyometrics and sport-specific exercises. *PT Protocol:* Full AROM. OK to initiate stretching. Initiate and gradually progress eccentric loading exercises. Initiate cross friction soft tissue mobilization to injected tissues. Progress exercises and functional mobility. May continue to utilize modalities for tissue proliferation: non-thermal US, cold laser, Russian E-stim. If patient is not experiencing improvement or making expected progress by the end of this phase, contact referring MD.
Phase V GOALS: Restore normal tissue integrity; prepare for return to prior level of function and sport PT Protocol: Strengthening, Function, and Sport-Specific Training Phase	Weeks 6–12	• With sport-specific training, keep level of intensity: ○ Below 50% effort up to week 8 ○ Below 75% effort up to week 10 ○ Below 90% effort up to week 12 • Do not return to contact sport prior to week 10.	• Prepare for return to sport at 6–12 wk. • Consult your physical therapist regarding progression of eccentric exercise, proprioceptive training, plyometrics and sport-specific exercises. • Sprinting can begin after week 10 at 75% effort. • Patient should be at 100% effort with sport-specific training at the completion of this phase.

If you had a PRP injection to a ligament, the following protocol may be delayed 2–4 weeks due to decreased blood supply in ligaments.

Credits Podesta L, Honbo E. Clinical Applications for Platelet Rich Plasma Therapy. In: Rehabilitation for the Postsurgical Orthopedic Patient. 3rd edition. St Louis (MO): Elsevier Health Sciences; 2013. p. 171–92; Mautner K, Mason RA. Post PRP & Stem Cell Rehabilitation. Emory Sports Medicine Center. Accessed January 20, 2015; University of Wisconsin Health Sports Rehabilitation. Platelet-Rich Plasma Rehabilitation Guidelines. 2014. Available at: http://www.uwhealth.org/sports-medicine/physical-therapy-athletic-training/sports-medicine-rehabilitation-guidelines/20398. Accessed 2014.

tenocyte proliferation from 2.0×10^6 PLT/µL to 4.0×10^5 PLT/µL.[183] Thrombin and calcium have a dose-response effect on growth factor release from platelets, with higher concentrations leading to immediate and significantly greater anabolic growth factor release, and lower concentrations leading to delayed and reduced release.[189] Compared with thrombin, collagen activation results in a more sustained growth factor release.[190] Although activation can accelerate growth factor release, this may not be ideal to optimize therapeutic effect, as thrombin-activated compared with unactivated PRP has been shown to be less effective for wound healing.[11]

PLRA Classification System

The lack of standardized protocols for PRP preparation and the subsequent interproduct variability among PRP formulations[191] contribute to variability in clinical outcomes. The inconsistent and insufficient quantification of PRP components in clinical studies further contributes to confusion over results. The lack of accepted standards for reporting PRP in research has limited the interpretation of data, comparison of results, translation of findings to clinical practice, and progress of further investigations, prompting classification schemes to be developed to clarify use and communication of PRP therapy. Earlier classification schemes were proposed, including those by Dohan Ehrenfest and colleagues,[192] DeLong and colleagues,[24] and Mishra and colleagues,[27] but none were widely adopted nor do they now adequately capture all of the PRP attributes that may affect efficacy based on current knowledge.

Most recently, in 2015, Mautner and colleagues[26] proposed the PLRA classification, a new standard reporting system for PRP, which accounts for platelet count, leukocyte presence, RBC presence, and activation. Recommendations are to document the following when reporting PRP treatments: (1) concentration of platelets, total number of platelets, and injected volume delivered to a target tissue; (2) concentration of leukocytes, and if present, the percentage of neutrophils; (3) concentration of RBCs; and (4) type of exogenous activation applied, if used (**Table 3**).

Postprocedure Rehabilitation Protocol

PRP administration is recommended to be accompanied by a postprocedure rehabilitation and PT program that gradually incorporates range-of-motion exercises and weight-bearing to avoid reinjury (**Table 4**).[193]

SUMMARY

This is an exciting era for regenerative sports medicine. We are beyond infancy and now toddling as we strive to optimize platelet-based therapies. Research on PRP continues to advance. Presently, moderate-quality evidence supports the use of PRP for lateral epicondylosis and knee OA. Low-quality evidence suggests safety and benefit of PRP for ankle and hip OA; patellar and Achilles tendinopathy; and injuries of the ulnar collateral ligament of the elbow, ankle ligaments, and possibly medial meniscus. For the next phase of advancement, further investigations are needed to optimize platelet dosing, cellular composition, and postprocedure rehabilitation protocols for PRP. Patient physiologic and genetic factors that influence response to treatment should also be considered and investigated. Precise outcome measures as well as follow-up over years, not weeks to months, are required to accurately evaluate efficacy. PRP is a therapy for and investment in long-term connective tissue health and should not be regarded as a short-term pain management strategy. Until research consistently accounts for and measures this scope of therapeutic benefit, results will likely continue to mislead and frustrate.

ACKNOWLEDGMENTS

The authors wish to formally acknowledge the Spaulding Rehabilitation Hospital in Wellesley Sports Physical Therapy Team.** This team has optimized our post PRP Rehabilitation protocol with contributions from: Dr Luga Podesta, Dr Kenneth Mautner and the Emory Sports Medicine Center as well as the University of Wisconsin Health Sports Medicine center.

**SRH WELLESLEY SPORTS PT TEAM:
Tessa Taylor, PT, DPT, OCS
Christine Roy, PT, MS
Elisabeth St. George, PT, MS
Tessa Rowin, PT, DPT, OCS
Jennifer Spitz, PT, CN, IMTC

REFERENCES

1. Malanga GA, Goldin M. PRP: review of the current evidence for musculoskeletal conditions. Curr Phys Med Rehabil Rep 2014;2:1–5.
2. Davis VL, Abukabda AB, Radio NM, et al. Platelet-rich preparations to improve healing. Part I: workable options for every size practice. J Oral Implantol 2014;40(4):500–10.
3. DelRossi AJ, Cernaianu AC, Vertrees RA, et al. Platelet-rich plasma reduces postoperative blood loss after cardiopulmonary bypass. J Thorac Cardiovasc Surg 1990;100(2):281–6.
4. Ferrari M, Zia S, Valbonesi M, et al. A new technique for hemodilution, preparation of autologous platelet-rich plasma and intraoperative blood salvage in cardiac surgery. Int J Artif Organs 1987;10(1):47–50.
5. Anitua E. Plasma rich in growth factors: preliminary results of use in the preparation of future sites for implants. Int J Oral Maxillofac Implants 1999;14(4):529–35.
6. Marx RE, Carlson ER, Eichstaedt RM, et al. Platelet-rich plasma: growth factor enhancement for bone grafts. Oral Surg Oral Med Oral Pathol Oral Radiol Endod 1998;85(6):638–46.
7. Nguyen RT, Borg-Stein J, McInnis K. Applications of platelet-rich plasma in musculoskeletal and sports medicine: an evidence-based approach. PM R 2011;3(3):226–50.
8. Boswell SG, Cole BJ, Sundman EA, et al. Platelet-rich plasma: a milieu of bioactive factors. Arthroscopy 2012;28(3):429–39.
9. Sanchez M, Anitua E, Azofra J, et al. Comparison of surgically repaired Achilles tendon tears using platelet-rich fibrin matrices. Am J Sports Med 2007;35(2):245–51.
10. Broughton G 2nd, Janis JE, Attinger CE. Wound healing: an overview. Plast Reconstr Surg 2006;117(7 Suppl):1e-S–32e-S.
11. Scherer SS, Tobalem M, Vigato E, et al. Nonactivated versus thrombin-activated platelets on wound healing and fibroblast-to-myofibroblast differentiation in vivo and in vitro. Plast Reconstr Surg 2012;129(1):46e–54e.
12. Blair P, Flaumenhaft R. Platelet alpha-granules: basic biology and clinical correlates. Blood Rev 2009;23(4):177–89.
13. Hoemann CD, Chen G, Marchand C, et al. Scaffold-guided subchondral bone repair: implication of neutrophils and alternatively activated arginase-1+ macrophages. Am J Sports Med 2010;38(9):1845–56.

14. Assirelli E, Filardo G, Mariani E, et al. Effect of two different preparations of platelet-rich plasma on synoviocytes. Knee Surg Sports Traumatol Arthrosc 2015;23(9):2690–703.
15. Braun HJ, Kim HJ, Chu CR, et al. The effect of platelet-rich plasma formulations and blood products on human synoviocytes: implications for intra-articular injury and therapy. Am J Sports Med 2014;42(5):1204–10.
16. Dragoo JL, Braun HJ, Durham JL, et al. Comparison of the acute inflammatory response of two commercial platelet-rich plasma systems in healthy rabbit tendons. Am J Sports Med 2012;40(6):1274–81.
17. McCarrel TM, Minas T, Fortier LA. Optimization of leukocyte concentration in platelet-rich plasma for the treatment of tendinopathy. J Bone Joint Surg Am 2012;94(19). e143(1–8).
18. Boswell SG, Schnabel LV, Mohammed HO, et al. Increasing platelet concentrations in leukocyte-reduced platelet-rich plasma decrease collagen gene synthesis in tendons. Am J Sports Med 2014;42(1):42–9.
19. Hooiveld M, Roosendaal G, Wenting M, et al. Short-term exposure of cartilage to blood results in chondrocyte apoptosis. Am J Pathol 2003;162(3):943–51.
20. Madhok R, Bennett D, Sturrock RD, et al. Mechanisms of joint damage in an experimental model of hemophilic arthritis. Arthritis Rheum 1988;31(9):1148–55.
21. Roosendaal G, Vianen ME, Marx JJ, et al. Blood-induced joint damage: a human in vitro study. Arthritis Rheum 1999;42(5):1025–32.
22. Castillo TN, Pouliot MA, Kim HJ, et al. Comparison of growth factor and platelet concentration from commercial platelet-rich plasma separation systems. Am J Sports Med 2011;39(2):266–71.
23. Filardo G, Kon E, Pereira Ruiz MT, et al. Platelet-rich plasma intra-articular injections for cartilage degeneration and osteoarthritis: single- versus double-spinning approach. Knee Surg Sports Traumatol Arthrosc 2012;20(10):2082–91.
24. DeLong JM, Russell RP, Mazzocca AD. Platelet-rich plasma: the PAW classification system. Arthroscopy 2012;28(7):998–1009.
25. Dohan Ehrenfest DM, Andia I, Zumstein MA, et al. Classification of platelet concentrates (Platelet-Rich Plasma-PRP, Platelet-Rich Fibrin-PRF) for topical and infiltrative use in orthopedic and sports medicine: current consensus, clinical implications and perspectives. Muscles Ligaments Tendons J 2014;4(1):3–9.
26. Mautner K, Malanga GA, Smith J, et al. A call for a standard classification system for future biologic research: the rationale for new PRP nomenclature. PM R 2015;7(4 Suppl):S53–9.
27. Mishra A, Harmon K, Woodall J, et al. Sports medicine applications of platelet rich plasma. Curr Pharm Biotechnol 2012;13(7):1185–95.
28. Roh YH, Kim W, Park KU, et al. Cytokine-release kinetics of platelet-rich plasma according to various activation protocols. Bone Joint Res 2016;5(2):37–45.
29. Jeon YR, Jung BK, Roh TS, et al. Comparing the effect of nonactivated platelet-rich plasma, activated platelet-rich plasma, and bone morphogenetic protein-2 on calvarial bone regeneration. J Craniofac Surg 2016;27(2):317–21.
30. Varon D, Spectre G. Antiplatelet agents. Hematology Am Soc Hematol Educ Program 2009;267–72.
31. Schippinger G, Pruller F, Divjak M, et al. Autologous platelet-rich plasma preparations: influence of nonsteroidal anti-inflammatory drugs on platelet function. Orthop J Sports Med 2015;3(6). 2325967115588896.
32. Mongan J, Mieszczanska HZ, Smith BH, et al. Pioglitazone inhibits platelet function and potentiates the effects of aspirin: a prospective observation study. Thromb Res 2012;129(6):760–4.

33. Moraes VY, Lenza M, Tamaoki MJ, et al. Platelet-rich therapies for musculoskel-etal soft tissue injuries. Cochrane Database Syst Rev 2014;(4):CD010071.
34. Edwards SG, Calandruccio JH. Autologous blood injections for refractory lateral epicondylitis. J Hand Surg Am 2003;28(2):272–8.
35. Connell DA, Ali KE, Ahmad M, et al. Ultrasound-guided autologous blood injec-tion for tennis elbow. Skeletal Radiol 2006;35(6):371–7.
36. Hechtman KS, Uribe JW, Botto-vanDemden A, et al. Platelet-rich plasma injec-tion reduces pain in patients with recalcitrant epicondylitis. Orthopedics 2011; 34(2):92.
37. Mishra A, Pavelko T. Treatment of chronic elbow tendinosis with buffered platelet-rich plasma. Am J Sports Med 2006;34(11):1774–8.
38. Peerbooms JC, Sluimer J, Bruijn DJ, et al. Positive effect of an autologous platelet concentrate in lateral epicondylitis in a double-blind randomized controlled trial: platelet-rich plasma versus corticosteroid injection with a 1-year follow-up. Am J Sports Med 2010;38(2):255–62.
39. Gosens T, Peerbooms JC, van Laar W, et al. Ongoing positive effect of platelet-rich plasma versus corticosteroid injection in lateral epicondylitis: a double-blind ran-domized controlled trial with 2-year follow-up. Am J Sports Med 2011;39(6):1200–8.
40. Creaney L, Wallace A, Curtis M, et al. Growth factor-based therapies provide additional benefit beyond physical therapy in resistant elbow tendinopathy: a prospective, single-blind, randomised trial of autologous blood injections versus platelet-rich plasma injections. Br J Sports Med 2011;45(12):966–71.
41. Thanasas C, Papadimitriou G, Charalambidis C, et al. Platelet-rich plasma versus autologous whole blood for the treatment of chronic lateral elbow epicondylitis: a randomized controlled clinical trial. Am J Sports Med 2011;39(10):2130–4.
42. Krogh TP, Fredberg U, Stengaard-Pedersen K, et al. Treatment of lateral epicon-dylitis with platelet-rich plasma, glucocorticoid, or saline: a randomized, double-blind, placebo-controlled trial. Am J Sports Med 2013;41(3):625–35.
43. Mishra AK, Skrepnik NV, Edwards SG, et al. Efficacy of platelet-rich plasma for chronic tennis elbow: a double-blind, prospective, multicenter, randomized controlled trial of 230 patients. Am J Sports Med 2014;42(2):463–71.
44. Raeissadat SA, Rayegani SM, Hassanabadi H, et al. Is platelet-rich plasma su-perior to whole blood in the management of chronic tennis elbow: one year ran-domized clinical trial. BMC Sports Sci Med Rehabil 2014;6:12.
45. Chiavaras MM, Jacobson JA, Carlos R, et al. IMpact of Platelet Rich plasma OVer alternative therapies in patients with lateral Epicondylitis (IMPROVE): protocol for a multicenter randomized controlled study: a multicenter, randomized trial comparing autologous platelet-rich plasma, autologous whole blood, dry needle tendon fenestration, and physical therapy exercises alone on pain and quality of life in patients with lateral epicondylitis. Acad Radiol 2014;21(9):1144–55.
46. Schepull T, Kvist J, Norrman H, et al. Autologous platelets have no effect on the healing of human Achilles tendon ruptures: a randomized single-blind study. Am J Sports Med 2011;39(1):38–47.
47. Gaweda K, Tarczynska M, Krzyzanowski W. Treatment of Achilles tendinopathy with platelet-rich plasma. Int J Sports Med 2010;31(8):577–83.
48. Monto RR. Platelet rich plasma treatment for chronic Achilles tendinosis. Foot Ankle Int 2012;33(5):379–85.
49. Ferrero G, Fabbro E, Orlandi D, et al. Ultrasound-guided injection of platelet-rich plasma in chronic Achilles and patellar tendinopathy. J Ultrasound 2012;15(4): 260–6.

50. Deans VM, Miller A, Ramos J. A prospective series of patients with chronic Achilles tendinopathy treated with autologous-conditioned plasma injections combined with exercise and therapeutic ultrasonography. J Foot Ankle Surg 2012;51(6):706–10.
51. Volpi P, Quaglia A, Schoenhuber H, et al. Growth factors in the management of sport-induced tendinopathies: results after 24 months from treatment. A pilot study. J Sports Med Phys Fitness 2010;50(4):494–500.
52. Finnoff JT, Fowler SP, Lai JK, et al. Treatment of chronic tendinopathy with ultrasound-guided needle tenotomy and platelet-rich plasma injection. PM R 2011;3(10):900–11.
53. Oloff L, Elmi E, Nelson J, et al. Retrospective analysis of the effectiveness of platelet-rich plasma in the treatment of Achilles tendinopathy: pretreatment and posttreatment correlation of magnetic resonance imaging and clinical assessment. Foot Ankle Spec 2015;8(6):490–7.
54. Kearney RS, Parsons N, Costa ML. Achilles tendinopathy management: a pilot randomised controlled trial comparing platelet-rich plasma injection with an eccentric loading programme. Bone Joint Res 2013;2(10):227–32.
55. Murawski CD, Smyth NA, Newman H, et al. A single platelet-rich plasma injection for chronic midsubstance Achilles tendinopathy: a retrospective preliminary analysis. Foot Ankle Spec 2014;7(5):372–6.
56. Owens RF Jr, Ginnetti J, Conti SF, et al. Clinical and magnetic resonance imaging outcomes following platelet rich plasma injection for chronic midsubstance Achilles tendinopathy. Foot Ankle Int 2011;32(11):1032–9.
57. Mautner K, Colberg RE, Malanga G, et al. Outcomes after ultrasound-guided platelet-rich plasma injections for chronic tendinopathy: a multicenter, retrospective review. PM R 2013;5(3):169–75.
58. Filardo G, Kon E, Di Matteo B, et al. Platelet-rich plasma injections for the treatment of refractory Achilles tendinopathy: results at 4 years. Blood Transfus 2014; 12(4):533–40.
59. de Vos RJ, Weir A, van Schie HT, et al. Platelet-rich plasma injection for chronic Achilles tendinopathy: a randomized controlled trial. JAMA 2010;303(2):144–9.
60. de Jonge S, de Vos RJ, Weir A, et al. One-year follow-up of platelet-rich plasma treatment in chronic Achilles tendinopathy: a double-blind randomized placebo-controlled trial. Am J Sports Med 2011;39(8):1623–9.
61. de Vos RJ, Weir A, Tol JL, et al. No effects of PRP on ultrasonographic tendon structure and neovascularisation in chronic midportion Achilles tendinopathy. Br J Sports Med 2011;45(5):387–92.
62. Krogh TP, Bartels EM, Ellingsen T, et al. Comparative effectiveness of injection therapies in lateral epicondylitis: a systematic review and network meta-analysis of randomized controlled trials. Am J Sports Med 2013;41(6):1435–46.
63. Rabago D, Best TM, Zgierska AE, et al. A systematic review of four injection therapies for lateral epicondylosis: prolotherapy, polidocanol, whole blood and platelet-rich plasma. Br J Sports Med 2009;43(7):471–81.
64. Gross CE, Hsu AR, Chahal J, et al. Injectable treatments for noninsertional Achilles tendinosis: a systematic review. Foot Ankle Int 2013;34(5):619–28.
65. Kon E, Filardo G, Delcogliano M, et al. Platelet-rich plasma: new clinical application: a pilot study for treatment of jumper's knee. Injury 2009;40(6):598–603.
66. Gosens T, Den Oudsten BL, Fievez E, et al. Pain and activity levels before and after platelet-rich plasma injection treatment of patellar tendinopathy: a prospective cohort study and the influence of previous treatments. Int Orthop 2012;36(9):1941–6.

67. Charousset C, Zaoui A, Bellaiche L, et al. Are multiple platelet-rich plasma injections useful for treatment of chronic patellar tendinopathy in athletes? A prospective study. Am J Sports Med 2014;42(4):906–11.

68. Filardo G, Kon E, Di Matteo B, et al. Platelet-rich plasma for the treatment of patellar tendinopathy: clinical and imaging findings at medium-term follow-up. Int Orthop 2013;37(8):1583–9.

69. Filardo G, Kon E, Della Villa S, et al. Use of platelet-rich plasma for the treatment of refractory jumper's knee. Int Orthop 2009;34(6):909–15.

70. Kaux JF, Bruyere O, Croisier JL, et al. One-year follow-up of platelet-rich plasma infiltration to treat chronic proximal patellar tendinopathies. Acta Orthop Belg 2015;81(2):251–6.

71. Vetrano M, Castorina A, Vulpiani MC, et al. Platelet-rich plasma versus focused shock waves in the treatment of jumper's knee in athletes. Am J Sports Med 2013;41(4):795–803.

72. Zayni R, Thaunat M, Fayard JM, et al. Platelet-rich plasma as a treatment for chronic patellar tendinopathy: comparison of a single versus two consecutive injections. Muscles Ligaments Tendons J 2015;5(2):92–8.

73. Dragoo JL, Wasterlain AS, Braun HJ, et al. Platelet-rich plasma as a treatment for patellar tendinopathy: a double-blind, randomized controlled trial. Am J Sports Med 2014;42(3):610–8.

74. de Almeida AM, Demange MK, Sobrado MF, et al. Patellar tendon healing with platelet-rich plasma: a prospective randomized controlled trial. Am J Sports Med 2012;40(6):1282–8.

75. Cervellin M, de Girolamo L, Bait C, et al. Autologous platelet-rich plasma gel to reduce donor-site morbidity after patellar tendon graft harvesting for anterior cruciate ligament reconstruction: a randomized, controlled clinical study. Knee Surg Sports Traumatol Arthrosc 2012;20(1):114–20.

76. Randelli PS, Arrigoni P, Cabitza P, et al. Autologous platelet rich plasma for arthroscopic rotator cuff repair. A pilot study. Disabil Rehabil 2008;30(20–22): 1584–9.

77. Hak A, Rajaratnam K, Ayeni OR, et al. A double-blinded placebo randomized controlled trial evaluating short-term efficacy of platelet-rich plasma in reducing postoperative pain after arthroscopic rotator cuff repair: a pilot study. Sports Health 2015;7(1):58–66.

78. Jo CH, Kim JE, Yoon KS, et al. Does platelet-rich plasma accelerate recovery after rotator cuff repair? A prospective cohort study. Am J Sports Med 2011; 39(10):2082–90.

79. Randelli P, Arrigoni P, Ragone V, et al. Platelet rich plasma in arthroscopic rotator cuff repair: a prospective RCT study, 2-year follow-up. J Shoulder Elbow Surg 2011;20(4):518–28.

80. Castricini R, Longo UG, De Benedetto M, et al. Platelet-rich plasma augmentation for arthroscopic rotator cuff repair: a randomized controlled trial. Am J Sports Med 2011;39(2):258–65.

81. Antuna S, Barco R, Martinez Diez JM, et al. Platelet-rich fibrin in arthroscopic repair of massive rotator cuff tears: a prospective randomized pilot clinical trial. Acta Orthop Belg 2013;79(1):25–30.

82. Malavolta EA, Gracitelli ME, Ferreira Neto AA, et al. Platelet-rich plasma in rotator cuff repair: a prospective randomized study. Am J Sports Med 2014;42(10): 2446–54.

83. Rodeo SA, Delos D, Williams RJ, et al. The effect of platelet-rich fibrin matrix on rotator cuff tendon healing: a prospective, randomized clinical study. Am J Sports Med 2012;40(6):1234–41.

84. Gumina S, Campagna V, Ferrazza G, et al. Use of platelet-leukocyte membrane in arthroscopic repair of large rotator cuff tears: a prospective randomized study. J Bone Joint Surg Am 2012;94(15):1345–52.

85. Chahal J, Van Thiel GS, Mall N, et al. The role of platelet-rich plasma in arthroscopic rotator cuff repair: a systematic review with quantitative synthesis. Arthroscopy 2012;28(11):1718–27.

86. Carr AJ, Murphy R, Dakin SG, et al. Platelet-rich plasma injection with arthroscopic acromioplasty for chronic rotator cuff tendinopathy: a randomized controlled trial. Am J Sports Med 2015;43(12):2891–7.

87. Kesikburun S, Tan AK, Yilmaz B, et al. Platelet-rich plasma injections in the treatment of chronic rotator cuff tendinopathy: a randomized controlled trial with 1-year follow-up. Am J Sports Med 2013;41(11):2609–16.

88. Rha DW, Park GY, Kim YK, et al. Comparison of the therapeutic effects of ultrasound-guided platelet-rich plasma injection and dry needling in rotator cuff disease: a randomized controlled trial. Clin Rehabil 2013;27(2):113–22.

89. Orrego M, Larrain C, Rosales J, et al. Effects of platelet concentrate and a bone plug on the healing of hamstring tendons in a bone tunnel. Arthroscopy 2008; 24(12):1373–80.

90. Sanchez M, Anitua E, Azofra J, et al. Ligamentization of tendon grafts treated with an endogenous preparation rich in growth factors: gross morphology and histology. Arthroscopy 2010;26(4):470–80.

91. Vogrin M, Rupreht M, Crnjac A, et al. The effect of platelet-derived growth factors on knee stability after anterior cruciate ligament reconstruction: a prospective randomized clinical study. Wien Klin Wochenschr 2010;122(Suppl 2):91–5.

92. Mirzatolooei F, Alamdari MT, Khalkhali HR. The impact of platelet-rich plasma on the prevention of tunnel widening in anterior cruciate ligament reconstruction using quadrupled autologous hamstring tendon: a randomised clinical trial. Bone Joint J 2013;95-B(1):65–9.

93. Vadala A, Iorio R, De Carli A, et al. Platelet-rich plasma: does it help reduce tunnel widening after ACL reconstruction? Knee Surg Sports Traumatol Arthrosc 2013;21(4):824–9.

94. Seijas R, Ares O, Catala J, et al. Magnetic resonance imaging evaluation of patellar tendon graft remodelling after anterior cruciate ligament reconstruction with or without platelet-rich plasma. J Orthop Surg (Hong Kong) 2013;21(1): 10–4.

95. Nin JR, Gasque GM, Azcarate AV, et al. Has platelet-rich plasma any role in anterior cruciate ligament allograft healing? Arthroscopy 2009;25(11):1206–13.

96. Silva A, Sampaio R. Anatomic ACL reconstruction: does the platelet-rich plasma accelerate tendon healing? Knee Surg Sports Traumatol Arthrosc 2009;17(6): 676–82.

97. Figueroa D, Melean P, Calvo R, et al. Magnetic resonance imaging evaluation of the integration and maturation of semitendinosus-gracilis graft in anterior cruciate ligament reconstruction using autologous platelet concentrate. Arthroscopy 2010;26(10):1318–25.

98. Rupreht M, Vogrin M, Hussein M. MRI evaluation of tibial tunnel wall cortical bone formation after platelet-rich plasma applied during anterior cruciate ligament reconstruction. Radiol Oncol 2013;47(2):119–24.

99. Rupreht M, Jevtic V, Sersa I, et al. Evaluation of the tibial tunnel after intraoperatively administered platelet-rich plasma gel during anterior cruciate ligament reconstruction using diffusion weighted and dynamic contrast-enhanced MRI. J Magn Reson Imaging 2013;37(4):928–35.

100. Vogrin M, Rupreht M, Dinevski D, et al. Effects of a platelet gel on early graft revascularization after anterior cruciate ligament reconstruction: a prospective, randomized, double-blind, clinical trial. Eur Surg Res 2010;45(2):77–85.

101. Radice F, Yanez R, Gutierrez V, et al. Comparison of magnetic resonance imaging findings in anterior cruciate ligament grafts with and without autologous platelet-derived growth factors. Arthroscopy 2010;26(1):50–7.

102. Valenti Azcarate A, Lamo-Espinosa J, Aquerreta Beola JD, et al. Comparison between two different platelet-rich plasma preparations and control applied during anterior cruciate ligament reconstruction. Is there any evidence to support their use? Injury 2014;45(Suppl 4):S36–41.

103. Eirale C, Mauri E, Hamilton B. Use of platelet rich plasma in an isolated complete medial collateral ligament lesion in a professional football (soccer) player: a case report. Asian J Sports Med 2013;4(2):158–62.

104. Griffin JW, Hadeed MM, Werner BC, et al. Platelet-rich plasma in meniscal repair: does augmentation improve surgical outcomes? Clin Orthop Relat Res 2015;473(5):1665–72.

105. Martinelli N, Marinozzi A, Carni S, et al. Platelet-rich plasma injections for chronic plantar fasciitis. Int Orthop 2013;37(5):839–42.

106. Kumar V, Millar T, Murphy PN, et al. The treatment of intractable plantar fasciitis with platelet-rich plasma injection. Foot (Edinb) 2013;23(2–3):74–7.

107. Ragab EM, Othman AM. Platelets rich plasma for treatment of chronic plantar fasciitis. Arch Orthop Trauma Surg 2012;132(8):1065–70.

108. Mahindra P, Yamin M, Selhi HS, et al. Chronic plantar fasciitis: effect of platelet-rich plasma, corticosteroid, and placebo. Orthopedics 2016;39(2):e285–9.

109. Say F, Gurler D, Inkaya E, et al. Comparison of platelet-rich plasma and steroid injection in the treatment of plantar fasciitis. Acta Orthop Traumatol Turc 2014; 48(6):667–72.

110. Omar AS, Ibrahim ME, Ahmed AS, et al. Local injection of autologous platelet rich plasma and corticosteroid in treatment of lateral epicondylitis and plantar fasciitis: randomized clinical trial. Egypt Rheumatol 2012;34:43–9.

111. Jain K, Murphy PN, Clough TM. Platelet rich plasma versus corticosteroid injection for plantar fasciitis: a comparative study. Foot (Edinb) 2015;25(4):235–7.

112. Monto RR. Platelet-rich plasma efficacy versus corticosteroid injection treatment for chronic severe plantar fasciitis. Foot Ankle Int 2014;35(4):313–8.

113. Shetty VD, Dhillon M, Hegde C, et al. A study to compare the efficacy of corticosteroid therapy with platelet-rich plasma therapy in recalcitrant plantar fasciitis: a preliminary report. Foot Ankle Surg 2014;20(1):10–3.

114. Aksahin E, Dogruyol D, Yuksel HY, et al. The comparison of the effect of corticosteroids and platelet-rich plasma (PRP) for the treatment of plantar fasciitis. Arch Orthop Trauma Surg 2012;132(6):781–5.

115. Lee TG, Ahmad TS. Intralesional autologous blood injection compared to corticosteroid injection for treatment of chronic plantar fasciitis. A prospective, randomized, controlled trial. Foot Ankle Int 2007;28(9):984–90.

116. Kim E, Lee JH. Autologous platelet-rich plasma versus dextrose prolotherapy for the treatment of chronic recalcitrant plantar fasciitis. PM R 2013;6(2):152–8.

117. Chew KT, Leong D, Lin CY, et al. Comparison of autologous conditioned plasma injection, extracorporeal shockwave therapy, and conventional treatment for plantar fasciitis: a randomized trial. PM R 2013;5(12):1035–43.

118. Rowden A, Dominici P, D'Orazio J, et al. Double-blind, randomized, placebo-controlled study evaluating the use of platelet-rich plasma therapy (PRP) for acute ankle sprains in the Emergency Department. J Emerg Med 2015;49(4): 546–51.

119. Laver L, Carmont MR, McConkey MO, et al. Plasma rich in growth factors (PRGF) as a treatment for high ankle sprain in elite athletes: a randomized control trial. Knee Surg Sports Traumatol Arthrosc 2015;23(11):3383–92.

120. Podesta L, Crow SA, Volkmer D, et al. Treatment of partial ulnar collateral ligament tears in the elbow with platelet-rich plasma. Am J Sports Med 2013; 41(7):1689–94.

121. Wetzel RJ, Patel RM, Terry MA. Platelet-rich plasma as an effective treatment for proximal hamstring injuries. Orthopedics 2013;36(1):e64–70.

122. Bubnov R, Yevseenko V, Semeniv I. Ultrasound guided injections of platelets rich plasma for muscle injury in professional athletes. Comparative study. Med Ultrason 2013;15(2):101–5.

123. Ekstrand J, Healy JC, Walden M, et al. Hamstring muscle injuries in professional football: the correlation of MRI findings with return to play. Br J Sports Med 2012; 46(2):112–7.

124. Orchard JW, Seward H, Orchard JJ. Results of 2 decades of injury surveillance and public release of data in the Australian Football League. Am J Sports Med 2013;41(4):734–41.

125. A. Hamid M, Mohamed Ali MR, Yusof A, et al. Platelet-rich plasma injections for the treatment of hamstring injuries: a randomized controlled trial. Am J Sports Med 2014;42(10):2410–8.

126. Hamilton B, Tol JL, Almusa E, et al. Platelet-rich plasma does not enhance return to play in hamstring injuries: a randomised controlled trial. Br J Sports Med 2015;49(14):943–50.

127. Reurink G, Goudswaard GJ, Moen MH, et al. Platelet-rich plasma injections in acute muscle injury. N Engl J Med 2014;370(26):2546–7.

128. Reurink G, Goudswaard GJ, Moen MH, et al. Rationale, secondary outcome scores and 1-year follow-up of a randomised trial of platelet-rich plasma injections in acute hamstring muscle injury: the Dutch Hamstring Injection Therapy Study. Br J Sports Med 2015;49(18):1206–12.

129. Martinez-Zapata MJ, Orozco L, Balius R, et al. Efficacy of autologous platelet-rich plasma for the treatment of muscle rupture with haematoma: a multicentre, randomised, double-blind, placebo-controlled clinical trial. Blood Transfus 2016;14(2):245–54.

130. Filardo G, Kon E, Buda R, et al. Platelet-rich plasma intra-articular knee injections for the treatment of degenerative cartilage lesions and osteoarthritis. Knee Surg Sports Traumatol Arthrosc 2011;19(4):528–35.

131. Kon E, Buda R, Filardo G, et al. Platelet-rich plasma: intra-articular knee injections produced favorable results on degenerative cartilage lesions. Knee Surg Sports Traumatol Arthrosc 2010;18(4):472–9.

132. Napolitano M, Matera S, Bossio M, et al. Autologous platelet gel for tissue regeneration in degenerative disorders of the knee. Blood Transfus 2012; 10(1):72–7.

133. Wang-Saegusa A, Cugat R, Ares O, et al. Infiltration of plasma rich in growth factors for osteoarthritis of the knee short-term effects on function and quality of life. Arch Orthop Trauma Surg 2010;131(3):311–7.

134. Sanchez M, Anitua E, Azofra J, et al. Intra-articular injection of an autologous preparation rich in growth factors for the treatment of knee OA: a retrospective cohort study. Clin Exp Rheumatol 2008;26(5):910–3.

135. Lai LP, Stitik TP, Foye PM, et al. Use of platelet-rich plasma in intra-articular knee injections for osteoarthritis: a systematic review. PM R 2015;7(6):637–48.

136. Li M, Zhang C, Ai Z, et al. Therapeutic effectiveness of intra-knee-articular injection of platelet-rich plasma on knee articular cartilage degeneration. Zhongguo Xiu Fu Chong Jian Wai Ke Za Zhi 2011;25(10):1192–6 [in Chinese].

137. Raeissadat SA, Rayegani SM, Babaee M, et al. The effect of platelet-rich plasma on pain, function, and quality of life of patients with knee osteoarthritis. Pain Res Treat 2013;2013:165967.

138. Gobbi A, Karnatzikos G, Mahajan V, et al. Platelet-rich plasma treatment in symptomatic patients with knee osteoarthritis: preliminary results in a group of active patients. Sports Health 2012;4(2):162–72.

139. Rayegani SM, Raeissadat SA, Taheri MS, et al. Does intra articular platelet rich plasma injection improve function, pain and quality of life in patients with osteoarthritis of the knee? A randomized clinical trial. Orthop Rev (Pavia) 2014;6(3):5405.

140. Sampson S, Reed M, Silvers H, et al. Injection of platelet-rich plasma in patients with primary and secondary knee osteoarthritis: a pilot study. Am J Phys Med Rehabil 2010;89(12):961–9.

141. Vaquerizo V, Plasencia MA, Arribas I, et al. Comparison of intra-articular injections of plasma rich in growth factors (PRGF-Endoret) versus Durolane hyaluronic acid in the treatment of patients with symptomatic osteoarthritis: a randomized controlled trial. Arthroscopy 2013;29(10):1635–43.

142. Spakova T, Rosocha J, Lacko M, et al. Treatment of knee joint osteoarthritis with autologous platelet-rich plasma in comparison with hyaluronic acid. Am J Phys Med Rehabil 2012;91(5):411–7.

143. Raeissadat SA, Rayegani SM, Hassanabadi H, et al. Knee osteoarthritis injection choices: platelet-rich plasma (PRP) versus hyaluronic acid (a one-year randomized clinical trial). Clin Med Insights Arthritis Musculoskelet Disord 2015;8:1–8.

144. Sanchez M, Fiz N, Azofra J, et al. A randomized clinical trial evaluating plasma rich in growth factors (PRGF-Endoret) versus hyaluronic acid in the short-term treatment of symptomatic knee osteoarthritis. Arthroscopy 2012;28(8):1070–8.

145. Kon E, Mandelbaum B, Buda R, et al. Platelet-rich plasma intra-articular injection versus hyaluronic acid viscosupplementation as treatments for cartilage pathology: from early degeneration to osteoarthritis. Arthroscopy 2011;27(11): 1490–501.

146. Gormeli G, Gormeli CA, Ataoglu B, et al. Multiple PRP injections are more effective than single injections and hyaluronic acid in knees with early osteoarthritis: a randomized, double-blind, placebo-controlled trial. Knee Surg Sports Traumatol Arthrosc 2015. [Epub ahead of print].

147. Cerza F, Carni S, Carcangiu A, et al. Comparison between hyaluronic acid and platelet-rich plasma, intra-articular infiltration in the treatment of gonarthrosis. Am J Sports Med 2012;40(12):2822–7.

148. Filardo G, Kon E, Di Martino A, et al. Platelet-rich plasma vs hyaluronic acid to treat knee degenerative pathology: study design and preliminary results of a randomized controlled trial. BMC Musculoskelet Disord 2012;13:229.

149. Filardo G, Di Matteo B, Di Martino A, et al. Platelet-rich plasma intra-articular knee injections show no superiority versus viscosupplementation: a randomized controlled trial. Am J Sports Med 2015;43(7):1575–82.

150. Patel S, Dhillon MS, Aggarwal S, et al. Treatment with platelet-rich plasma is more effective than placebo for knee osteoarthritis: a prospective, double-blind, randomized trial. Am J Sports Med 2013;41(2):356–64.

151. Forogh B, Mianehsaz E, Shoaee S, et al. Effect of single injection of platelet-rich plasma in comparison with corticosteroid on knee osteoarthritis: a double-blind randomized clinical trial. J Sports Med Phys Fitness 2016;56(7–8):901–8.

152. Sanchez M, Guadilla J, Fiz N, et al. Ultrasound-guided platelet-rich plasma injections for the treatment of osteoarthritis of the hip. Rheumatology (Oxford) 2012;51(1):144–50.

153. Battaglia M, Guaraldi F, Vannini F, et al. Efficacy of ultrasound-guided intra-articular injections of platelet-rich plasma versus hyaluronic acid for hip osteoarthritis. Orthopedics 2013;36(12):e1501–8.

154. Battaglia M, Guaraldi F, Vannini F, et al. Platelet-rich plasma (PRP) intra-articular ultrasound-guided injections as a possible treatment for hip osteoarthritis: a pilot study. Clin Exp Rheumatol 2011;29(4):754.

155. Mei-Dan O, Carmont MR, Laver L, et al. Platelet-rich plasma or hyaluronate in the management of osteochondral lesions of the talus. Am J Sports Med 2012;40(3):534–41.

156. Angthong C, Khadsongkram A, Angthong W. Outcomes and quality of life after platelet-rich plasma therapy in patients with recalcitrant hindfoot and ankle diseases: a preliminary report of 12 patients. J Foot Ankle Surg 2013;52(4):475–80.

157. Guney A, Akar M, Karaman I, et al. Clinical outcomes of platelet rich plasma (PRP) as an adjunct to microfracture surgery in osteochondral lesions of the talus. Knee Surg Sports Traumatol Arthrosc 2013;23(8):2384–9.

158. Blanke F, Vavken P, Haenle M, et al. Percutaneous injections of platelet rich plasma for treatment of intrasubstance meniscal lesions. Muscles Ligaments Tendons J 2015;5(3):162–6.

159. Pujol N, Salle De Chou E, Boisrenoult P, et al. Platelet-rich plasma for open meniscal repair in young patients: any benefit? Knee Surg Sports Traumatol Arthrosc 2015;23(1):51–8.

160. Shen W, Li Y, Tang Y, et al. NS-398, a cyclooxygenase-2-specific inhibitor, delays skeletal muscle healing by decreasing regeneration and promoting fibrosis. Am J Pathol 2005;167(4):1105–17.

161. Anitua E. The use of plasma-rich growth factors (PRGF) in oral surgery. Pract Proced Aesthet Dent 2001;13(6):487–93 [quiz: 487–93].

162. Leitner GC, Gruber R, Neumuller J, et al. Platelet content and growth factor release in platelet-rich plasma: a comparison of four different systems. Vox Sang 2006;91(2):135–9.

163. Dohan DM, Choukroun J, Diss A, et al. Platelet-rich fibrin (PRF): a second-generation platelet concentrate. Part I: technological concepts and evolution. Oral Surg Oral Med Oral Pathol Oral Radiol Endod 2006;101(3):e37–44.

164. Oh JH, Kim W, Park KU, et al. Comparison of the cellular composition and cytokine-release kinetics of various platelet-rich plasma preparations. Am J Sports Med 2015;43(12):3062–70.

165. Arora S, Doda V, Kotwal U, et al. Quantification of platelets and platelet derived growth factors from platelet-rich-plasma (PRP) prepared at different centrifugal force (g) and time. Transfus Apher Sci 2016;54(1):103–10.

166. Weibrich G, Kleis WK, Hafner G. Growth factor levels in the platelet-rich plasma produced by 2 different methods: curasan-type PRP kit versus PCCS PRP system. Int J Oral Maxillofac Implants 2002;17(2):184–90.

167. Weibrich G, Kleis WK, Buch R, et al. The harvest smart PRePTM system versus the Friadent-Schutze platelet-rich plasma kit. Clin Oral Implants Res 2003;14(2): 233–9.

168. Weibrich G, Kleis WK, Hafner G, et al. Comparison of platelet, leukocyte, and growth factor levels in point-of-care platelet-enriched plasma, prepared using a modified Curasan kit, with preparations received from a local blood bank. Clin Oral Implants Res 2003;14(3):357–62.

169. Weibrich G, Kleis WK, Hitzler WE, et al. Comparison of the platelet concentrate collection system with the plasma-rich-in-growth-factors kit to produce platelet-rich plasma: a technical report. Int J Oral Maxillofac Implants 2005;20(1): 118–23.

170. Magalon J, Bausset O, Serratrice N, et al. Characterization and comparison of 5 platelet-rich plasma preparations in a single-donor model. Arthroscopy 2014; 30(5):629–38.

171. Aydin F, Pancar Yuksel E, Albayrak D. Platelet collection efficiencies of three different platelet-rich plasma preparation systems. J Cosmet Laser Ther 2015; 17(3):165–8.

172. Dohan Ehrenfest DM, de Peppo GM, Doglioli P, et al. Slow release of growth factors and thrombospondin-1 in Choukroun's platelet-rich fibrin (PRF): a gold standard to achieve for all surgical platelet concentrates technologies. Growth Factors 2009;27(1):63–9.

173. Dohan Ehrenfest DM, Bielecki T, Jimbo R, et al. Do the fibrin architecture and leukocyte content influence the growth factor release of platelet concentrates? An evidence-based answer comparing a pure platelet-rich plasma (P-PRP) gel and a leukocyte- and platelet-rich fibrin (L-PRF). Curr Pharm Biotechnol 2012;13(7):1145–52.

174. Dohan DM, Choukroun J, Diss A, et al. Platelet-rich fibrin (PRF): a second-generation platelet concentrate. Part II: platelet-related biologic features. Oral Surg Oral Med Oral Pathol Oral Radiol Endod 2006;101(3):e45–50.

175. Schar MO, Diaz-Romero J, Kohl S, et al. Platelet-rich concentrates differentially release growth factors and induce cell migration in vitro. Clin Orthop Relat Res 2015;473(5):1635–43.

176. Passaretti F, Tia M, D'Esposito V, et al. Growth-promoting action and growth factor release by different platelet derivatives. Platelets 2014;25(4):252–6.

177. Gassling VL, Acil Y, Springer IN, et al. Platelet-rich plasma and platelet-rich fibrin in human cell culture. Oral Surg Oral Med Oral Pathol Oral Radiol Endod 2009;108(1):48–55.

178. Zumstein MA, Berger S, Schober M, et al. Leukocyte- and platelet-rich fibrin (L-PRF) for long-term delivery of growth factor in rotator cuff repair: review, preliminary results and future directions. Curr Pharm Biotechnol 2012;13(7):1196–206.

179. He L, Lin Y, Hu X, et al. A comparative study of platelet-rich fibrin (PRF) and platelet-rich plasma (PRP) on the effect of proliferation and differentiation of rat osteoblasts in vitro. Oral Surg Oral Med Oral Pathol Oral Radiol Endod 2009;108(5):707–13.

180. Braune S, Walter M, Schulze F, et al. Changes in platelet morphology and function during 24 hours of storage. Clin Hemorheol Microcirc 2014;58(1):159–70.
181. Giusti I, Rughetti A, D'Ascenzo S, et al. Identification of an optimal concentration of platelet gel for promoting angiogenesis in human endothelial cells. Transfusion 2009;49(4):771–8.
182. Giusti I, Rughetti A, D'Ascenzo S, et al. The effects of platelet gel-released supernatant on human fibroblasts. Wound Repair Regen 2013;21(2):300–8.
183. Jo CH, Kim JE, Yoon KS, et al. Platelet-rich plasma stimulates cell proliferation and enhances matrix gene expression and synthesis in tenocytes from human rotator cuff tendons with degenerative tears. Am J Sports Med 2012;40(5): 1035–45.
184. Bielecki T, Dohan Ehrenfest DM, Everts PA, et al. The role of leukocytes from L-PRP/L-PRF in wound healing and immune defense: new perspectives. Curr Pharm Biotechnol 2012;13(7):1153–62.
185. Yoshida R, Murray MM. Peripheral blood mononuclear cells enhance the anabolic effects of platelet-rich plasma on anterior cruciate ligament fibroblasts. J Orthop Res 2013;31(1):29–34.
186. Zimmermann R, Arnold D, Strasser E, et al. Sample preparation technique and white cell content influence the detectable levels of growth factors in platelet concentrates. Vox Sang 2003;85(4):283–9.
187. Pifer MA, Maerz T, Baker KC, et al. Matrix metalloproteinase content and activity in low-platelet, low-leukocyte and high-platelet, high-leukocyte platelet rich plasma (PRP) and the biologic response to PRP by human ligament fibroblasts. Am J Sports Med 2014;42(5):1211–8.
188. Sundman EA, Cole BJ, Fortier LA. Growth factor and catabolic cytokine concentrations are influenced by the cellular composition of platelet-rich plasma. Am J Sports Med 2011;39(10):2135–40.
189. Martineau I, Lacoste E, Gagnon G. Effects of calcium and thrombin on growth factor release from platelet concentrates: kinetics and regulation of endothelial cell proliferation. Biomaterials 2004;25(18):4489–502.
190. Harrison S, Vavken P, Kevy S, et al. Platelet activation by collagen provides sustained release of anabolic cytokines. Am J Sports Med 2011;39(4):729–34.
191. Amable PR, Carias RB, Teixeira MV, et al. Platelet-rich plasma preparation for regenerative medicine: optimization and quantification of cytokines and growth factors. Stem Cell Res Ther 2013;4(3):67.
192. Dohan Ehrenfest DM, Rasmusson L, Albrektsson T. Classification of platelet concentrates: from pure platelet-rich plasma (P-PRP) to leucocyte- and platelet-rich fibrin (L-PRF). Trends Biotechnol 2009;27(3):158–67.
193. Wu PI, Meleger A, Witkower A, et al. Nonpharmacologic Options for Treating Acute and Chronic Pain. Pm R 2015;7(11 Suppl):S278–94.

Stem Cell Considerations for the Clinician

Karen A. Hasty, PhD*, Hongsik Cho, PhD

KEYWORDS

- Mesenchymal stem cells • Adipose-derived stem cells
- Bone marrow–derived stem cells • Nonunions • Osteoarthritis • Autologous
- Allogeneic • Paracrine

KEY POINTS

- Mesenchymal stem cells (MSCs) isolated from different tissues share many characteristics, such as the capability for multilineage differentiation, absence of HLA-DR expression, and possession of the markers CD105, CD73, and CD90, but may vary in expression of other markers, such as CD36 and CD106.
- In the United States, unpurified stem cells from bone marrow and other tissues can meet minimally manipulated classification as 361 tissue with exemption from Food and Drug Administration premarket review and regulation; however, enzymatic harvesting and culture expansion of MSCs are exclusive of 361 classification.
- Harvesting of MSCs from different anatomic sites yields varying cell numbers and proliferation rates, as exemplified by comparison of MSCs isolated from bone marrow and adipose tissues. Age and sex differences were observed with decreased proliferation and differentiation and increased senescence markers.
- Paracrine effects of soluble mediators and cell-to-cell interactions of MSCs affect innate and adaptive immunity and decrease inflammation.

INTRODUCTION

Over the past 60 years, evidence has accumulated supporting the existence of a multipotent adult stem cell population in the body that has the potential to differentiate into bone, cartilage, tendon, ligament, adipocytes, dermis, muscle, and connective tissue. These cells are now collectively grouped under the term mesenchymal stem cells (MSCs) or multipotent mesenchymal stromal cells. A large proportion of the studies on MSCs have involved the role of these cells in the development and repair of bone and cartilage, heightening interest in the clinical orthopaedic community. In 1966, intraperitoneal diffusion chambers implanted with mouse bone marrow cells

Department of Orthopaedic Surgery and Biomedical Engineering, Campbell Clinic/UTHSC, VA Medical Center, Research Service 151, 1030 Jefferson Avenue, Memphis, TN 38104, USA
* Corresponding author.
E-mail address: khasty@uthsc.edu

Phys Med Rehabil Clin N Am 27 (2016) 855–870
http://dx.doi.org/10.1016/j.pmr.2016.06.004
1047-9651/16/Published by Elsevier Inc.

demonstrated that undifferentiated "stem" cells were present and resulted in osteogenic foci of cells producing alkaline phosphatase (AlkP) and fibroblasts while hematopoietic cells were lost.[1] Interestingly, orthopaedic surgeons were already using viable cancellous bone chips containing these cells in fracture repair. In the first edition of *Campbell's Operative Orthopaedics* (1939), a recommended treatment of nonunions included a combination of stable fixation and packing of cancellous bone chips from the proximal tibia.[2] Even though the concept of stem cells as we know today was unknown at the time, early orthopaedic surgeons recognized the osteogenic effect of cancellous bone and bone marrow.

Today it is clear that stem cell supplementation offers a valuable tool for correcting some of the clinical challenges in treatment of musculoskeletal diseases and injury. Between 2006 and 2012, there was a threefold increase in the number of MSC product Investigational New Drug (IND) submissions to the Food and Drug Administration (FDA), resulting in clinical trials initiated worldwide (246 trials; source: http://www. clinicaltrials.gov). Although much of the initial research focused on bone marrow–derived MSCs (bmMSCs) with umbilical or placental sources serving as secondary sources, an increasing trend of adipose-derived MSC-based product INDs has occurred since 2011.[3] Many of these new INDs deal with MSCs destined for allogeneic use, with more than 80% using cryopreservation for storage of the MSC products to facilitate transport to the clinical site where they are used. Cell banking of cultured MSCs (35%) in these endeavors has also been denoted; however, one report showed reduced immunomodulatory function of thawed cryopreserved MSCs immediately after thawing that was recovered after subsequent in vitro culture.[4] The bioactivity of these products in the IND is variably described with molecular markers such as "secreted factors or expression of proteins on the surface of either the MSC or target cells (eg, T cells) that may be related to a given biological activity."[3]

MESENCHYMAL STEM CELL DEFINITION

What is the definition of this stem cell population and what are the differences between stem cell populations isolated from different tissues (bone marrow, adipose tissues, cord blood, muscle, synovium, dental pulp, muscle, and others)? Caplan[5,6] has stated that "All or most MSC arise in vivo from perivascular cells (pericytes) that are released from the damaged or inflamed blood vessels at the site of injury." If this is so, then tissues that have a poor vascular supply would heal poorly or not at all and this is supported by clinical observations of the mid to inner portions of the meniscal and articular cartilages. However, healing by fibroblast proliferation and scar formation and the regrowth of differentiated cells originating from stem cells that are specific to the function of the damage tissue are separate issues. Are stem cells from different tissues equivalent?

Review of the published literature on this question gives evidence to support shared characteristics of MSCs from different tissues, but also supports that variations are present as well. Perivascular MSCs from both bone marrow (BM) and dental pulp (DP) tissues localized immunohistochemically or isolated by immunoselection document that these cells do show expression of STRO1 an early marker of stem cells and CD146 an endothelial marker, but that a 3G5 antigen marker of pericytes was predominantly in the DP population and only in a small portion of the BM cells.[7] Another report observed that the MSC population derived from veins, artery, perivascular cells, or fibroblasts showed similarity of cell morphology and phenotypes established with 22 markers with heterogeneous expression of genes related to angiogenesis.[8] According to criteria set up by the Mesenchymal and Tissue Stem Cell Committee of the International Society for Cellular Therapy, MSCs are adherent cells that have the capacity to differentiate in vitro into osteoblasts, chondrocytes, and adipocytes and must express CD105, CD73, and CD90 and lack expression of CD45, CD34, CD14, CD11b, CD79α, CD19, and HLA-DR surface molecules.[9] A joint statement of the International Federation for Adipose Therapeutics and Science and the International Society for Cellular Therapy, identified CD90+, CD73+, CD105+, and CD44+ as adipose tissue stem cell markers with absence of CD45− and CD31−. The adipose-derived MSCs are different from BM MSCs in being positive for CD36 and negative for CD106.[10]

FOOD AND DRUG ADMINISTRATION REGULATORY GUIDELINES

The harvesting of BM or adipose tissue from the patient for autologous transplantation results in a heterogeneous mixture of cells including the desired stem cell population. Differential centrifugation and erythrocyte lysis accomplish some concentration of the stem cells, but this population still includes hematopoietic stem cells, endothelial cells, erythrocytes, fibroblasts, lymphocytes, monocyte/macrophages, and pericytes, among other nucleated cells. These relatively unpurified cells from BM can meet in many cases the "minimally manipulated" classification as 361 tissue with exemption from premarket review and regulation by US FDA regulations. For adipose tissue, this stromal vascular fraction has been estimated to contain 15% to 30% stromal cells and 3% to 5% pericytes, with hematopoietic-related and endothelial-related cells making up 20% to 45% and 10% to 20%, respectively, of the remainder.[10] However, enzymatic harvesting or mechanical release of the cells from adipose tissue currently disqualifies them from the 361 classification.[11] Expansion of the adherent stem cells in culture in vitro allows another purification step and also permits differentiation of the cells, but also may be considered disqualification from 361 status dependent on culture conditions.[12]

HARVESTING AND CHARACTERIZATION OF MESENCHYMAL STEM CELLS FROM DIFFERENT TISSUES

Review of the literature for the use of human MSCs identified 4 major harvest sites from placental, adipose, BM, and umbilical cord tissues.[11] Although other tissues have been used, reports of these tissues are not as common. Comparisons of the yield of MSCs from the major sites were difficult due to the large variations among different techniques, but adipose tissue consistently yielded higher levels of MSCs, ranging from 4.7×10^3 to 1.5×10^6 cells/mL of tissue compared with BM ranges of 1 to 30 cells/mL to 3.2×10^5 cells/mL and umbilical cord tissues yielding 1.0×10^4 to 4.7×10^6. The number of MSCs from placental tissues and synovium ranged from 1.0 to 30.0×10^3 cells per milliliter. Quantitation of the connective-tissue progenitor yield was conducted in the primary tissue isolate principally by limited dilution fibroblast colony-forming unit (CFU) assay and enumeration of the colonies (ranging from 20–50 cells per colony) forming in vitro. This allows comparison from various studies or of the yields from different tissues, but does not evaluate the capability of these cells to undergo other types of differentiation. Some investigations have reported the findings with respect to the number of phenotypic CFUs when cultured under conditions whereby multilineage differentiation occurs.[13] Information for selective differentiation of cultures is reported as Alizarin Red staining CFUs for osteogenesis, Alcian Blue–positive staining CFUs for chondrogenesis or Oil Red O–staining CFUs for adipogenesis (**Fig. 1**). These numbers are more relevant to the MSC population than the nucleated cell counts of the primary cells isolated as they make up such a minority of the total cells. It has been estimated that there is a mean of 55 osteoblastic

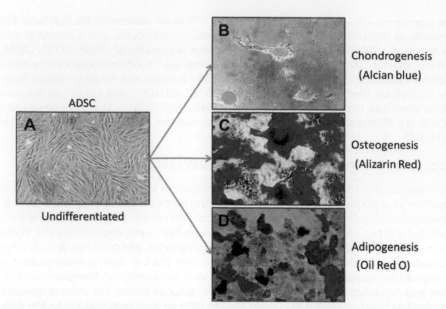

Fig. 1. In vitro differentiation of porcine MSCs derived from subcutaneous adipose tissue. The adipose-derived MSCs (ADSCs) were isolated from dorsal subcutaneous fat. Following 24 hours in culture, the nonadherent hematopoietic cells were removed and the cells differentiated or cultured undifferentiated (A) for 14 days. The Alcian Blue staining was performed for (B) chondrogenic cultures (StemPro Chondrogenesis Differentiation Kit; Thermo Fisher Scientific, Waltham, MA), Alizarin Red staining was performed for (C) osteogenic differentiation (StemPro Osteogenesis Kit; Thermo Fisher Scientific) and the Oil Red O Staining was performed for (D) adipogenic cultures (StemPro Adipogenesis kit; Thermo Fisher Scientific).

progenitors per 10^6 nucleated cells from the BM,[14] with a cautionary note for risk of variation due to blood contamination.[11]

Not only did MSCs vary dependent on the tissue source, the anatomic location was important. The MSCs from subcutaneous fat proliferate in vitro at a higher rate and differentiate better than those from visceral fat.[15] Human MSCs from different adipose anatomic sites showed that the yield was site dependent with higher frequencies of MSCs from the abdomen than the hip or thigh. In this study, abdominal adipose tissue was determined to contain 2.6 to 10.2×10^6 MSCs from 100 g of adipose tissue. The anatomic site of BM harvesting also associated with significant variation with up to twofold difference in the yield. Pierini and colleagues[13] analyzed MSC yield from the posterior or anterior iliac crest and the subchondral knee sites and concluded that the posterior iliac crest was preferable, although no differences were found for viability, phenotype, expansion kinetics, or multilineage differentiation. Hernigou and colleagues[16] studied the risk of complications when harvesting from the iliac crest and determined that higher risks, such as trocar contact with the external iliac artery, were observed with aspiration in the 4 most anterior sections with a higher risk in women. Placement of the trocar deeper than 6 cm in the posterior iliac crest was at risk for sciatic nerve and gluteal vessel damage.

Pittenger and colleagues[17] showed only 0.001% to 0.01% of the cells in the iliac crest aspirate of normal adults exhibited the capacity for CFUs in vitro. This low number mandates larger collection volumes or culture expansion. Although the iliac crest has been the traditional site of harvest for BM, the intramedullary cavities of the long bone offers another resource, with high numbers of stem cells present in the BM.[18] The number of stem cells that can be obtained has been enormously increased by the adaptation of a Reamer-Irrigator-Aspirator (RIA) (Synthes, Westchester, PA), consisting of a cutting head on a drive shaft with an attached irrigating and aspirating system.[19] Comparisons were made for MSCs harvested using a traditional 10-mL iliac crest BM aspiration (ICBMA) and MSCs collected during the reaming of the femur to remove 1.5 mm at the isthmus. The material obtained during the reaming was divided into liquid (RIA liquid) and that which was strained out of the liquid through a cell strainer (RIA solid) and further digested with collagenase. Manual white cell count and in vitro culture of the cells under conditions of differentiation showed that colony formation was equivalent in ICBMA and RIA liquid fractions, although the volume of the RIA liquid was 70 times that of the ICBMA. The RIA solid had almost 4 times more colonies than the ICBMA sample and had approximately 2.5 times the volume. The ability to collect such high amounts of these stem cells suggests that this methodology could provide 50,000 MSCs in a BM concentrate, a number that has been effective in nonunions, without culture expansion.[20]

EFFECTS OF AGE AND GENDER ON MESENCHYMAL STEM CELLS

Other variables to be considered for autologous stem cell supplementation concern the age and gender of the patient. What is the impact of age on stem cell number in an individual? A decrease in stem cell number with aging could contribute to delayed or incomplete repair in older individuals and would be a factor for consideration of supplementing with allogeneic versus autologous MSC. The data are somewhat controversial for an age-related change in the number of MSCs in BM, but the bulk of the evidence supports that aging decreases MSC numbers in the BM and increases markers of senescence. In studies of healthy volunteers, both the number and the proliferative capacity of bmMSCs from aged donors (>40 years) decreased compared with young or adult individuals.[21] Cells from older individuals showed increased levels of radical oxygen species and senescence markers, such as p53 and p21, while AlkP-positive CFUs were reduced. These data agree with a similar study in which comparisons of MSCs harvested from young (18 years) and older (59–75 years) donors showed that the number of AlkP-positive colonies were decreased in older individuals as well as their proliferation. The decreased proliferation of the older cells was associated with a shorter telomere restriction fragment. Telomere length of a cell positively correlates with replicative ability.[22]

A study of MSCs (STRO-1+ cells) taken from BM from discarded femoral tissues from 57 subjects, ages ranging from 17 to 90 years old, undergoing hip arthroplasty for osteoarthritis (OA) showed that the number of STRO-1+ cells in the marrow did not change with age. However, significant age-associated effects were observed, such as delayed proliferation due to prolongation of the duration of cell cycling, increased apoptosis, a fourfold greater senescence-associated β-galactosidase (SA-β-gal) in the group 55 years or older, and decreased osteoblast differentiation in terms of alkaline phosphatase activity and in the number of AlkP-positive cells.[23] The levels of p53, a negative regulator of osteoblast differentiation, showed an age-related increase in p53. In contrast, an earlier study of BM aspirates in orthopedic patients ranging in age from 13 to 83 years showed a significant decline of nucleated cells with age, but only the female patients showed a significant decline in AlkP-positive CFUs with age, possibly relevant to osteoporosis in older women.[14]

Tissue-dependent effects were obtained comparing the MSCs of old and young rabbits. The bone marrow–derived stem cells from old rabbits showed reduced proliferation and chondrogenic response whereas muscle-derived stem and adipose-derived stem cells exhibited no negative effects although the yield from all tissues were lower in the older animals.[24] Although bmMSCs show detrimental changes with aging, this may not be the case for adipose-derived MSCs. The number of MSCs derived from adipose tissue or their differentiation capacity did not correlate with age of the donor in several studies,[15,25] although the androgenic status of the pre-adipocytes at different locations influences the proliferation and differentiation of these cells.[25] Another factor that has been shown to affect the stem cell population is previous treatment with steroids. Corticosteroid treatment results in decreased stem cells in the BM of the iliac crest.[26]

MODE OF ACTION OF MESENCHYMAL STEM CELL SUPPLEMENTATION

Although much of the initial enthusiasm for the use of MSCs pertained to their function as a precursor population for a more differentiated phenotype and their plasticity and multipotency in giving rise to different reparative cell types, it is apparent that these cells can also function to impact local resident cells and to decrease the immune response of both innate and adaptive immune cells and reduce inflammation.[27] The MSCs that are present in an initial injury inhibit the immune system early in the reparative process possibly as an attempt to forestall autoimmune reactions to components of the damaged tissue.[28] In addition, they also produce molecules that stimulate replication of progenitor cells, stimulate formation of new blood vessels, and inhibit the apoptosis of cells due to ischemia. Building on this hypothesis, investigations of the downregulation of the immune response by MSCs have been undertaken in a variety of autoimmune diseases. This immunomodulatory influence of MSCs has been used in the treatment of lupus erythematosus,[29] multiple sclerosis,[30] systemic sclerosis,[31] and graft-versus-host disease.[32] Many of the beneficial effects on autoimmunity and the reparative function are elicited by production of soluble mediators and through cell-to-cell interaction (Table 1). Cocultures of MSCs suppress proliferation of stimulated mononuclear cells[33] or T-lymphocytes[34,35] and Fas ligand–mediated apoptosis of T cells.[36] The interaction of T1 or T17 lymphocytes upregulates adenosine production by MSCs that suppresses these lymphocyte populations[37,38] and leads to new blood vessel formation through stimulation of vascular endothelial growth factor.[39] The interaction of MSCs and monocytes results in their production of interleukin-10 and an anti-inflammatory phenotype.[40]

In addition to the immune suppressive properties of MSCs, their ability to give rise to more differentiated cell types needed for damaged tissues such as cartilage, bone, and cardiac muscle are equally important. Interestingly, these cells have been reported to express HLA class I but very little HLA class II molecules. This suggests that the cells can be used in an allogeneic as well as an autologous setting, an attractive alternative supplying an available off-the-shelf supply of well-characterized, healthier MSCs. However, recently other studies have shown MHC II expression presents following stimulation with interferon gamma,[41] after chondrogenic differentiation[42–44] or osteogenic differentiation.[45] Others have found that immunosuppressive therapy is needed for differentiated MSCs to survive and evade infiltrating immune cells.[46,47] This has raised concern for the longevity of allogeneic cells in the donor recipient,[48] particularly for therapies in which the differentiated cell type is important, such as cartilage replacement in OA.

Table 1
Immunomodulatory molecules produced by MSCs

Source	Factor	Action	Reference
Mouse bmMSC	IL-1ra	Decreased inflammatory response to bleomycin in the lung	64
Human bmMSC	Soluble TNF receptor −1	Attenuated systemic inflammatory response to intraperitoneal injection of lipopolysaccharide	65
Human bmMSC	TNF-α stimulated gene/protein 6	Reduced early inflammatory response to permanent ligation of the anterior descending coronary artery and size of the myocardial infarcts	66
Human MSC	TNF-α stimulated gene/protein 6	Reduced inflammation in a model of sterile cornea injury	67
Human bmMSC	TNF-α stimulated gene/protein 6	Reduction of neutrophils and macrophages in model of zymosan-induced peritonitis	68
Mouse bmMSC	PGE$_2$	Mouse model of sepsis induced by cecal ligation and puncture	69
Human bmMSC	PGE$_2$	Increased numbers of anti-inflammatory M2 phenotype in human macrophages in vitro cocultures	70
Mouse MSC	Adenosine	Suppression of T-cell proliferation	37
Human bmMSC	Adenosine	Suppresses immune responses of Th17 cells	38
Human bmMSC	IL-6	Skew monocytes to an IL-10 producing phenotype	40

Abbreviations: bmMSC, bone marrow–derived mesenchymal stem cell; IL, interleukin; MSC, mesenchymal stem cell; PGE2, prostaglandin E2; TNF, tumor necrosis factor.

Indeed, monitoring the in vivo survival of implanted autologous MSCs that undergo differentiation in vivo is difficult, as the implanted cells do not differ from the adjacent resident cells and do not have identifying markers. One way of marking stem cells is by labeling them with fluorescent dyes, bioluminescent reporters, radionucleotides, or paramagnetic particles before implantation (for review see Ref.[49]). We have used fluorescently labeled rabbit bmMSCs for implantation into a surgically created partial defect in the physis in young growing rabbits.[50] Fluorescent microscopy of histologic sections of the implanted cells in the rabbit physis shows their persistence in the tissue at 3 weeks after implantation (**Fig. 2**) and their phenotypic appearance in histologic stained sections as newly formed chondrocytes organized as proliferating isogenous groups that were contiguous with the remaining physis (**Fig. 3**). If left untreated in this model, the animals develop an angular deformity due to the unequal growth across the physis. Angular deformity was significantly different from the untreated control group I in all groups receiving MSCs with the greatest reduction in angular deformity in the groups that received MSCs cultured on Gelfoam with transforming growth factor beta 3 (TGF-β3), a growth factor that enhances the chondrogenic differentiation of MSCs (**Fig. 4**).

USE OF MESENCHYMAL STEM CELLS FOR ORTHOPEDIC PROBLEMS

The current expectations are very high for the benefits of using stem cell therapy for diverse diseases and traumatic injuries. The largest body of data on the clinical use

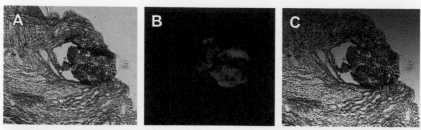

Fig. 2. ADSCs transplanted into a physeal defect in the rabbit hind limb. Allogeneic ADSCs were labeled with the fluorescent dye, dialkylcarbocyanine (DiI) before transplantation into a surgically created partial defect in the epiphyseal growth plate of young rabbits. Histologic sections of implanted cells in the growth plate after a 3-week interval. (*A*) Without fluorescent imaging, (*B*) with fluorescent imaging, (*C*) merged images. (*Reprinted from Ahn JI, Canale TS, Butler SD, et al. Stem cell repair of physeal cartilage. J Orthop Res 2004;22:1220; with permission.*)

of these cells is within the orthopaedic clinical setting, although the use of these cells within the United States has been under the more restrictive guidelines of the FDA than those outside the United States. Coverage of trials worldwide is beyond the scope of this report, but the most common applications are described in the following sections.

Fracture Repair and Nonunions

Nonunions following stabilization and treatment of a fracture of a long bone are problematic and can be exacerbated by previous drug treatment and ongoing comorbidities of the patient. Many of these fractures occur in aging patients with osteoporosis with compromised fracture repair. Treatment with autologous bmMSCs was evaluated in patients of varying ages with atrophic tibial diaphyseal nonunions.[20] Percutaneous grafting with BM concentrates harvested from the iliac crest showed a positive

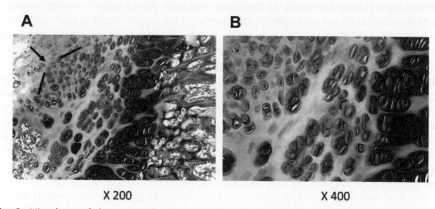

X 200   X 400

Fig. 3. Histology of the surgically damaged site of a growth plate in a rabbit treated with cells cultured on Gelfoam in medium containing 10 ng/mL of transforming growth factor (TGF)-β3 in group C analyzed in **Fig. 4**. Images at (*A*) ×200 and (*B*) ×400 magnification show differentiated chondrocytes and isogenous columns (denoted by black bars and *arrow*) irregularly arranged in the matrix and contiguous with the damaged growth plate (hematoxylin-eosin stain). (*Reprinted from Ahn JI, Canale TS, Butler SD, et al. Stem cell repair of physeal cartilage. J Orthop Res 2004;22:1218; with permission.*)

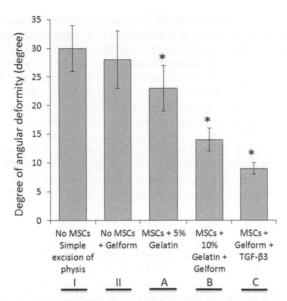

Fig. 4. Differences in angular deformity in the treated and untreated rabbits. Deformity measured as the angle formed between perpendiculars from the distal femoral and distal tibial articular surfaces in radiographs. No cells were implanted into the control groups, group I (4 rabbits) the physeal defect was left untreated and group II (3 rabbits) the physeal defect was treated with Gelfoam. Experimental groups with approximately 2 to 4 million MSCs per implant: Group A (5 rabbits), the defect was filled with 5% gelatin containing cultured MSCs; Group B (3 rabbits), the defect was filled with 10% gelatin containing the same cells and a Gelfoam resorbable sponge plug placed at the periphery of physeal defect to prevent leakage of the cells; Group C (5 rabbits), the defect was filled with cells cultured on Gelfoam in medium containing 10 ng/mL of TGF-β3 to enhance chondrogenesis. Angular deformity was significantly different (*asterisk*) from control group I in all animal groups receiving MSCs with the most reduction of ($P<.001$) in deformity seen in group C (MSCs + Gelfoam + TGF-β3). (*Reprinted from* Ahn JI, Canale TS, Butler SD, et al. Stem cell repair of physeal cartilage. J Orthop Res 2004;22:1217; with permission.)

correlation between the volume of the mineralized callus at 4 months and the number and concentration of the fibroblast CFUs that were injected. Sixty patients with non-unions, defined as a failure of the fracture to heal within 6 months and considered to be atrophic due to minimal callus formation, were treated with BM concentrates averaging a total of 50,000 CFUs. Fifty-three of the grafted patients obtained bone union with radiographic evidence of callus formation on average at 12 weeks. The 7 patients who did not achieve union received lower concentrations of progenitor cells.

Osteonecrosis of the Hip

Osteonecrosis of the femoral head was one of the first conditions of the hip in which cellular therapies showed good clinical outcomes (for review see Ref.[51]). Many of these patients have been previously treated with steroids, a drug that results in adipo-cyte differentiation of BM stem cells. Extensive osteocyte death and the observation that reduced MSC numbers are seen in the BM of the iliac crest[26] form a logical basis for this treatment and possibly recommend the use of allogeneic MSCs. Another likely benefit may result from angiogenic cytokines secreted by the mononuclear BM cells.[51] Interestingly, the BM concentrate can be percutaneously injected with a small trocar into the necrotic head.[52] In some cases, autologous bmMSCs were combined with beta-tricalcium phosphate ceramic composites[53] or mixed with allogeneic MSCs before implantation. Recently, good results were shown with harvested osteoprogenitor cells for grafting secondary osteonecrosis of the knee.[54] In another study of patients with sickle cell disease, decompression and autologous BM grafting proved effective with a reduced incidence (only 12.5%) of collapse after 5 years of follow-up compared with 87% collapse seen historically. Two recent reviews of the literature on core decompression with autologous stem cell injection determined that addition of stem cells was superior to core decompression alone in osteonecrotic femoral heads by different investigations, several with long-term follow-up.[55] Approximation of the number of stem cells needed for loading in an osteonecrotic femoral head was calculated by evaluation of the number of MSCs in a normal femoral head. A total of 35,000 bmMSCs is considered as a useful approximation of the number of MSCs present in a femoral head.[26,56]

Cartilage Repair

One of the most difficult challenges in the future for tissue engineering with MSCs will be to undertake the reconstruction of articular cartilage. Although this tissue is composed of only one cell type and lacks innervation and vascularization, the chondrocytes and their matrix components are stratified in their phenotype from the articular surface to the subchondral underpinning in apparent response to the ratio of the different types of mechanical stresses exerted on the layers. It is clear that MSCs cultured in vitro under chondrogenic conditions express differentiated cartilage components, but do not display the stratified appearance of articular chondrocytes. Even MSCs differentiating at the articular surface with microfracture; the drilling through the osteochondral boundary and the subsequent upgrowth and chondrogenic differentiation of the stem cells from the marrow cavity, do not achieve a mature hyaline cartilage phenotype.[57] The new cartilage that forms under this condition initially looks promising, but gradually progresses to a fibrocartilage phenotype with an unknown half-life.[58] As it is known that the expressive phenotype of the chondrocyte is responsive to mechanical stress, it is clear that more information is needed regarding the impact of physical rehabilitation and the long-term response to weight bearing on newly formed or implanted cartilage tissue.

The phenotype of articular cartilage in the joint often modifies with aging displaying hypertrophic markers, such as type X collagen and matrix metalloproteinase expression typical of the hypertrophic zone of the physis. These markers are thought to signal the onset of OA (for a review see Ref.[59]). It is unknown if these changes are inherent in the chondrocytes themselves or arise from the response of the chondrocyte to changes in their milieu whether it be to soluble factors or mechanical forces. If an external factor is the primary impetus eliciting the hypertrophic changes, would newly implanted chondrocytes be resistant to such changes or would the same sequela develop over time? If hypertrophy develops due to inherent properties of the aging chondrocytes, would autologous MSCs used for tissue engineering of the cartilage replacement be subject to early degeneration as well? Alternatively, do MSCs exert a beneficial modification of the inflammatory milieu through paracrine effects in addition to their role as chondrocyte precursors? Clinical trials going forward in this area should incorporate some of the guidelines for "detailed methodological recommendations...developed for the statistical study design, patient recruitment, control group considerations, study endpoint definition, documentation of results, use of validated patient-reported outcome instruments, and inclusion and exclusion criteria for the design and conduct of scientifically sound cartilage repair study protocols" developed by the International Cartilage Repair Society.[60]

Homologous use of MSCs is their implantation in a tissue for a condition in which the cells would normally participate. An example of this is the use of bmMSCs for nonunion of bone fractures. The use of bmMSCs or adipose-derived MSCs for cartilage repair is considered nonhomologous use by the FDA, a classification inhibiting clinical application of their use in the United States; however, clinical investigations outside the United States show promising results with these cells. Patients with unilateral OA have been treated with autologous BM stem cells expanded in autologous serum for 3 weeks and supplemented by intra-articular injection into the knees of 56 patients (<55 years of age) who had previously undergone microfracture and medial opening-wedge high tibial osteotomy.[61] Those patients receiving MSCs showed more improvement in short-term clinical and longer-term MRI findings at 1 year than patients similarly treated who did not receive the cells. However, the investigators stated that a limitation of this study was that the injected MSCs could not be followed to the desired regeneration site, raising the question if the beneficial effects were due to paracrine factors from the MSCs or their direct participation as chondrogenic precursor cells. In another study, Jo and colleagues[62] injected enzymatically isolated, culture-expanded adipose-derived MSCs into the knee joint of 18 patients with arthroscopically graded OA lesions. Significantly improved WOMAC scores and decreased knee pain were observed compared with baseline in only patients receiving the highest number of 1×10^8 cells. MRI evaluations at 3 months showed a thick layer of articular cartilage that was thickened at 6 months. Arthroscopic measurement of the original cartilage lesion in the lateral femoral and tibial condyles at 6 months postinjection showed a significant decrease in the high-dose group, but not the other groups. Histologic evaluations of biopsies at 6 months showed a hyaline-like cartilage in the mid to deep zones, but the upper half of the mid zone and the superficial zone demonstrated that type I collagen–positive fibrocartilage was present. Although this study injected the cells in the solution, implantation of such cells or autologous chondrocytes in various scaffolds is now second generation for cartilage replacement engineering. However, utilization of a scaffold requires 2 invasive procedures: one for harvesting of the autologous stem cells from tissues with possible expansion in culture or cell/scaffold preparation and another surgery for implantation of this tissue. Comparison of treatments with autologous BM stem cells and autologous chondrocytes showed equivalent results, although the stem cell treatments were less expensive.[63]

SUMMARY

Although there is ample evidence that beneficial results can be obtained from the use of MSCs, several questions regarding their use remain to be answered. Several questions are in regard to the mechanism or mechanisms by which the MSCs are eliciting the positive outcome of their use, whether it be paracrine factors that are made by the MSCs that affect the innate or adaptive immunity or impact the metabolism of resident cells or by their contribution as precursor cells giving rise to reparative cells. If paracrine factors are the paramount impetus, then commercial sources of allogeneic MSCs could possibly provide an easily obtainable, well-characterized reagent for the clinician if such can be suitably standardized. Tissue engineering of MSCs contained within a suitable scaffold also has value for stabilizing and localizing these cells within the implantation site. However, in their function as reparative cells, the longevity and fate of allogeneic MSCs need to be further evaluated on a longer-term basis. Does the fact that allogeneic cells have the potential to express their own inherent HLA protein under certain stimuli impair their desirability for serving as reparative cells for cartilage, ligaments, and bone; tissues that may be subject on occasion to inflammation or the activity of innate and acquired immune cells?

Alternatively, the use of autologous cells has both advantages and its own inherent disadvantages involving additional procedures for collection, preparation, and characterization of the MSCs. It is apparent that a critical number of MSCs are necessary for implantation to effect an optimal outcome. This underscores the importance of deciding if tissues such as adipose tissue provide more MSCs than BM and if the capability for differentiation is the same for MSCs isolated from different tissue sources. If autologous MSCs are limited, what are the conditions for optimal culture expansion and are there benefits for initiating differentiation pathways before reimplantation? Also, we need to better understand how individual patient factors, such as age, sex, drug regimens, and comorbidities influence the MSC population. Do some conditions presuppose for administration of allogeneic cells? For many of these questions, preclinical models will be helpful, but in the final analysis, the task of evaluating and implementing these findings for orthopaedic patients falls onto the shoulders of clinical researchers.

REFERENCES

1. Friedenstein AJ, Piatetzky S II, Petrakova KV. Osteogenesis in transplants of bone marrow cells. J Embryol Exp Morphol 1966;16:381–90.
2. Campbell WC. Delayed union and nonunion of fractures [Chapter 15]. St Louis (MO): C.V. Mosby Co; 1939. p. 648–725.
3. Mendicino M, Bailey AM, Wonnacott K, et al. MSC-based product characterization for clinical trials: an FDA perspective. Cell Stem Cell 2014;14:141–5.
4. Francois M, Copland IB, Yuan S, et al. Cryopreserved mesenchymal stromal cells display impaired immunosuppressive properties as a result of heat-shock response and impaired interferon-gamma licensing. Cytotherapy 2012;14: 147–52.
5. Caplan AI. MSCs: the sentinel and safe-guards of injury. J Cell Physiol 2016;231: 1413–6.
6. Caplan AI. All MSCs are pericytes? Cell Stem Cell 2008;3:229–30.
7. Shi S, Gronthos S. Perivascular niche of postnatal mesenchymal stem cells in human bone marrow and dental pulp. J Bone Miner Res 2003;18:696–704.
8. Covas DT, Panepucci RA, Fontes AM, et al. Multipotent mesenchymal stromal cells obtained from diverse human tissues share functional properties and gene-expression profile with CD146+ perivascular cells and fibroblasts. Exp Hematol 2008;36:642–54.
9. Dominici M, Le Blanc K, Mueller I, et al. Minimal criteria for defining multipotent mesenchymal stromal cells. The International Society for Cellular Therapy position statement. Cytotherapy 2006;8:315–7.
10. Bourin P, Bunnell BA, Casteilla L, et al. Stromal cells from the adipose tissue-derived stromal vascular fraction and culture expanded adipose tissue-derived stromal/stem cells: a joint statement of the International Federation for Adipose Therapeutics and Science (IFATS) and the International Society for Cellular Therapy (ISCT). Cytotherapy 2013;15:641–8.
11. Vangsness CT Jr, Sternberg H, Harris L. Umbilical cord tissue offers the greatest number of harvestable mesenchymal stem cells for research and clinical application: a literature review of different harvest sites. Arthroscopy 2015;31:1836–43.

12. US Food and Drug Administration. Guidance for industry and FDA staff: Minimal manipulation of structural tissue (jurisdictional update). 2016. Available at: http://www.fda.gov/regulatoryinformation/guidances/ucm126197.htm.

13. Pierini M, Di Bella C, Dozza B, et al. The posterior iliac crest outperforms the anterior iliac crest when obtaining mesenchymal stem cells from bone marrow. J Bone Joint Surg Am 2013;95:1101–7.

14. Muschler GF, Nitto H, Boehm CA, et al. Age- and gender-related changes in the cellularity of human bone marrow and the prevalence of osteoblastic progenitors. J Orthop Res 2001;19:117–25.

15. Jurgens WJ, Oedayrajsingh-Varma MJ, Helder MN, et al. Effect of tissue-harvesting site on yield of stem cells derived from adipose tissue: implications for cell-based therapies. Cell Tissue Res 2008;332:415–26.

16. Hernigou J, Picard L, Alves A, et al. Understanding bone safety zones during bone marrow aspiration from the iliac crest: the sector rule. Int Orthop 2014;38:2377–84.

17. Pittenger MF, Mackay AM, Beck SC, et al. Multilineage potential of adult human mesenchymal stem cells. Science 1999;284:143–7.

18. Cox G, Boxall SA, Giannoudis PV, et al. High abundance of CD271(+) multipotential stromal cells (MSCs) in intramedullary cavities of long bones. Bone 2012;50:510–7.

19. Cox G, McGonagle D, Boxall SA, et al. The use of the reamer-irrigator-aspirator to harvest mesenchymal stem cells. J Bone Joint Surg Br 2011;93:517–24.

20. Hernigou P, Poignard A, Beaujean F, et al. Percutaneous autologous bone-marrow grafting for nonunions. Influence of the number and concentration of progenitor cells. J Bone Joint Surg Am 2005;87:1430–7.

21. Stolzing A, Jones E, McGonagle D, et al. Age-related changes in human bone marrow-derived mesenchymal stem cells: consequences for cell therapies. Mech Ageing Dev 2008;129:163–73.

22. Baxter MA, Wynn RF, Jowitt SN, et al. Study of telomere length reveals rapid aging of human marrow stromal cells following in vitro expansion. Stem Cells 2004;22:675–82.

23. Zhou S, Greenberger JS, Epperly MW, et al. Age-related intrinsic changes in human bone-marrow-derived mesenchymal stem cells and their differentiation to osteoblasts. Aging Cell 2008;7:335–43.

24. Beane OS, Fonseca VC, Cooper LL, et al. Impact of aging on the regenerative properties of bone marrow-, muscle-, and adipose-derived mesenchymal stem/stromal cells. PLoS One 2014;9:e115963.

25. Lacasa D, Garcia E, Henriot D, et al. Site-related specificities of the control by androgenic status of adipogenesis and mitogen-activated protein kinase cascade/c-fos signaling pathways in rat preadipocytes. Endocrinology 1997;138:3181–6.

26. Hernigou P, Beaujean F. Treatment of osteonecrosis with autologous bone marrow grafting. Clin Orthop Relat Res 2002;(405):14–23.

27. Prockop DJ, Oh JY. Mesenchymal stem/stromal cells (MSCs): role as guardians of inflammation. Mol Ther 2012;20:14–20.

28. Caplan AI, Sorrell JM. The MSC curtain that stops the immune system. Immunol Lett 2015;168:136–9.

29. Liang J, Zhang H, Hua B, et al. Allogenic mesenchymal stem cells transplantation in refractory systemic lupus erythematosus: a pilot clinical study. Ann Rheum Dis 2010;69:1423–9.

30. Karussis D, Karageorgiou C, Vaknin-Dembinsky A, et al. Safety and immunological effects of mesenchymal stem cell transplantation in patients with multiple sclerosis and amyotrophic lateral sclerosis. Arch Neurol 2010;67:1187–94.
31. Keyszer G, Christopeit M, Fick S, et al. Treatment of severe progressive systemic sclerosis with transplantation of mesenchymal stromal cells from allogeneic related donors: report of five cases. Arthritis Rheum 2011;63:2540–2.
32. Prasad VK, Lucas KG, Kleiner GI, et al. Efficacy and safety of ex vivo cultured adult human mesenchymal stem cells (Prochymal) in pediatric patients with severe refractory acute graft-versus-host disease in a compassionate use study. Biol Blood Marrow Transplant 2011;17:534–41.
33. Aggarwal S, Pittenger MF. Human mesenchymal stem cells modulate allogeneic immune cell responses. Blood 2005;105:1815–22.
34. Di Nicola M, Carlo-Stella C, Magni M, et al. Human bone marrow stromal cells suppress T-lymphocyte proliferation induced by cellular or nonspecific mitogenic stimuli. Blood 2002;99:3838–43.
35. Rasmusson I, Ringden O, Sundberg B, et al. Mesenchymal stem cells inhibit the formation of cytotoxic T lymphocytes, but not activated cytotoxic T lymphocytes or natural killer cells. Transplantation 2003;76:1208–13.
36. Akiyama K, Chen C, Wang D, et al. Mesenchymal-stem-cell-induced immunoregulation involves FAS-ligand-/FAS-mediated T cell apoptosis. Cell Stem Cell 2012;10:544–55.
37. Sattler C, Steinsdoerfer M, Offers M, et al. Inhibition of T-cell proliferation by murine multipotent mesenchymal stromal cells is mediated by CD39 expression and adenosine generation. Cell Transplant 2011;20:1221–30.
38. Lee JJ, Jeong HJ, Kim MK, et al. CD39-mediated effect of human bone marrow-derived mesenchymal stem cells on the human Th17 cell function. Purinergic Signal 2014;10:357–65.
39. Adair TH. Growth regulation of the vascular system: an emerging role for adenosine. Am J Physiol Regul Integr Comp Physiol 2005;289:R283–96.
40. Melief SM, Geutskens SB, Fibbe WE, et al. Multipotent stromal cells skew monocytes towards an anti-inflammatory interleukin-10-producing phenotype by production of interleukin-6. Haematologica 2013;98:888–95.
41. Le Blanc K, Tammik C, Rosendahl K, et al. HLA expression and immunologic properties of differentiated and undifferentiated mesenchymal stem cells. Exp Hematol 2003;31:890–6.
42. Technau A, Froelich K, Hagen R, et al. Adipose tissue-derived stem cells show both immunogenic and immunosuppressive properties after chondrogenic differentiation. Cytotherapy 2011;13:310–7.
43. Ryan AE, Lohan P, O'Flynn L, et al. Chondrogenic differentiation increases antidonor immune response to allogeneic mesenchymal stem cell transplantation. Mol Ther 2014;22:655–67.
44. Chen X, McClurg A, Zhou GQ, et al. Chondrogenic differentiation alters the immunosuppressive property of bone marrow-derived mesenchymal stem cells, and the effect is partially due to the upregulated expression of B7 molecules. Stem Cells 2007;25:364–70.
45. Liu H, Kemeny DM, Heng BC, et al. The immunogenicity and immunomodulatory function of osteogenic cells differentiated from mesenchymal stem cells. J Immunol 2006;176:2864–71.
46. Kotobuki N, Katsube Y, Katou Y, et al. In vivo survival and osteogenic differentiation of allogeneic rat bone marrow mesenchymal stem cells (MSCs). Cell Transplant 2008;17:705–12.

47. Chatterjea A, LaPointe VL, Alblas J, et al. Suppression of the immune system as a critical step for bone formation from allogeneic osteoprogenitors implanted in rats. J Cell Mol Med 2014;18:134–42.

48. Lohan P, Coleman CM, Murphy JM, et al. Changes in immunological profile of allogeneic mesenchymal stem cells after differentiation: should we be concerned? Stem Cell Res Ther 2014;5:99.

49. Srinivas M, Aarntzen EH, Bulte JW, et al. Imaging of cellular therapies. Adv Drug Deliv Rev 2010;62:1080–93.

50. Ahn JI, Terry Canale S, Butler SD, et al. Stem cell repair of physeal cartilage. J Orthop Res 2004;22:1215–21.

51. Hernigou P, Trousselier M, Roubineau F, et al. Stem cell therapy for the treatment of hip osteonecrosis: a 30-year review of progress. Clin Orthop Surg 2016;8:1–8.

52. Hernigou P, Daltro G, Filippini P, et al. Percutaneous implantation of autologous bone marrow osteoprogenitor cells as treatment of bone avascular necrosis related to sickle cell disease. Open Orthop J 2008;2:62–5.

53. Kawate K, Yajima H, Ohgushi H, et al. Tissue-engineered approach for the treatment of steroid-induced osteonecrosis of the femoral head: transplantation of autologous mesenchymal stem cells cultured with beta-tricalcium phosphate ceramics and free vascularized fibula. Artif Organs 2006;30:960–2.

54. Goodman SB, Hwang KL. Treatment of secondary osteonecrosis of the knee with local debridement and osteoprogenitor cell grafting. J Arthroplasty 2015;30:1892–6.

55. Hernigou P, Flouzat-Lachaniette CH, Delambre J, et al. Osteonecrosis repair with bone marrow cell therapies: state of the clinical art. Bone 2015;70:102–9.

56. Homma Y, Kaneko K, Hernigou P. Supercharging allografts with mesenchymal stem cells in the operating room during hip revision. Int Orthop 2014;38:2033–44.

57. Steadman JR, Briggs KK, Rodrigo JJ, et al. Outcomes of microfracture for traumatic chondral defects of the knee: average 11-year follow-up. Arthroscopy 2003;19:477–84.

58. Hannon CP, Murawski CD, Fansa AM, et al. Microfracture for osteochondral lesions of the talus: a systematic review of reporting of outcome data. Am J Sports Med 2013;41:689–95.

59. Somoza RA, Welter JF, Correa D, et al. Chondrogenic differentiation of mesenchymal stem cells: challenges and unfulfilled expectations. Tissue Eng Part B Rev 2014;20:596–608.

60. Mithoefer K, Saris DB, Farr J, et al. Guidelines for the design and conduct of clinical studies in knee articular cartilage repair: international cartilage repair society recommendations based on current scientific evidence and standards of clinical care. Cartilage 2011;2:100–21.

61. Wong KL, Lee KB, Tai BC, et al. Injectable cultured bone marrow-derived mesenchymal stem cells in varus knees with cartilage defects undergoing high tibial osteotomy: a prospective, randomized controlled clinical trial with 2 years' follow-up. Arthroscopy 2013;29:2020–8.

62. Jo CH, Lee YG, Shin WH, et al. Intra-articular injection of mesenchymal stem cells for the treatment of osteoarthritis of the knee: a proof-of-concept clinical trial. Stem Cells 2014;32:1254–66.

63. Nejadnik H, Hui JH, Feng Choong EP, et al. Autologous bone marrow-derived mesenchymal stem cells versus autologous chondrocyte implantation: an observational cohort study. Am J Sports Med 2010;38:1110–6.

64. Ortiz LA, Dutreil M, Fattman C, et al. Interleukin 1 receptor antagonist mediates the antiinflammatory and antifibrotic effect of mesenchymal stem cells during lung injury. Proc Natl Acad Sci U S A 2007;104:11002–7.
65. Yagi H, Soto-Gutierrez A, Navarro-Alvarez N, et al. Reactive bone marrow stromal cells attenuate systemic inflammation via sTNFR1. Mol Ther 2010;18:1857–64.
66. Lee RH, Pulin AA, Seo MJ, et al. Intravenous hMSCs improve myocardial infarction in mice because cells embolized in lung are activated to secrete the anti-inflammatory protein TSG-6. Cell Stem Cell 2009;5:54–63.
67. Roddy GW, Oh JY, Lee RH, et al. Action at a distance: systemically administered adult stem/progenitor cells (MSCs) reduce inflammatory damage to the cornea without engraftment and primarily by secretion of TNF-alpha stimulated gene/protein 6. Stem Cells 2011;29:1572–9.
68. Choi H, Lee RH, Bazhanov N, et al. Anti-inflammatory protein TSG-6 secreted by activated MSCs attenuates zymosan-induced mouse peritonitis by decreasing TLR2/NF-kappaB signaling in resident macrophages. Blood 2011;118:330–8.
69. Nemeth K, Leelahavanichkul A, Yuen PS, et al. Bone marrow stromal cells attenuate sepsis via prostaglandin E(2)-dependent reprogramming of host macrophages to increase their interleukin-10 production. Nat Med 2009;15:42–9.
70. Kim J, Hematti P. Mesenchymal stem cell-educated macrophages: a novel type of alternatively activated macrophages. Exp Hematol 2009;37:1445–53.

Biocellular Regenerative Medicine

Use of Adipose-Derived Stem/Stromal Cells and It's Native Bioactive Matrix

Robert W. Alexander, MD, DMD, FICS

KEYWORDS

• Stem cells • Stromal cells • PRP • Regenerative medicine • Nanofat
• Mesenchymal cells • Fat grafts • SVF

KEY POINTS

• Autologous Stem/Stromal Cells and Platelet Concentrates Guided to Targets.
• Combination of Cells & PRP concentrates work better than either alone.
• Biocellular Combination Is Believed To Facilitate Patient's Own Wound Healing/ Regeneration.

EVOLUTION OF CELL-BASED THERAPIES

Over the past decade, great strides have been made in the understanding and potential of targeted cell-based therapies. Starting decades ago, use of an irritant solution to stimulate inflammatory reactions has been replaced in the past few years with transition to injecting various platelet-rich plasma (PRP) concentrates for supporting an effective inflammatory reaction at damaged or degenerative sites. Use of the contained growth factors and signal proteins became recognized as offering a significant improvement in tissue healing responses but seemed limited by incomplete repair while requiring a series (often 4–6) to achieve long-term clinical improvement. Current evolution of combining these trophic growth factors and signal proteins with concentrated undifferentiated cellular/stromal populations seemed like a logical and effective modality, moving into the forefront since 2000. Aesthetic and reconstructive applications led the way, because constant challenges of injury, loss of circulatory capabilities, degenerative, repair, and so forth demanded an optimal approach to regenerative needs. In-depth examination of how the body maintains itself revealed that undesignated cells were integrally important to replacing aging cells (such as

There are no conflicts of interest reported in this article or its content.
Department of Surgery, University of Washington, Institute of Regenerative Medicine, 715 Main Street, Suite B, Stevensville, MT 59870, USA
E-mail address: rwamd@cybernet1.com

Phys Med Rehabil Clin N Am 27 (2016) 871–891
http://dx.doi.org/10.1016/j.pmr.2016.06.005
1047-9651/16/© 2016 Published by Elsevier Inc.

skin, hair, bowel lining, and so forth). Early on, fat was not thought of as undergoing such homeostatic mechanisms, because typical mitotic activities were not observed. Now it is recognized that rather than a static number of cells varying only in size, mature adipocytes actually undergo total replacement at a rate of 10% to 20% per year but do so in a different form of cell division known as asymmetric cell division. The ability to have resident precursor cells that are capable of responding to local site signals and the ability of providing a replacement cell of the needed type result in potential replacement cell differentiation, while retaining a single precursor cell type. Without that mechanism eventually there would be an uncontrollable stem/stromal cell population.[1]

With the advent of Food and Drug Administration (FDA)–approved tabletop devices for high platelet concentrations via a closed system, use of a simple blood draw yielded more than 4 to 6 times a patient's own circulating baselines levels. It has been well shown that the higher the achieved concentrations, the proportionally higher delivery of important factors intrinsically involved in all wound healing and repair.

It has become clear that certain tissue characteristics are most favorable for use in cell-based therapies, including easy and safe access and plentiful autologous stores of a group of cells possessing multipotent potential. Multipotency is important in that such cells have the capability of responding to local signals and possess the ability to transform or replenish signals needed at damaged or diseased sites for repair or regeneration.

Research has confirmed that a vast majority of such undesignated cells are associated and stored in proximity to the microvascular capillary system (**Fig. 1**). Essentially all tissues (with blood supply) have some of these multipotent cells available to deal with local and isolated demands. The body retains the ability to chemotactically attract and mobilize cells from local and remote storage points in response to chemical and physical signaling in the body. Approximately 15 years ago, an important scientific advance was made by researchers in finding that adipose tissue (fat) contained high numbers of such cells.[2,3] This is not totally surprising considering that fat also represents the largest microvascular organ in the body.

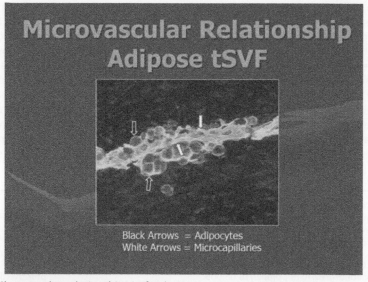

Fig. 1. Microvascular relationships in fetal pig.

Enhancement of cellular and biological therapies comes directly with the ability for providers to be able to identify, target, and guide the cellular-biological combination to areas of injury or degeneration. In that regard, ultrasonography has become a major feature of clinical responses and success. As an example, in medium and deep targets, or those difficult to access, guided musculoskeletal (MSK) ultrasound capabilities offer the optimal integral part of successful responses. Over the past decade, thousands of treatments using biocellular regenerative medicine techniques have proved safe and remarkably effective. The information provided in this article is intended as an introduction to important concepts and describes the current logic believed involved. Major steps have been taken, moving from the laboratory to the bedside. Today, MSK and aesthetic–plastic surgical patients are routinely treated with this combination of biocellular elements.[4–6]

WHAT IS BIOCELLULAR MEDICINE?

The term, *biocellular*, refers to the combination of important biological chemicals (such as growth factors, signal proteins, and chemicals important to wound healing) with undesignated cells (often referred to as adult stem/stromal cells) found widely spread within the body and which participate in tissue maintenance, repair, and regeneration. Science and medicine have recently entered a translational phase, where proved laboratory science has demonstrated important contributions join the clinical application of the science in human applications in the past decade. There has been controversy concerning the use of the term, *stem cells*, in current practice of medicine. Unfortunately, these arguments typically occur with the use of stem cell interpreted as uses of pure embryonic or fetal stem cells, implying destruction of embryo or fetal tissues. In the past decade, the recognition of the safety and efficacy of using a person's own (autologous) adult stem/stromal cells has advanced to the point that it is widely documented and published (**Box 1**).

Cellular Components

Biocellular regenerative medicine within the United States currently refers to use of autologous, adult (nonembryonic) multipotent cells capable of participating in maintaining tissues (homeostasis), healing, and regeneration. Since 2006, the number of scientific studies demonstrating the values of the highly variable stromal cell populations has exploded, to the point that active reports and studies of component cells of adipose origin exceed the study of nonhematopoietic stromal cells in bone marrow in MSK and aesthetic–plastic surgical applications. The importance of such studies, and

---

Box 1
Basic goals in biocellular regenerative medicine

- Return to full form or function
- Eliminate or markedly decrease pain
- Resist recurrence of injury
- Reverse, stabilize, resist degeneration
- Use autologous tissues for repair
- Restore tissues with minimal scar
- Accelerate healing processes

an understanding that adipose tissue deposits have gained such recognition due to the greater numbers of stem/stromal cells (other than blood forming element) in the body, is coupled with the important overlap of potential cellular functions. Essentially every tissue in the body that contains microvascular supply maintains a reservoir of such cells. That said, it is recognized that adipose tissues possess the greatest microvascular organ in the body. Many peer-reviewed scientific reports suggest that adipose-derived (AD) stem/stromal cells of mesodermal origin provide between 1000 and 2500 times the actual numbers found in bone marrow.[7] With the easy collection of adipose tissue, less penetration, widely heterogeneous cellular populations, and important immune-privileged properties, subdermal fat deposits serve as a primary source for gathering stem/stromal cells (**Box 2**, **Fig. 2**).

The small nucleated cells found closely associated within the vascular tissues are recognized as serving important roles in maintaining normal tissue content (homeostasis) plus having the ability to respond to injury or disease processes in a constant effort to heal or repair damaged cells (as in aging, arthritis, MSK tissues, neurologic disorders, and so forth). The remarkable design of the human body uses these reservoirs of available, nondifferentiated multipotent cells as the tissue first responders in the situations of major trauma, microtrauma, and aging. By secretion of certain chemicals from an injured site, these multipotent cells (ie, can become various types of cells) can be called on to participate in the repairs needed to restore tissues and functions. There are many peer-reviewed publications that provide examples of how the cells involved in this process can be enhanced by combined provision of the cellular, native scaffolding, and biologically active components (**Box 3**).

Biological Components

The biological components in this context refer specifically to the availability of a diverse and important variety of growth factors and signal proteins that interact with the cells of degenerative or damaged sites to help recruit needed reparative cells and materials to repair the area. There are 2 major biological components in common use. One is found within recognized contents of platelets, which store and release a wide variety of needed growth factors and proteins to act on available cells to begin the wound healing processes.[8] For many years, the only important role of platelets was believed to become "sticky," that is, adhere to each other and participate in clotting mechanisms. It is now realized that this may be their least important contribution to wounds and wound healing (with exception of providing a fibrin clot to permit gradual release of platelet contents). Platelets represent a storehouse of small granules, each containing important growth factors and signal proteins that serve to

---

Box 2
Optimal cellular source features

- Ease to get
- High quantity of cells
- Minimum morbidity of donor site
- Safety after implantation (own cells)
- Multipotent and proliferative cell groups
- Secrete immunomodulatory factors
- Immunoprivileged cells preferred

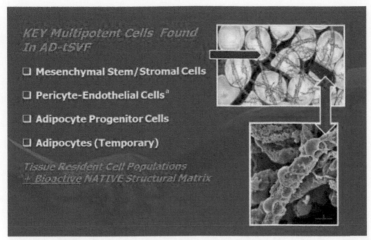

Fig. 2. Locations and components of AD-tSVF. [a] Pericyte & Endothelial Cells may be the origin of all MSCs. Microvasculature (*red arrows*); Highlights pericyte cell attachments (*blue arrows*).

quarterback the healing cascade and do this for a prolonged time during the healing phases. For example, an important chemical available from these granules is essential for blood vessel replacement and repair to improve the circulation ability critical to healing of all wounds. Without adequate blood flow, needed oxygen can neither reach the area of damage nor permit migration of a variety of cells from nearby or distant cell sites (**Figs. 3** and **4**).

The second source of biological contributors is found in bone marrow aspirates. Bone marrow has been used for many decades, and it is common use in blood-related disorders. Bone marrow does demonstrate microvasculature and therefore does have some undesignated cells (stem/stromal cells). They are, however, in very low numbers compared with adipose tissues. Therefore, many regenerative practitioners consider bone marrow as primarily a valuable biologic and platelet source. To become a valuable cell contributor, it is required that bone marrow aspirates be isolated, concentrated, and culture-expanded to achieve meaningful numbers needed in regenerative and healing applications. This source is technically more invasive to obtain, poses higher complication-sequelae rates, and is significantly more expensive to the patients. In addition to the undesignated stem/stromal cells, content considered of value (such as mesenchymal, periadventitial, and endothelial) is more scarce

---

Box 3
Ideal cell-based therapy

- Use your own cells (autologous)
- Safe and easy harvest via closed system
- Optimal to include native matrix
- Transplant in same surgical session
- Predictable and reproducible outcomes
- Optional ability to use parenteral uses for systemic disorders
- Require minimal manipulation (offer optional culture/expansion)

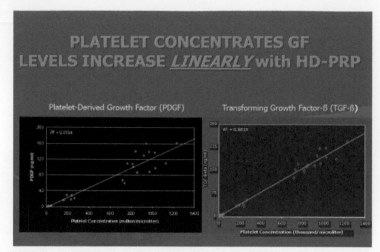

Fig. 3. Platelet concentrations of growth factors linear increase.

compared with millions of resident hematopoietic cells. The primary difference between concentrated platelets from peripheral blood versus marrow concentrates is a large store of hematopoietic stem cells (HSCs) while offering an almost identical platelet content. At this time there is little evidence of significant contribution to the platelet regeneration process of MSK tissues derived from the HSC group.

Concentrates primary importance and value is the ability to provide important growth factors and cytokines/chemokines to optimize earlier healing conditions and abilities. Of even more importance in the cellular therapeutic-based effects seems to be their important paracrine secretory influences rather than contributions of individual cellular components and physical engraftment. Furthermore, it well established

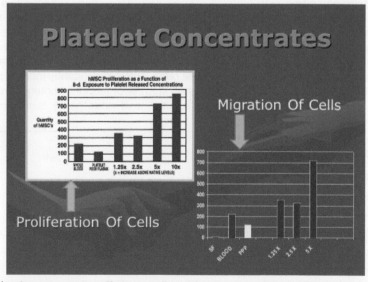

Fig. 4. Platelet concentrate effects on cell proliferation/migration. hMSC, human mesenencymal cells; PPP, platelet poor plasma.

that the mesenchymal group (MSC) of multipotent cells may originate from the pericyte-endothelial cell groups.[9] Stromal cellular elements offer a great amount of overlapping capabilities in vitro, suggesting that all tissues having some microvasculature and have resident stem/stromal elements capable of providing first responders to sites of damage or degenerative effects. It is suggested that the MSC groups overlap at greater than 95% in their capabilities. Host site interaction with these cells, growth factors, and signal proteins seem to create a complex, heterogeneous precursor population that is considered site specific in many of their responses.[10]

HOW DID BIOLOGIC AND CELLULAR THERAPEUTIC CONCEPTS EVOLVE?

Aesthetic and plastic surgeons traditionally have dealt with wound healing and scarring issues for many years. During that time, careful study of the processes of homeostasis, remodeling, and repair led to a better understanding of how the body tissues manage to maintain themselves. For many years, the importance of biologics as a derivative part of platelets become appreciated not only for clotting functions but also for the gradual release of critical chemical components essential to the healing processes with individual sites. These biocellular concentrates are thought to immediately begin to participate in secretions capable of site specific repair and regeneration, while local cells begin to actively contribute. In addition to these elements, appreciation of the importance of the native adipose (3-D) scaffolding (matrix) in provision of essential contact points, which serve to encourage microenvironment changes, including cellular proliferation and chemotactic migration, has come to the forefront.[11–13] Site specificity greatly influences cellular changes within the nondesignated, heterogeneous multipotent populations found in essentially all tissues that have microvasculature. In addition, appreciation of the importance of cellular secretions (paracrine and autocrine) within these undifferentiated cell groups has been reported to be as great, or greater in some instances, as the multipotent cellular differentiation effects.[14]

Once the complex processes of repair and regeneration were examined closely, it became apparent that determination of specific interactions of any single cell or chemical is not able to be determined. At this time, the ability to create an in vitro situation that can clinically duplicate the in vivo microenvironment, making selection of optimal components impossible.

Key adult multipotent cells are found in essentially every tissue and organ in the body. Determination that some of the highest concentrations of these adult stem/stromal cell populations were found within adipose tissue complex (ATC) has led to a major trend shift to more closely evaluate the activities of such tissues and how they can be easily and safely acquired and concentrated for uses in wound healing and repair. Early on, because adipocytes within the ATC were not thought to cell divide, it was assumed that these were static in number and only changed in size according to lipid storage droplets. At this point, it is clear that adipocytes do have a life cycle, replacing all mature adipocytes every 5 to 10 years.[15] Examination of how they accomplish this replacement, via a process of asymmetric cell division, was found that the precursor cell population reacting to secretions from a senescent adipocyte. This replication by cell division results in a replacement immature adipocyte, whereas the other portion retains its precursor form and abilities. This is logical, in that if otherwise, a massive number of precursor cells would accumulate in the tissues (Box 4, Fig. 5).

Zuk and colleagues[16] identified the multipotent capabilities of AD–tissue stromal vascular fraction (tSVF), with capabilities of differentiation to a variety of tissues, including bone, cartilage, tendon-ligament, muscle, fat, nerve, and so forth (Fig. 6).

> **Box 4**
> **Tissue stromal vascular fraction: adult stem/stromal cell elements**
>
> *Stromal vascular fraction AD-tSVF — very heterogeneous*
>
> - Mesenchymal stem cells (a key cell group)
> - Pericytes/endothelial cells and adventitial cells
> - Preadipocytes (adipose progenitors)
> - Fibroblasts
> - Macrophages
> - Vascular smooth muscle cells
> - Miscellaneous native blood derived cells
> - Extensive bioactive-secreting ECM

Once this capability was identified, efforts to isolate specific cell types started. This has proved difficult in that it is currently impossible to imitate the in vivo microenvironment in the laboratory. Over the past decade, exploration of concentrating the identified ATC undifferentiated cell population coupled with high-density (HD) platelet concentrates (HD-PRP) has received a great deal of attention. Identifying stem/stromal cells that can participate in the processes has revealed what an ideal cell-based therapy may represent (see **Box 4**).

In the early 1990s, a method of closed syringe lipoaspiration was patented, permitting a less traumatic and efficient means of acquiring ATC for use as a structural graft.[17] This has evolved to a disposable, microcannula option that permits safe and efficacious low-pressure acquisition of AD-tSVF. In the past 15 years, clinicians and laboratory researchers have identified several important cell types, which interact to provide remarkable contributions in tissue repair and regeneration. These have

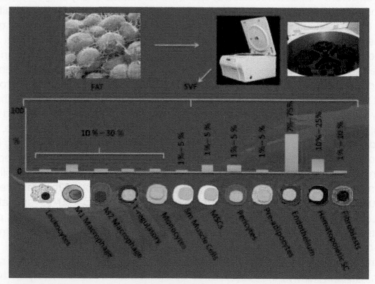

Fig. 5. Range of cellular components in AD-tSVF.

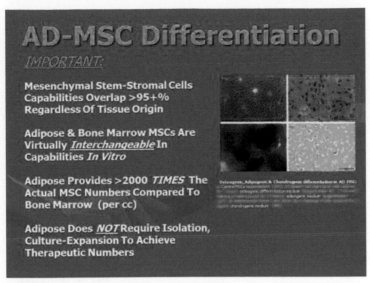

Fig. 6. Examples of tissue differentiation from AD-cSVF.

been identified as a complex and heterogeneous population, closely related to cellular, adventitial areas and extracellular matrix contacts. At first, mesenchymal cell group (MSC or AD stem cell) was thought the most important multipotent stem cell. Further examination, however, suggests that it may serve a sentry capacity and that the actual cell group is known as pericyte/endothelial stem/stromal cells[18] (**Box 5, Figs. 7** and **8**).

There is confusion in interpretation of the scientific and clinical published materials caused by a lack of explanation of the difference between tSVF and cellular stromal vascular fraction (cSVF) (**Box 6**). For clarification, cSVF is the isolated cellular elements in the ATC created via use of certain collagenase-enzyme blends to separate the attachment comprising the cell-to-cell or cell-to-matrix connections. The use of such cSVF is the subject of multiple clinical trial applications (see clinicaltrial.gov) and is heavily used in cell isolation, culture expansion, and cell characterization studies. This creates an information gap between clinical applications and those strictly of research value. If clinicians read only the peer-reviewed clinical journals,

---

Box 5
Advantages of closed syringe microcannula use

- Disposable system (prevents contamination)
- Reasonably priced, many optional openings
- Maintains closed harvest and uses
- Ability to reduce vacuum pressures
- Cell-friendly surfaces protect tissues
- SuperLuerLok (Tulip Medical, San Diego CA) provides optimal vacuum
- Easily permits additives (HD-PRP or bone marrow aspirate)
- Has decades of clinical experiences that prove safety and efficacy

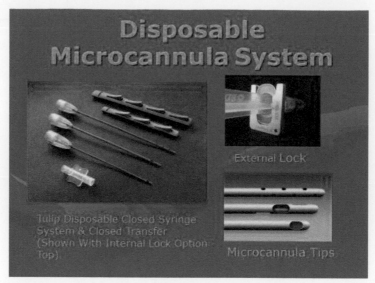

Fig. 7. GEMs (Tulip), microcannula closed aspiration syringe system.

they miss up to 85% of the pertinent information and data evolving on almost a daily basis, because the important advances appear in basic scientific and engineering publications.

In clinical applications, use of AD-tSVF has taken the primary role in aesthetic and regenerative uses, because it is a product that provides the full complement of structural (stroma and extracellular matrix [ECM]) elements plus the resident cellular population of the AD-cSVF. The existing native stroma of ATC is considered of great importance due not only to the available attachment sites but also to the actual secretory bioactivity of the tissue. This dual role is considered of importance, making use of existing native scaffolding of ATC to positively contribute to the local recipient sites in need.

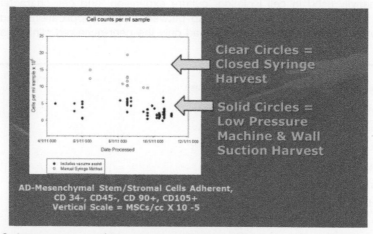

Fig. 8. Syringe versus machine pump aspiration. (*Courtesy of* R. Mandle, PhD and R. Alexander, MD, Harvard BSR Lab 2011, Cambridge, MA.)

Box 6
Understanding terms: tissue stromal vascular fraction and cellular stromal vascular fraction

Tissue stromal vascular fraction (tSVF)

- Includes all cellular components of tissue
- Includes all biologic components
- Includes native bioactive matrix (secretive)
- Requires no manipulation

Cellular stromal vascular fraction (cSVF)

- Requires digestion, incubation, isolation
- Common uses reported in research settings
- Does not have native matrix component
- Often used as cell-enrichment protocols

In biological aspects, it is important to recognize that not all PRP preparations and concentrates are the same. The amount of growth factors, signal proteins, and important chemical agents has a direct linear relationship to the concentration of platelets actually achieved. It is confusing to follow the variety of processes used in creating what is called PRP, particularly because most practitioners do not have the capability of confirming actual patient measured baselines to compare with achieved concentrations. To qualify as a true HD- PRP, the minimal concentrations used are 4 to 6 times an actual measured baseline, not a calculated extrapolation. This is important based on the correlation of such concentration to cellular proliferation and migration capabilities (see **Fig. 4**).

Use of centrifugation has increased in biocellular applications, because it creates an effective gravity density separation, which avoids cellular debris, unwanted fluids and local anesthetics, and isolation of the unwanted free lipid layer from the upper portions of the lipoaspirate. In addition, it permits decrease of the interstitial fluid load, a factor requiring overcorrection of grafts or small joint placements. This unneeded load is thought to potentially have an impact on site perfusion, a factor of importance in many plastic surgical reconstructive wounds and MSK applications.[19,20]

The final area of importance in MSK applications relates to the ability of optimal targeting of areas of damage, degeneration, or inflammation. Without use of high-definition ultrasonography, it is virtually impossible to assure accurate placement of the biocellular therapeutic modality. With the use of ultrasonography, coupled with compressed and thoroughly mixed biocellular components, patients respond more rapidly, show metrics of responses, and achieve earlier final outcome than when placed via palpation only.[21]

Within the past 2 years, an option of removing the unwanted mature adipocytes from the AD-tSVF has become available. It is well documented that the large, mature adipocytes do not contribute significant value to an injection site (including when performing structural fat grafting in aesthetic surgery) because they are gradually lost and removed after their anoxic exposure. It is likewise clear that the stem/stromal cells in the ATC are not as susceptible to those conditions and may be stimulated in low oxygen tension environments. Recent publication of viability and numbers of stem/stromal cells remaining after emulsification process confirms that the relative numbers of such cells remain statistically the same as those not submitted for emulsification.

One of the advantages of this process is that the AD-tSVF not only retains valuable stromal tissue but also the entire specimen (mixed with HD-PRP) can be easily injected through small-bore needles (25–30 gauge). This facilitates uses in scars, radiated damage skin, and hair loss plus permits more patient comfort in MSK injections (including small joint targets).[22]

In regenerative medicine, the main goals are well established (see **Box 1**). Likewise, description of optimal features of cellular-based therapy in both aesthetic and regenerative applications is becoming standardized. The combination of platelet concentrates and AD-tSVF seems more effective than either of the entities by themselves.

"WORKERS AND BRICKS" ANALOGY

A simple analogy is helpful in understanding the importance of both the biological and the cellular elements to achieve more rapid and complete healing and repair.

If a brick wall is beginning to break down, some of the mortar holding the bricks together is lost or crumbling. What is needed to repair the wall is hiring workers to come in, clean up the site, and repair and replace the damaged mortar. Once completed, the wall is repaired and functions as originally intended. These workers are found in great quantities in platelet concentrates and comprise the biological contribution of the biocellular regenerative treatments.

Imagine, however, that the wall not only is losing mortar holding the bricks in place but also many of the bricks in the wall are lost or broken. This would require not only the workers but also bricks to replace the lost and damaged ones. The bricks in this analogy come from the cellular source. Combining biologics and cell source has proved more successful than use of either of the agents by themselves (**Box 7**).

It is well established that there are many more of these undifferentiated cells located in the largest microvascular organ of the body, within the adipose (fat) matrix. Therefore, the readily available and safely accessible cellular contributor of choice has become adipose tissue retrieved from subdermal fat deposits in the abdomen and thigh areas. These are gently removed via closed syringe lipoaspiration, compressed by centrifugation, and mixed the platelet concentrates (>4–6 times patient circulating platelets) to form the therapeutic mixture known as biocellular regenerative matrix.

This mixture is in current use in aesthetic (plastic), reconstructive, sports, and pain medicine, orthopedic medicine and surgery, neurologic disorders, MSK and arthritic applications, and a wide area of overlapping disorders.

WHAT ARE ADIPOSE-DERIVED ADULT STEM/STROMAL CELLS?

AD adult stem/stromal cells are a diverse group of nondesignated cells found throughout the tissues of the body. They serve as a reservoir of replacement and repair cells, which react to injury, aging, or disease. Adult cells in this category are often referred to as stem/stromal cells or stromal cells and should be clearly separated from embryonic cells. They are also called progenitor or precursor cells, which means

---

Box 7
"Workers and bricks" analogy

It is important to note that use of combined cellular and biologic elements work better than either cellular or biologic alone.

they have the capability to differentiate into different types of cells via responses to growth factors and signal proteins within the microenvironment where they are located. For example, with a muscle or ligament tear, local and the nondifferentiated cells are thought to participate in healing or repairing the damage providing replacement muscle or ligament tissues rather than resulting in scarified tissue. Scar tissue is not as functional or tolerant of future stresses and is not the ideal goal in wound healing. By providing the needed elements to such a site, the body is given the opportunity to fully repair damaged areas, often by cellular and biological events (**Figs. 9** and **10**).[16,23,24]

There are many experiences of such cases over the past 10 years in MSK area and for more than 25 years in aesthetic surgical practice. These are often reported in small case series or case reports of treatment and outcome and are being further studied in many clinical trials.[25,26] Evolving clinical trials include not only guided placement of stem/stromal elements and biological agents in orthopedic medicine and surgery but also intravenous and central nervous system placement in a variety of complex disorders that do not respond to conventional therapy (such as diabetes, multiple sclerosis, Alzheimer disease, Parkinson disease, severe limb ischemia, traumatic brain injuries, and so forth). Early reports of improvement in chronic conditions, including pain, arthritis, damaged tendons/ligaments, and so forth, are driving many to select this option to improve surgical outcomes or avoid surgical interventions and shorten the demands for physical therapy.

Many clinicians and researchers remained confused about the potentials or best source of stem cells, often believing only refers to use of embryonic tissues. In the past 10 to 15 years, evidence has led to understanding that the body's own fat may be a more plentiful and optimal cell source, avoiding the need to destroy fetal or embryonic tissues or undergo more invasive marrow access to acquire cells and culture-expand them to achieve optimal potential.

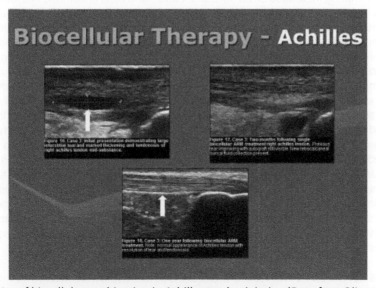

Fig. 9. Use of biocellular combination in Achilles tendon injuries. (*Data from* Oliver K, Alexander RW. Combination of autologous adipose-derived tissue stromal vascular fraction plus high-density platelet-rich plasma or bone marrow concentrates in achilles tendon tears. Journal of Prolotherapy 2013;5;e895–912)

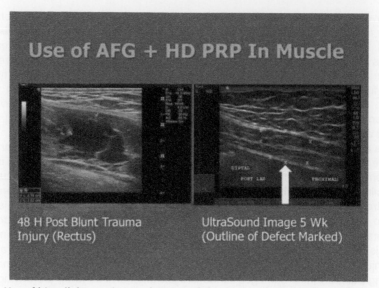

Fig. 10. Use of biocellular use in muscle tears, abdominal wall. Note: Minimal Scar Evidence Residual.

Considering the ready availability of fat, minimally invasive access (using closed syringe liposuction, for example) adipose has become an optimal source for these cells with a high safety profile for patients. As previously described, ATC is the largest microvascular organ in the body and, as such, has become well recognized as the largest depository of undifferentiated stem/stromal cells in the entire body. The ease of gathering fat tissues on an outpatient basis and local anesthetic has led to evolution of biocellular therapy (sometimes called cell-based therapy) for a wide variety of disorders and conditions. It is most common for these procedures to be performed in outpatient ambulatory surgical centers or dedicated clinic procedural facilities.

Specific key cells needed to promote healing and repair reside in tissue microenvironments, where they comprise parts of tissues and organ systems remain elusive. The complex components within the AD-tSVF may be considered to offer a smorgasbord of elements that can become available to any site or tissue. Analyses of growth factors and signal chemicals suggests that the intact AD-tSVF may offer contributions over and above those as isolated elements.[8] The cell groups participating in the healing or repair are subject to important contributions of native cell components in vascularized tissues and, by introduction of concentrates of cells and biologics, seem to autoenhance the site controls and effects. These native site cell groups are also called niches and are the locations where injury or disease must be addressed to permit the body to repair or regenerate itself. It is believed that when that process is under way, addition of needed cell types and biological elements specifically targeted (via ultrasound guidance for example) can effectively use the body's own tissues to heal themselves in a more efficient and effective manner.

WHAT IS INVOLVED IN PROVIDING BIOCELLULAR REGENERATIVE THERAPY?

Because the platelets are appreciated as key contributors in provision of critical healing growth factors and signal proteins, the author recommends striving for greater concentrations achieved translates directly with linear increases of those elements.

Acting as a central component in the inflammatory and healing cascade, they help begin and maintain the healing processes in conjunction with the local site stroma and cells. This effect is recognized as an autoamplification effect, wherein the site specific needs are boosted in response during the most important regenerative or healing processes. Factors such as vascular-endothelial growth factor contribute to this process with encouragement of microvessel formation and improved perfusion. Thousands of patients have undergone treatments using these concentrates with quality results in many inflammatory or aging conditions.

Next, the autologous cellular sample is harvested from subdermal fat deposits under sterile protocols, using the patented closed syringe system for minimal tissue disruption. This is often referred to as microcannula lipoaspiration or lipoharvesting.[27] ATC may be cleaned and compressed (centrifuged) and unwanted liquid layers separated by centrifugation (**Box 8**). This process not only helps with removal of unwanted liquids but also compresses the adipose cellular components to provide a more effective cell and bioactive matrix with less intercellular fluid load (**Fig. 11**). By effectively reducing the volume of injection materials, earlier recovery of comfort and ambulation is common. Biologics, such as HD-PRP, are then added via closed, sterile luer-to-luer transfer to create a mixture of cells and the important growth factors/signal proteins provided from within the platelet alpha-granules. There is a direct correlation between concentration achieved and the delivery to targets (RW Alexander, unpublished data, 2012).[28]

There are now the capabilities to submit some volumes of the fat harvested (AD-tSVF) that can be separated into another syringe, expose the ATC to certain digestive agents, incubated, shaken to permit cellular isolation, and then neutralized, rinsed, and recentrifuged to create a cellular pellet (AD-cSVF). Enzymatic release of cell-to-cell and cell-to-matrix contacts forms a concentrate of the heterogeneous, mononuclear undifferentiated cellular collection. Once created, these cells are available for intravascular uses or be added back to adipose graft (AD-tSVF) (which still has its bioactive matrix). This cellular additive has been studied and reported in preclinical and clinical trials. This is termed *cell-enrichment* when simply added back to the AD-tSVF, mixed with HD PRP, and carefully guided into identified target sites to assist tissue healing using autologous tissues. This is commonly performed in many areas outside the United States, while FDA suggested guidelines discussed currently are confusing these issues regarding "manipulation" when employing digestive enzymes. Many sites are actively providing these services in the United States, often within controlled Institutional Review Board (IRB) trials or study groups within specialties. The author currently provides both options, following multiple institutional

---

Box 8
Advantages of centrifugation of adipose derived–tissue stromal vascular fraction

- Creates a density gradient of SVF
- Markedly improved layer separation of
  - Infranatant fluids
  - Red blood cells and cellular debris
  - Lipids, proteases, and lipases (separator disk)
- Optimal centrifugation 800 g to 1000 g for 3 to 4 minutes
- Favors transplantation of maximum stroma
- Decreases fluid load to site and reduces exposure to local anesthetics

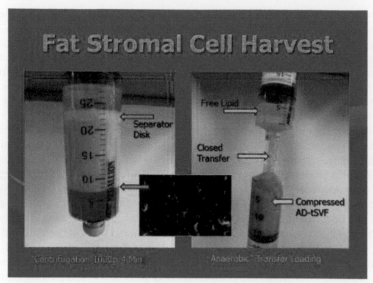

Fig. 11. Centrifuged (compressed) adipose graft layered separation.

and organizational IRB guidelines using specific trial studies by providing the approved trial protocols, both within the United States and internationally.

Termed AD-cSVF, the cellular isolates are currently used for a wide variety of human clinical applications on a global basis. After myriad basic research studies, animal models were tested and reported in the bioscientific literature and gradually reported in translational clinical journals in the medical literature. The parenteral uses (including intravenous, intra-arterial, intrathecal, and intraperitoneal) are reported on a regular basis. Because the cellular group is well recognized as favoring immune privilege, those systemic and autoimmune issues are included in many clinical studies (**Box 9**).

WHAT IS THE FUTURE IN STEM/STROMAL CELLULAR AND BIOCELLULAR TREATMENTS?

There are now capabilities of closed isolation of the large numbers of stem and stromal cells from the adipose tissues. Within such semiautomated and automated closed

---

Box 9
Current biocellular regenerative therapeutic applications

- Antiaging, unstable scarring and aesthetic surgery
- Skin, hair, radiation applications
- MSK - musculoskeletal uses, joints and structures
- Wound and chronic pain care
- Neurodegenerative diseases
- Disorders - Chonic obstructive pulmonary disease (COPD)
- Crohn's disease and ulcerative bowel disorders

systems, this ability is becoming practical even in outpatient procedural rooms and carefully prepared within sterile protocols. Once this was exclusively possible only in costly laboratory settings, requiring extensive equipment and technician costs. Today such isolation is done in the United States under IRB settings to ensure reporting of patient safety and effectiveness. Clinical trials are gradually being released, many requiring several years to acquire data, compile, and report. A vast majority of such reports are providing clear clinical evidence of patient safety and effective clinical treatment outcomes.

Isolation of these cells permits creation of what is termed, *cell-enriched biocellular grafts*. These grafts, higher in numbers of the heterogeneous undifferentiated cells, are believed to provide an even more potent guided injectable therapy. For example, there are many peer-reviewed clinical articles providing strong evidence of enhanced outcomes within the aesthetic–plastic surgical literature. Over the past decade, there are estimated numbers of use of biocellular therapies in MSK application exceeding 150,000 human clinical uses, with a remarkable efficacy and safety profile. These are reported in case series or reports and should not be discarded out of hand, simply because they are not participating in specific trial settings. It remains a pivotal value to insure that accurate diagnostics and guided placement to defined targets. Ultrasonography, with its dynamic abilities during examination, will remain a needed core competency for those taking care of MSK and chronic wound cases.

In the future, it is likely that such isolated cells will provide parenteral (intravenous, intra-arterial, intrathecal, intraperitoneal, and so forth) pathways and become effective for an expansive treatment in disorders, such as neurodegenerative diseases (multiple sclerosis, Alzheimer disease, amyotrophic lateral sclerosis, Parkinson disease, brain injuries/stroke, and so forth), diabetes, chronic lung disease, heart disease and damage, chronic wound healing, fibromyalgia/causalgia, ulcerative bowel disease, Crohn disease, colitis, and so forth (**Box 10**).

A RECENT ADVANCE IN USE OF BIOCELLULAR USES: NANOFAT (EMULSIFIED ADIPOSE DERIVED–TISSUE STROMAL VASCULAR FRACTION)

Over the past 2 years, major advances in processing the lipoaspirated AD-tSVF via mechanical emulsification has evolved. Although still favoring the same biocellular product creation, including use of additive advantages offered by addition of HD-PRP concentrates while retaining small-fragment AD-tSVF capable of injection via small-bore needles. Recent published evidence has shown that creation of the mechanically emulsified nanofat does not have a detrimental impact on stem/stromal cellular numbers or viabilities while markedly reducing the volume of ATC provided by mature adipocytes (**Fig. 12**).

Box 10
Trends in stem/stromal biocellular uses

- Targeted applications cells + HD-PRP
  - Skin, hair restoration, and scarring
  - MSK injuries and regenerative needs
- Cell-enrichment potentials increasing
- Emulsified AD-tSVF and systemic uses
- Culture/expansion and cryopreservation of AD-cSVF
- Increased uses in devascularized wounds and tissues

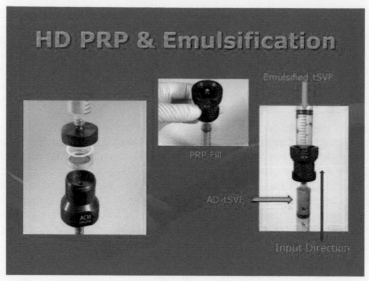

Fig. 12. ACM emulsification system (Healeon Medical, Newport Beach, CA) AD-tSVF with HD-PRP additive.

With the ability to inject through small-bore needles, patient comfort is enhanced along with offering a range of intradermal and small joint–targeted applications. The abilities of biocellular modalities to promote wound healing and regenerative capabilities via intradermal placement have created opportunities to permit improved skin circulation and texture, skin aging and radiation damage, and hair regeneration and participate in chronic wound applications as well as many small joint and superficial targets in MSK applications (**Fig. 13**).

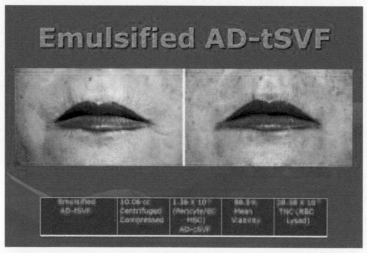

Fig. 13. Emulsified AD-tSVF intradermal injection use. EC, endothelial cells; MSC, mesenchymal stromal cell; TNC, total nuclear count; RBC, red blood cell. (*Courtesy of* Tonnard P, 2012.)

Box 11
Biocellular success is a three-legged stool

- Highest-quality graft harvest
- Achieve a high density of PRP
- Exact placement in target sites

WHO PROVIDES BIOCELLULAR TREATMENT?

Patients and providing doctors (eg, primary care health care providers, internists/neurologists, aesthetic–plastic surgeons, general surgeons, orthopedic surgeon, emergency/sports medical specialist, pain management specialists, wound care centers, and so forth) decide whether candidates have a condition that has reasonable potential for improvement through use of combinations of biologic and stem/stromal cellular treatment (see **Fig. 10**). Thorough physical and pretreatment evaluations are essential in diagnostic and treatment planning. Circulatory, neurologic, and indicated systemic conditions should be documented. In cases orthopedic applications, use of metrics, such as range of motion, indicated MRI studies, and high-quality ultrasonographic imaging, combine to determine the specific locations of problems and guide proper placement (see **Fig. 9**). Use of high-quality MSK ultrasonography is considered a key part of such evaluation, particularly considering that this modality plays a central role for providers to effectively hit the desired targets. Palpation may provide fairly accurate placement with experienced providers; targeted and tracked therapy consistently correlates with earlier and improved clinical outcomes. Use of metrics that are more objective and successful monitoring of many patients, including range of motion, remodeling of tissues in repeated interval ultrasound studies, and return of strength, provide valuable informative standards. For many years, prolotherapy major benchmarks were limited to patient-reported pain levels, activity levels, and perceived improvement as their primary metrics (**Box 11**).

Most times these procedures are completed on outpatient, ambulatory basis using local anesthesia, nitrous oxide, or occasionally light sedation depending on patient needs and desires. These cases are designed and planned to be completed within the same day. Providers handle tissues using standard aseptic protocols. Since the advent of using a mechanical emulsification system, which permits guided injections through very small-bore needles (25 gauge–30 gauge) without statistically reduced viabilities, the ability to provide improved patient comfort and access to small joints is rapidly becoming an appealing option (**Box 12**).

Box 12
Biocellular therapies change treatment paradigm

Things have changed

- Biocellular therapy
  - Combination more potent than either alone
  - Shown to be the most potent regimen
  - Offers reduction toxic inflammation
  - Effectively heal with minimal scar formation
  - Provides needed cells for specific site
- Parenteral applications for systemic issues rapidly evolving

---

SUMMARY

"Using your own tissues to heal" represents a major health care paradigm change and is one of the most exciting minimally invasive options currently available. Biocellular regenerative therapies are rapidly improving in documentation and cellular analyses and are gaining good safety and efficacy profiles. Once considered purely experimental, they have entered into an accepted, translational period to clinical providers, backed by improving science supporting the basic hypotheses. It is a well-recognized and reported alternative to many traditional medical/ interventions.

ACKNOWLEDGMENTS

The author wishes to thank the clinical and laboratory staff, Mrs Nancy L. Smith and Ms Susan Riley, for their endless hours and efforts to facilitate patients, sample gathering, and testing. Without such devotees, clinical articles cannot be reported.

REFERENCES

1. Alexander RW. Understanding adipose-derived stromal vascular fraction (AD-SVF) cell biology and use on the basis of cellular, chemical, structural and paracrine components: a concise review. Journal of Prolotherapy 2012;4(1):e855–69.
2. Zuk PA, Zhu M, Mizuno H, et al. Multi-lineage cells from human adipose tissue: implications for cell-based therapies. Tissue Eng 2001;7(2):211–28.
3. Zuk P. Adipose-Derived Stem Cells in Tissue Regeneration: A Review. Cells 2013; 35. ID 713959.
4. Alexander RW. Understanding Adipose-Derived Stromal Vascular Fraction (SVF) Cell Biology In Reconstructive and Regenerative Applications On the Basis of Mononucleated Cell Components. Journal of Prolotherapy 2013;10:15–29.
5. Alderman D, Alexander RW, Harris G. Stem cell prolotherapy in regenerative medicine: background, research, and protocols. Journal of Prolotherapy 2011; 3(3):689–708.
6. Sadati KS, Corrado AC, Alexander RW. Platelet-rich plasma (PRP) utilized to promote greater graft volume retention in autologous fat grafting. Am J Cosmet Surg 2006;23(4):627–31.
7. Alexander RW. Author textbook, use of PRP in autologous fat grafting. In: Shiffman M, editor. Autologous fat grafting, textbook, vol. 14. Berlin: Springer; 2010. p. 87–112.
8. Blaber S, Webster R, Cameron J, et al. Analysis of in vitro secretion profiles from adipose-derived cell populations. J Transl Med 2012;10:172.
9. Crisan M, Yap S, Casteilla L, et al. A perivascular origin for mesenchymal stem cells in multiple human organs. Cell Stem Cell 2008;3:301–13.
10. Guilak F, Cohen DM, Estes BT, et al. Control of stem cell fate by physical interactions with the extracellular matrix. Cell Stem Cell 2009;5(1):17–26.
11. Brizzi M, Tarone G, Defilippi P. Extracellular matrix, integrins, and growth factors as tailors of stem cell niche. Curr Opin Cell Biol 2012;24(5):645–51.
12. Soo-Yyun K, Turnbull J, Guimond S. Extracellular matrix and cell signaling: the dynamic cooperation of integrin, proteoglycan, and growth factor receptor. J Endocrinol 2011;209:139–51.
13. Alexander RW. Fat transfer with platelet-rich plasma for breast augmentation. In: Shiffman M, editor. Breast augmentation: principles and practice. Berlin: Springer; 2009. p. 451–70.

14. Kato H. Short- and long-term cellular events in adipose tissue remodel-ing after non-vascularized grafting. Paper presented at the International Federation for Adipose Therapeutics and Science Miami, 9th Annual Symposium on Adipose Stem Cells and Clinical Applications of Adipose Tissue. Miami, Florida, USA, November 4–6, 2011.
15. Alexander RW. Liposculpture in the superficial plane: closed syringe system for improvement in fat removal and free fat transfer. Am J Cosmet Surg 1994; 11(2):127–34.
16. Albano J, Alexander RW. Autologous fat grafting as a mesenchymal stem cell source and living bioscaffold in a patellar tendon tear. Am J Sports Med 2011; 21(4):359–61.
17. Crisan M, Yap S, Casteilla L, et al. A Perivascular Origin For Mesenchymal Stem Cells In Multiple Human Organs. Cell Stem Cell 2008;3:301–13.
18. Kurita M, Matsumoto D, Shigeura T, et al. Influences of centrifuga-tion on cells and tissues in liposuction aspirates: optimized cen-trifugation for lipotransfer and cell isolation. Plast Reconstr Surg 2008;121(3):1033–41.
19. Alexander RW, Harrell DB. Autologous fat grafting: use of closed syringe micro-cannula system for enhanced autologous structural grafting. Clin Cosmet Investig Dermatol 2013;6:91–102.
20. Alexander RW. Contributing author, textbook "introduction to biocellular medi-cine. In: Moore R, Editor, editors. Sonography of the extremities: techniques & protocols 4th Ed. Cincinnati (OH): General Musculoskeletal Imaging Inc.; 2015. p. 97–104.
21. Eto H, Suga H, Inoue K, et al. Adipose injury-associated factors miti-gate hypoxia in ischemic tissues through activation of adipose-derived stem/progenitor/stro-mal cells and induction of angiogenesis. Am J Pathol 2011;178(5):2322–32.
22. Alexander RW. Understanding Mechanical Emulsification (Nanofat) Versus Enzy-matic Isolation of Tissue Stromal Vascular Fraction (tSVF) Cells from Adipose Tis-sue: Potential Uses in Biocellular Regenerative Medicine. Journal of Prolotherapy 2016;8:e947–60.
23. Oliver K, Alexander RW. Combination of autologous adipose-derived tissue stro-mal vascular fraction plus high-density platelet-rich plasma or bone marrow con-centrates in achilles tendon tears. Journal of Prolotherapy 2013;5:e895–912.
24. Alderman D, Alexander RW. Advances in regenerative medicine: high-density platelet-rich plasma and stem cell prolotherapy. Journal of Pract Pain Manage-ment (PPM) 2011;10:49–90.
25. Alexander RW. Autologous fat grafts as mesenchymal stromal stem cell source for use in prolotherapy: a simple technique to acquire lipoaspirants. Journal of Prolotherapy 2011;3(3):680–8.
26. Bright, R., Bright, M., Bright, P. et al. Isolation of stem cells from adipose tissue by ultrasonic cavitation and methods of use. WO 2014; 2014000021a1.
27. Tobita M, Tajima S, Mizuno H. Adipose tissue-derived mesenchymal stem cells and platelet-rich plasma: stem cell transplantation methods that enhance stem-ness. Stem Cell Res Ther 2015;6:215–22.
28. Tonnard P, Verpaele A, Peeters G, et al. Nanofat grafting: basic research and clin-ical applications. Plast Reconstr Surg 2013;152:1017–26.

Autologous Conditioned Serum

Christopher H. Evans, PhD[a],*, Xavier Chevalier, MD[b], Peter Wehling, MD, PhD[c]

KEYWORDS

- Interleukin-1 receptor antagonist • Osteoarthritis • Radicular compression
- Intra-articular therapy • Anterior cruciate ligament • Tendinopathy • Muscle injury
- Pain

KEY POINTS

- Autologous conditioned serum is prepared by the incubation of whole blood with surface-treated glass beads within a special syringe.
- During incubation, the serum is enriched in products synthesized and released by peripheral blood platelets and leukocytes including, but not limited to, the interleukin-1 receptor antagonist.
- Randomized, controlled trials find that locally injected autologous conditioned serum is effective in treating osteoarthritis, radicular compression, and tunnel widening after reconstruction of the anterior cruciate ligament.
- Additional studies suggest utility in treating tendinopathies and muscle injuries.
- Further studies are required to confirm clinical effectiveness in specific indications, to determine the composition of autologous conditioned serum, to determine its mode of action, to understand individual responses to therapy, and to explore potential synergies with other therapeutic agents.

INTRODUCTION

Autologous conditioned serum (ACS) is an autologous blood product enriched in the interleukin-1 receptor antagonist (IL-1Ra), a naturally occurring inhibitor of interleukin-1 (IL-1).[1–4] ACS is administered locally to treat conditions in which IL-1 is thought to be an important agent of pathologic conditions. Several reviews have been written on this topic.[5–8]

Disclosure Statement: C.H. Evans is a member of the Supervisory Board of Orthogen, AG that sells a device for producing autologous conditioned serum; X. Chevalier has nothing to disclose; P. Wehling is founder and CEO of Orthogen AG.
a Rehabilitation Medicine Research Center, Mayo Clinic, 200, First Street Southwest, Rochester, MN 55905, USA; b Department of Rheumatology, Hopital Henri Mondor, UPEC Paris XII University, Bd De latter de Tassigny, Creteil 94010, France; c Orthogen AG, Ernst-Schneider-Platz 1, Düsseldorf 40212, Germany
* Corresponding author.
E-mail address: Evans.christopher@mayo.edu

Phys Med Rehabil Clin N Am 27 (2016) 893–908
http://dx.doi.org/10.1016/j.pmr.2016.06.003

IL-1Ra has been produced in *Escherichia coli* as the recombinant molecule ana-kinra, marketed as Kineret. Anakinra, in combination with methotrexate, is approved by the US Food and Drug Administration for the treatment of rheumatoid arthritis (RA), self-administered subcutaneously at a daily dose of 100 mg. However, the therapeutic efficacy of anakinra in RA has generally been disappointing, and it is not widely used in this context. Clinical responses in sepsis have also been weak. However, systemic anakinra is effective in systemic juvenile idiopathic arthritis and a variety of rare autoinflammatory disorders; it is also of benefit in gout and pseudogout.[9]

There is considerable interest in using anakinra intra-articularly in the treatment of osteoarthritis (OA) and injured joints. An initial, open-label clinical trial in patients with OA of the knee provided highly encouraging results with sustained clinical improvement after intra-articular injection of 100 mg of anakinra.[10] However, a subsequent multicenter, randomized controlled trial (RCT) showed no sustained benefit of intra-articular Anakinra.[11] Nevertheless, there was transient improvement, observed at day 4, in certain parameters, notably pain. The temporary nature of the beneficial effects probably reflects the rapidity with which proteins are removed from joints.[12] An additional clinical trial administered anakinra intra-articularly to patients after rupture of the anterior cruciate ligament (ACL) and again found improvement in certain parameters during the 2-week study period.[13] In a further small, uncontrolled, unblinded study of 6 patients with persistent postsurgical knee effusions, a single 200-mg injection of anakinra decreased pain and swelling, improved range of motion, and permitted return to sporting activities.[14]

There is, thus, optimism that IL-1Ra could prove efficacious in injured and arthritic joints if there were a way to maintain therapeutic concentrations intra-articularly. Gene delivery provides one technology for achieving this, and proof of principle has been established in animal models and human clinical trials for RA.[15–17] Genetic delivery of IL-1Ra into human knee joints with OA is at an advanced preclinical stage of development.[18]

AUTOLOGOUS CONDITIONED SERUM
Background

Wehling and colleagues developed ACS in the mid-1990s as an expeditious, practical, and relatively inexpensive means of generating IL-1Ra for local, therapeutic application in musculoskeletal diseases. ACS is based on studies that found that macrophages and monocytes are major endogenous sources of IL-1Ra.[19,20] Production of IL-1Ra can be enhanced by a variety of stimuli, including adhesion to certain surfaces. Based on this information, Meijer and colleagues[21] developed a method for stimulating IL-1Ra synthesis by whole human blood. According to their method, peripheral blood is drawn into a syringe containing treated glass beads to which blood monocytes and other adherent cells have the opportunity to attach. The syringe and its contents are then incubated at 37° for several hours, during which time platelets degranulate and mononuclear cells synthesize and secrete IL-1Ra along with a variety of additional anti-inflammatory products. During this period, synthesis of the inflammatory cytokines IL-1β and tumor necrosis factor-α (TNF-α) does not increase greatly. After incubation, the ACS is recovered and sterilized by filtration. ACS is then injected locally into sites of injury or disease.

Stimulation of blood cells by the glass beads is not specific to IL-1Ra, and ACS contains a variety of growth factors and cytokines (**Table 1**). Indeed, it has not been formally demonstrated that IL-1Ra is responsible for the therapeutic properties of ACS. The composition of ACS shown in **Table 1** is in rough agreement with that reported by Darabos and colleagues[22] and Rutgers and colleagues[23]; the only major discrepancy is the

Table 1
Cytokines and growth factors present in autologous conditioned serum

Cytokine	N	Basal Concentration	Concentration in ACS
IL-1Ra	224	236	2015
IL-1β	224	UD	7.9
IL-6	200	UD	28.7
TNF-α	92	UD	10.1
IL-10	92	UD	33.4
FGF-2	92	14.6	26.6
VEGF	92	61	508.6
HGF	92	431	1339
IGF-1	92	86,000	117,209
PDGF AB	92	205	39,026
TGF-β	80	1165	97,939

Concentrations are averages, given in picograms per milliliter before (basal) and after (ACS) incubation. N indicates the number of different samples tested.

Abbreviations: FGF, fibroblast growth factor; HGF, hepatocyte growth factor; IGF, insulin-like growth factor; PDGF, platelet-derived growth factor; TGF, transforming growth factor; UD, undetectable; VEGF, vascular endothelial growth factor.

Modified from Wehling P, Moser C, Frisbie D, et al. Autologous conditioned serum in the treatment of orthopedic diseases: the Orthokine therapy. BioDrugs 2007;21:326; with permission.

approximately 10-fold higher TNF-α concentrations noted by the latter investigators. These authors also reported the presence of osteoprotegerin, interferon-γ, and oncostatin M. The data in **Table 1**, including the TNF-α levels, are in agreement with the data of Wright-Carpenter and colleagues[24] who also noted the presence of IL-7. Darabos and colleagues[22] detected epidermal growth factor in ACS.

Clinical Development

ACS was first used clinically in 1997. Beginning in 2001, ACS was manufactured as Orthokine in a Good Manufacturing Process (GMP) facility. Participating physicians were provided with syringes, known as *Orthokine syringes*, containing treated glass beads. The beads are 3.5 mm in diameter, comprise borosilicate glass of maximum hydrolytic resistance, and are polished according to a proprietary process. Blood was drawn into Orthokine syringes and shipped to the GMP facility for the production of Orthokine. Typically, 6 injections of Orthokine, each 2 mL, were injected into knee joints over a period of 3 to 6 weeks. For epidural use, 3 injections, each 1 mL, were injected over a 3-week period. The number of injections and their timing were determined empirically.

This means of distribution proved cumbersome, time consuming, and geographically limiting and could not be performed in all markets because of regulatory hurdles. For these reasons, the system was changed in 2004 to one in which the physician was provided with a smaller, disposable Orthokine syringe and an incubator so that ACS could be produced locally in the individual clinic or physician's office. Although the original 50-mL syringe required a 24-hour incubation at 37° for optimal production of ACS, the newer 10-mL syringe allows a shorter incubation time of 6 to 9 hours.

Clinical Experience with Autologous Conditioned Serum —Intra-Articular Delivery

Baltzer and colleagues[25] published the first clinical use of ACS, describing treatment of 1000 patients with OA of the knee and Kellgren Lawrence (KL) scores of 1 to 3 (**Table 2**). In this prospective, nonrandomized, uncontrolled study, Western Ontario

Table 2
Clinical studies of intra-articular autologous conditioned serum

Indication	No of Patients	Study Design; Entry Criteria	Outcome Measures	Main Findings	Reference
Human knee OA	1000	Retrospective, uncontrolled, unblinded Established OA KL grades 1–3	WOMAC	WOMAC scores improved ≥50% in ≥70% of patients Improvement sustained for 3.5 y in ≥35% patients	25
Human knee OA	376	Randomized, placebo controlled ACS compared with saline and HA Established OA KL grades 2–3 Follow-up: 7 wk, 13 wk, 6 mo, and 2 y	WOMAC VAS SF-8 HRQL GPA	Sustained, statistically significant improvement in all outcome measures compared with saline and HA No severe adverse events	26
Human knee OA	167	Randomized, multicenter, placebo controlled ACS compared with saline KL grades 1–3 Follow-up: 3, 6, 9, 12 mo	WOMAC KOOS VAS KSCRS	Statistically significant improvements in KOOS symptoms and KOOS sport compared with saline No difference in WOMAC Trend toward improvement in other parameters Two severe adverse events, one of which attributed to ACS	27
Human knee OA	20	Patients who received placebo in the above study[27] were given ACS	WOMAC KOOS VAS KSCRS	Improvement to the same degree as previously[27] seen when receiving placebo	28
Human knee OA	118	Uncontrolled study; subjects received ACS (2 mL/wk for 4 wk) with physiotherapy Follow-up: 2 y Painful OA of knee, KL grades 1–4	WOMAC Pain	Rapid and sustained improvement in pain and WOMAC scores Only 1 patient progressed to total knee joint replacement	29
Human knee OA	30	Uncontrolled study; low-dose ACS (1 mL/wk for 3 wk) Follow-up: 3 mo Painful OA of knee, KL grades 1–3	WOMAC	Rapid and progressive improvement in WOMAC scores Maintained for at least 3 mo	30

Model	N	Study design	Outcome measure	Results	Ref
Human hip OA	119 (150 hips)	Retrospective, nonrandomized, no placebo; KL grades 2–4; ACS ± cortisone ± anakinra; Follow-up: 14 mo	VAS	Statistically significant improvement in VAS in all groups; No adverse events	[31]
Tunnel widening after single bundle ACL reconstruction (human)	62	Randomized, double blind, placebo controlled; Isolated ACL rupture; Outerbridge up to grade 2; Surgical reconstruction of ACL; Follow-up: 6 and 12 mo	CT; WOMAC; IKDC 2000	Statistically significant reduction in tunnel widening; Lower effusion at 6 mo; Improved range of motion; Improved WOMAC stiffness; No serious adverse events	[32]
Tunnel widening after double bundle ACL reconstruction (human)	62	Randomized, double blind, placebo controlled; Isolated ACL rupture; Outerbridge up to grade 2; Double-bundle surgical reconstruction of ACL; Follow-up: 6 and 12 mo	CT; Lysholm; IKDC 2000	Statistically significant reduction in tunnel widening; Better Lysholm and IKDC 2000 scores; No serious adverse events	[22]
Equine OA	262	Nonrandomized; no control; Lameness unresponsive to intra-articular glucocorticoid or HA; Follow-up: 6 and 12 wk	Lameness	Elimination or improvement in lameness in 221 horses at 6 wk; No lameness in 178 horses at 12 wk; No adverse events	[41]
Equine OA	20	Nonrandomized; Lameness unresponsive to intra-articular PSGAG or HA; Follow-up: 3 mo	Lameness	Full activity restored in 10/10 PSGAG failures and 7/10 HA failures	[43]
Equine OA	54	27 lame horses in each group received either ACS or a mixture of HA and betamethasone; Follow-up: 6 mo	Lameness	ACS produced a stronger reduction in lameness	[42] (abstract)
Canine OA	11 dogs 15 joints	OA confirmed by clinical examination and radiology; 2–4 injections of 1.4 mL ACS; Observational study; no control group	Lameness	Clinical signs improved within 1 wk of the first or second injection; Decrease in lameness in all dogs	[39] (abstract)

Abbreviations: CT, computed tomography; GPA, global patient assessment; KSCRS, Knee Society Clinical Rating System; SF-HRQL, Short-form 8 Health-related Quality-of-Life Survey.

MacMaster Universities (WOMAC) arthritis scores improved by ≥50% after 3 months in ≥70% of patients receiving intra-articular ACS. Each subcategory of the WOMAC scoring system improved, and improvements were maintained for 3.5 years in ≥35% of patients. There were no infections or allergic reactions to injection of ACS; 3.5% of patients reported joint swelling or pain immediately after injection, but these symptoms subsided spontaneously over the course of a few hours. Subsequently, there have been 2 large, double-blind RCTs evaluating the efficacy of ACS for the treatment of OA of the knee.

The first of these, also by Baltzer and colleagues,[26] compared ACS (6 injections, twice per week, 2 mL per injection) with standard of care (hyaluronic acid; HA) and placebo (saline). Subjects in the HA group received 1 injection (2 mL) per week for 3 weeks of a 1% solution of HA with a molecular weight of 1.4×10^6 Da (HYA-Ject Ormed, Freiburg, Germany). Entry criteria included age greater than 30 years, established OA of the knee, a KL score of 2 to 3, a pain score of at least 50 mm on a 100-mm visual analog scale (VAS), and a willingness to discontinue nonsteroidal anti-inflammatory drugs (NSAIDs) and other analgesics for 6 months. Outcome measures included VAS, WOMAC scores, Short-Form 8 Health-Related Quality-of-Life (SF-8 HRQL) survey, and the global patient assessment of treatment efficacy. Outcomes were measured at 7 weeks, 13 weeks, and 6 months; traceable patients were recalled after 2 years and reassessed in an observational, prospective, cohort study with a new, blinded observer.

A total of 376 patients were randomly assigned to 1 of the 3 study groups; 345 completed the initial, 6-month study, and 310 were traceable after 2 years. Patients receiving ACS experienced considerable, statistically significant improvement, beyond that obtained with placebo, in all outcome measures. Remarkably, these improvements were maintained for at least 2 years (**Fig. 1**). HA, in contrast, was no more effective than placebo. ACS produced no severe adverse events. At 3 months, 71% of subjects had greater than 50% reduction in VAS pain score; at 6 months, this response was 67%.

In the multicenter RCT of Yang and colleagues,[27] 176 patients with OA of the knee, KL scores 1 to 3, and VAS greater than 40 mm were randomly assigned to receive 6 injections of saline or ACS. Injections (2 mL) were given twice per week. Unlike the Baltzer and colleagues[26] study, continued use of NSAIDs and acetaminophen was permitted. Patients were assessed quarterly for 1 year. Efficacy was determined by VAS scores, the Knee Injury and Osteoarthritis Outcome Score (KOOS) and the Knee Society Clinical Rating System. WOMAC scores were calculated from components of the KOOS scores.

In this study, ACS did not improve the deduced WOMAC scores beyond placebo. However, ACS produced a statistically significant improvement in the KOOS symptom and KOOS sport scores. Moreover, use of ACS was associated with improvement in most other outcome measures, although these did not achieve statistical significance. Subgroup analysis found that participants who continued to take NSAIDs throughout the study had a superior response to ACS. This finding suggests that combination therapy including ACS could be an interesting option. Of note, the patients treated in this study had milder disease, as assessed by KL and VAS, than those recruited to the Baltzer study.[26] One serious adverse event, severe inflammation of the knee, was ascribed to ACS. In a follow-up study by the same group, ACS was administered to a subset of previous placebo patients without improvement beyond the previous placebo effect.[28]

A recent, nonblinded, 2-year prospective study by Baselga and Hernandez[29] showed promising results for highly symptomatic knee OA. Patients had mean

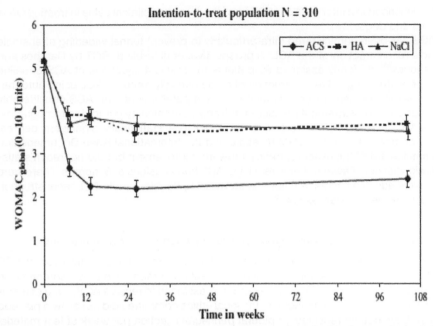

Fig. 1. WOMAC scores (0–10 scale) as a function of time after the last intra-articular injections of ACS into the knee joints of patients with OA. Figure shows mean ± standard error; P<.05 for the comparison ACS versus HA and saline; P>.05 for the comparison HA versus saline. (*From* Baltzer AW, Moser C, Jansen SA, et al. Autologous conditioned serum (Orthokine) is an effective treatment for knee osteoarthritis. Osteoarthritis and Cartilage 2009;17:157; with permission.)

VAS scores of 8.1 and mean WOMAC global scores of 81; they entered the clinic expecting surgery. One injection per week of ACS (2 mL) was administered intra-articularly to 118 patients over a 4-week period followed by 30 physiotherapy sessions spread over 10 weeks. Follow-up at 24 months found a 62% decrease in VAS scores and 56% decrease in WOMAC scores. Joint stiffness was the only WOMAC subcategory that did not improve. Of interest, there was no significant difference in response between patients with different KL scores. Only one patient progressed to joint replacement surgery during this study. This study suffered from the lack of a control group receiving physiotherapy alone. According to the authors, however, in their experience, physiotherapy alone produces a pain improvement of about 25%.

The optimum dose and frequency of ACS administration remains to be determined. A recent small, uncontrolled study[30] noted a strong clinical response in symptomatic knee joints with OA after the intra-articular injection of just 1 mL ACS once per week for 3 weeks. Clinical improvement was already noted 1 week after the first injection of ACS. However, follow-up was curtailed at 3 months.

Although nearly all interventional studies have been performed with OA of the knee, Baltzer and colleagues[31] recently reported efficacy when using ACS to treat OA of the hip. This retrospective, uncontrolled study involving 119 patients and 150 hips was based on just 1 outcome measure, pain, measured by VAS. Nevertheless, it suggested sustained improvement over a 14-month period with no adverse events. Co-administration of glucocorticoid or anakinra provided no additional clinical benefit.

As described in a later section, ACS has also proved of clinical value in treating OA in horses and dogs.

ACS has been administered intra-articularly to prevent tunnel widening after single bundle reconstruction of the ACL. A prospective, double-blind, RCT by Darabos and colleagues[32] randomly assigned 62 patients to receive 4 injections of ACS or saline (placebo) after surgical reconstruction of a traumatically ruptured ACL using autograft of the semitendinosus or gracilis tendon, or the patellar ligament. ACS considerably reduced tunnel enlargement measured at 6 and 12 months by computed tomography. WOMAC stiffness scores were also improved to a statistically significant degree. Other components of the WOMAC scale and the International Knee Documentation Committee (IKDC 2000) score, trended toward improvement but did not reach statistical significance. Fewer patients receiving ACS had effusions at 6 months. There were no severe adverse events. A follow-up study using double-bundle ACL reconstruction surgery showed similar results.[22]

Clinical Experience with Autologous Conditioned Serum—Other Indications

Becker and colleagues[33] conducted an RCT to determine the effectiveness of ACS versus nonsurgical standard of care in treating lumbar radicular compression (**Table 3**). A total of 84 patients were randomly assigned to receive ACS, 5 mg of triamcinolone, or 10 mg of triamcinolone; the local ethics committee did not allow a placebo group. Each patient received 1 epidural perineural injection per week of test material for 3 weeks. Patients were followed for 6 months and evaluated for pain (VAS) and by the Oswestry Disability Index (ODI).

Initially, all 3 treatments were equally effective, but the improvements in VAS produced by the glucocorticoid proved less durable and by the 6-month time point were separating from those produced by ACS, which remained high (**Fig. 2**). ODI improved to an equal degree in all 3 groups. There were no adverse events.

These findings were confirmed by Goni and colleagues,[34] who administered ACS or methylprednisone epidurally to patients with unilateral lumbar radiculopathy. ACS produced progressive improvements in pain and function scores during a 6-month follow-up. Although methylprednisone also improved these parameters initially, the scores were deteriorating by the 6-month time point.

Based on promising data from a muscle contusion model in mice,[35] Wright-Carpenter and colleagues[24] conducted a small pilot study in human athletes. Professional athletes with muscle injuries were treated with standard rehabilitation therapy involving the use of oral anti-inflammatories. One group of 18 individuals was also administered ACS, whereas a second group received Actovegin and Traumeel, a combination very commonly used in European sports medicine. In this study, 2.5 mL of ACS was diluted with 2.5 mL of serum, and 5 injections, each of 1 mL, were delivered into the damaged area. Injections were initiated 2 days after injury and repeated according to the clinical changes. There was a significant reduction in the recovery time for athletes treated with ACS.

Preclinical data in a rat model suggest a role for the local application of ACS in treating tendon injuries.[36,37] These studies used a model in which the Achilles tendon was transected and sutured. Rat ACS (170 µL) was injected percutaneously into the sutured area 24, 48, and 72 hours after surgery. Animals were euthanized after 1 week, 2 weeks, 4 weeks, and 8 weeks. The ACS-treated tendons were thicker, had more type I collagen, and displayed an accelerated recovery of tendon stiffness and histologic maturity of the repair tissue. Data consistent with these findings have been reported for horses with naturally occurring tendinopathies.[38]

Table 3
Clinical use of autologous conditioned serum in other musculoskeletal settings

Indication	No of Patients	Study Design; Entry Criteria	Outcome Measures	Main Findings	Reference
Lumbar radicular compression	84	Prospective, randomized, placebo-controlled study comparing ACS with triamcinolone. Unilateral lumbar radicular compression. ACS or steroid injected epidurally, perineurally. Follow-up: 6 mo	VAS ODI	Reduction in pain and disability, equal to glucocorticoid but more sustained	33
Unilateral cervical Radiculopathy	40	Prospective, randomized trial comparing ACS with methylprednisolone. Patients 30–60 y with neck pain >6 wk duration, pain VAS >7. ACS or steroid injected epidurally. Follow up: 6 mo	VAS Neck Disability Index SF-12	Improved outcome scores. Improvement more gradual with ACS, but sustained	34
Muscle injury	29	Unblinded, no control. ACS or Actovegin or Traumeel injected into lesion	MRI Recovery time	Reduction in recovery time in ACS group	24
Tendon healing (equine)	15 horses; 17 tendons	Intra-lesional ACS (n = 10) vs untreated or saline (n = 7). Follow up: 190 d	Swelling, ultrasonography, histology	More rapid recovery with ACS	38

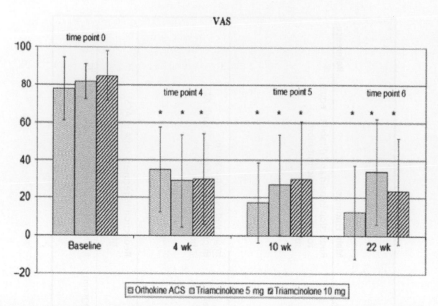

Fig. 2. Reduction in pain (VAS) after epidural injection of ACS or triamcinolone in patients with radicular compression. Mean, standard deviation, and median are given. Asterisks indicate significant difference from baseline. Time schedule is given in weeks after the first injection. (*From* Becker C, Heidersdorf S, Drewlo S, et al. Efficacy of epidural perineural injections with autologous conditioned serum for lumbar radicular compression: an investigator-initiated, prospective, double-blind, reference-controlled study. Spine (Phila Pa 1976) 2007;32:1805; with permission.)

Veterinary Applications of Autologous Conditioned Serum

ACS is widely used as an intra-articular injection for the treatment of OA in horses, whereas preliminary data suggest effectiveness in dogs.[39] Experimental studies conducted in an equine model of OA determined that ACS reduced lameness and synovial hyperplasia to a greater degree than saline.[40] There was also a trend toward improved cartilage morphology.

Although there have been no RCTs for the veterinary use of ACS, Weinberger[41] studied a large series of horses with OA whose lameness did not respond to either intra-articular glucocorticoids or HA. Remarkably, of these 262 horses treated with ACS, 178 were free from lameness at 12 weeks. These data are consistent with those of Jöstingmeier and colleagues[42] who found superiority of ACS over a combination of HA and betamethasone in treating aseptic arthritis of the coffin joint. A smaller study by Österdahl[43] injected ACS into the joints of horses that did not respond to intra-articular therapy with HA or polysulfated glycosaminoglycans (PSGAG). By 3 months, full activity was restored in 10 of 10 PSGAG failures and 7 of 10 HA failures. As noted earlier, ACS also shows promise as a treatment for equine tendinopathies.[38]

DISCUSSION
Safety and Efficacy of Autologous Conditioned Serum

From the combined experience of administering ACS to more than 100,000 human and 40,000 equine patients during a 15-year period it can be concluded that ACS is safe. Side effects are rare, the most common being a transient, local inflammatory response. The literature suggests that ACS can be effective in treating certain aspects of OA and radicular compression and in the postsurgical management of ACL reconstruction and certain other conditions.

Nevertheless, efficacy trials involving intra-articular therapies face certain challenges. Double blinding can be an issue, and, ideally, the injection syringes should be masked. When HA is used, its high viscosity reveals its identity. This obstacle can be addressed by separating the role of injection from that of evaluation. Because the patients' expectations of a new, safe treatment may be high, there is a marked placebo effect, the effect size of which is around 0.5 for OA in general and 0.7 with the intra-articular route of administration.[44] Thus, a placebo group is advised for such studies. When this is not possible, the test drug can be compared with that of standard of care. Finally, the interval between 2 injections, the volume injected, and the optimal number of injections are still empirical in intra-articular therapy studies.

Response rates of OA to ACS seem to be around 70%. However, there is disagreement about the specifics. For instance, Baltzer and colleagues[26] reported improvements in WOMAC scores for patients with OA receiving ACS, whereas Yang and colleagues[27] did not, although they did find improved KOOS scores. In a follow-up study delivering ACSs to a subset of previous placebo patients from this trial, Rutgers and colleagues[28] found no improvement beyond the previous placebo effect. Based on initial KL and VAS scores, patients entering the latter 2 studies had milder disease. This is interesting in light of the data of Baselga and Hernandez[29] reporting dramatic improvements in patients with highly symptomatic disease. However, these patients also received intensive physiotherapy. Although physiotherapy alone had only a small effect, there was no group that received only ACS. The concept of using ACS in synergy with other modalities merits further consideration. Patient selection may also be important, and ways to predict good responders would be helpful. Resolution of these issues and determination of the place of ACS in the musculoskeletal armamentarium should be accomplished with additional, well-powered, well-controlled studies.

In this context, it will be important to determine whether ACS has a disease-modifying effect in OA. The evidence so far suggests that ACS reduces pain and inflammation; in many patients symptomatic improvement is rapid and sustained. However, no clinical data address its effects on cartilage loss. In an in vitro study, Rutgers and colleagues[23] found no effect of ACS on the turnover of proteoglycans in fragments of cartilage recovered from human joints with end-stage OA. On the other hand, Frisbie and colleagues[40] noted a trend toward reduced cartilage fibrillation in an equine model of OA. This remains an unresolved issue.

Efficacy in Comparison with Alternative Intra-articular Treatments for Osteoarthritis

With the exception of the Baltzer study, which compared ACS with HA, there have been no direct comparisons between ACS and other intra-articular treatments for OA.[26] However, it is possible to calculate effect sizes from the published data (**Table 4**). This analysis suggests that ACS is superior to corticosteroids, HA, and platelet-rich plasma (PRP) in terms of pain and function.

Relationship to Other Autologous Blood Products

Since ACS was developed, there has been a rapid expansion in the popularity of autologous blood products, and variety of such products has become available for treating orthopedic conditions. There is now a bewildering array of choices including PRP,[45]

Table 4
Effect sizes of various intra-articular treatments for osteoarthritis

Treatment	Effect Size	
	Pain	Function
Corticosteroids (1–4 wk)	<0.50	0.06
HA (24 wk)	<0.46	0.33
PRP (24–52 wk)	<0.40	0.40
ACS (24–104 wk)	<0.73	0.54

Effect sizes were calculated from RCT data published before January 2016.
Effect sizes range from 0 to 1 and can be considered as follows: less than 0.1, no effect; 0.1–0.29, small effect; 0.3–0.49, moderate effect; greater than 0.5, large effect.

platelet-poor plasma,[46] autologous conditioned plasma,[47] autologous protein solution,[48] and plasma rich in growth factors.[49]

The incubation step and the absence of anticoagulants, activators such as Ca^{2+}, or cells, provide the main differences distinguishing ACS from these other products. Although they should all contain the contents of platelets, only ACS captures the products of blood mononuclear cells that are synthesized during prolonged in vitro incubation. The data of Meijer and colleagues,[21] for instance, show that a major portion of the IL-1Ra in ACS results from de novo synthesis. Other important products are also likely to be synthesized during this period.

Composition and Mode of Action

The sustained effectiveness of ACS when injected intra-articularly for OA is remarkable, given the rapid egress of molecules from the joint space[12] and the transient responses to intra-articular anakinra noted clinically.[11] Glycosylated, native IL-1Ra, as presumably present in ACS, has approximately the same potency as the recombinant form,[50] but it may have superior retention properties. However, it is more likely that other components within ACS are responsible for sustaining any effects of IL-1Ra, providing additional therapeutic signals, or both. Indeed, although the development of ACS was predicated on the induction of IL-1Ra, it remains to be shown that IL-1Ra is a key or important ingredient. It is clear that many other substances are induced, some of which may have therapeutic properties of their own. In this regard, attention has understandably focused on the growth factors contained within ACS, but the list shown in **Table 1** is almost certainly incomplete and does not even begin to address nonproteinaceous components that might be important therapeutically. Further analysis of the composition of ACS and its biological mode of action are required. Such information could lead to improving the qualities of ACS by addition or subtraction.[51,52]

Regulatory Status

The Orthokine syringe for producing ACS is an approved medical device in the European Union, Australia, and several other markets, but not in the United States. However, the Orthokine syringe is permitted for veterinary use in all markets, including the United States.

The World Anti-Doping Agency confirmed that the local application of ACS (Orthokine) is not considered doping.

SUMMARY

ACS is a safe and, based on the preponderance of evidence from a limited number of trials, effective treatment of a variety of orthopedic conditions including OA, radicular compression, tunnel widening after ACL reconstruction, and, possibly, soft tissue injuries. Further RCTs and laboratory studies are needed to refine and optimize its use and to provide more information concerning its composition, mode of action, and possible synergies with other treatments.

ACKNOWLEDGMENTS

The authors thank Prof. Sinclair Cleveland for calculating the effect sizes shown in **Table 4**. We thank Dr Julio Reinecke for review and comment on earlier drafts of this manuscript.

REFERENCES

1. Arend WP, Evans CH. Interleukin-1 receptor antagonist [IL-1F3]. In: Thompson AW, Lotze MT, editors. The Cytokine handbook. London: Academic Press; 2003. p. 669–708.
2. Bresnihan B. The prospect of treating rheumatoid arthritis with recombinant human interleukin-1 receptor antagonist. BioDrugs 2001;15:87–97.
3. Dinarello CA, Simon A, van der Meer JW. Treating inflammation by blocking interleukin-1 in a broad spectrum of diseases. Nat Rev Drug Discov 2012;11:633–52.
4. Gabay C, Lamacchia C, Palmer G. IL-1 pathways in inflammation and human diseases. Nat Rev Rheumatol 2010;6:232–41.
5. Wehling P, Moser C, Frisbie D, et al. Autologous conditioned serum in the treatment of orthopedic diseases: the orthokine therapy. BioDrugs 2007;21:323–32.
6. Fox BA, Stephens MM. Treatment of knee osteoarthritis with orthokine-derived autologous conditioned serum. Expert Rev Clin Immunol 2010;6:335–45.
7. Frizziero A, Giannotti E, Oliva F, et al. Autologous conditioned serum for the treatment of osteoarthritis and other possible applications in musculoskeletal disorders. Br Med Bull 2013;105:169–84.
8. Alvarez-Camino JC, Vazquez-Delgado E, Gay-Escoda C. Use of autologous conditioned serum (orthokine) for the treatment of the degenerative osteoarthritis of the temporomandibular joint. Review of the literature. Med Oral Patol Oral Cir Bucal 2013;18:e433–8.
9. Moll M, Kuemmerle-Deschner JB. Inflammasome and cytokine blocking strategies in autoinflammatory disorders. Clin Immunol 2013;147:242–75.
10. Chevalier X, Giraudeau B, Conrozier T, et al. Safety study of intraarticular injection of interleukin 1 receptor antagonist in patients with painful knee osteoarthritis: a multicenter study. J Rheumatol 2005;32:1317–23.
11. Chevalier X, Goupille P, Beaulieu AD, et al. Intraarticular injection of anakinra in osteoarthritis of the knee: a multicenter, randomized, double-blind, placebo-controlled study. Arthritis Rheum 2009;61:344–52.
12. Evans CH, Kraus VB, Setton LA. Progress in intra-articular therapy. Nat Rev Rheumatol 2014;10:11–22.
13. Kraus VB, Birmingham J, Stabler TV, et al. Effects of intraarticular IL1-Ra for acute anterior cruciate ligament knee injury: a randomized controlled pilot trial (NCT00332254). Osteoarthritis Cartilage 2012;20:271–8.
14. Brown C, Toth A, Magnussen R. Clinical benefits of intra-articular anakinra for persistent knee effusion. J Knee Surg 2011;24:61–5.

15. Evans CH, Ghivizzani SC, Robbins PD. Getting arthritis gene therapy into the clinic. Nat Rev Rheumatol 2011;7:244–9.
16. Wehling P, Reinecke J, Baltzer AW, et al. Clinical responses to gene therapy in joints of two subjects with rheumatoid arthritis. Hum Gene Ther 2009;20:97–101.
17. Evans CH, Robbins PD, Ghivizzani SC, et al. Gene transfer to human joints: progress toward a gene therapy of arthritis. Proc Natl Acad Sci U S A 2005;102: 8698–703.
18. Wang G, Evans CH, Benson JM, et al. Safety and biodistribution assessment of sc-rAAV2.5IL-1Ra administered via intra-articular injection in a mono-iodoacetate-induced osteoarthritis rat model. Mol Ther Methods Clin Dev 2016; 3:15052.
19. Hannum CH, Wilcox CJ, Arend WP, et al. Interleukin-1 receptor antagonist activity of a human interleukin-1 inhibitor. Nature 1990;343:336–40.
20. Carter DB, Deibel MR Jr, Dunn CJ, et al. Purification, cloning, expression and biological characterization of an interleukin-1 receptor antagonist protein. Nature 1990;344:633–8.
21. Meijer H, Reinecke J, Becker C, et al. The production of anti-inflammatory cytokines in whole blood by physico-chemical induction. Inflamm Res 2003;52:404–7.
22. Darabos N, Trsek D, Miklic D, et al. Comparison of double-bundle anterior cruciate ligament reconstruction with and without autologous conditioned serum application. Knee Surg Sports Traumatol Arthrosc 2014. [Epub ahead of print].
23. Rutgers M, Saris DB, Dhert WJ, et al. Cytokine profile of autologous conditioned serum for treatment of osteoarthritis, in vitro effects on cartilage metabolism and intra-articular levels after injection. Arthritis Res Ther 2010;12:R114.
24. Wright-Carpenter T, Klein P, Schaferhoff P, et al. Treatment of muscle injuries by local administration of autologous conditioned serum: a pilot study on sportsmen with muscle strains. Int J Sports Med 2004;25:588–93.
25. Baltzer AWA, Drever R, Granrath M, et al. Intraarticular treatment of osteoarthritis using autologous interleukin-1 receptor antagonist (IL-1Ra) conditioned serum. Dtsch Z Sportmed 2003;54:209–11.
26. Baltzer AW, Moser C, Jansen SA, et al. Autologous conditioned serum (orthokine) is an effective treatment for knee osteoarthritis. Osteoarthritis Cartilage 2009;17: 152–60.
27. Yang KG, Raijmakers NJ, van Arkel ER, et al. Autologous interleukin-1 receptor antagonist improves function and symptoms in osteoarthritis when compared to placebo in a prospective randomized controlled trial. Osteoarthritis Cartilage 2008;16:498–505.
28. Rutgers M, Creemers LB, Auw Yang KG, et al. Osteoarthritis treatment using autologous conditioned serum after placebo. Acta Orthop 2015;86:114–8.
29. Baselga Garcia-Escudero J, Miguel Hernandez Trillos P. Treatment of osteoarthritis of the knee with a combination of autologous conditioned serum and physiotherapy: a two-year observational study. PLoS One 2015;10:e0145551.
30. Motaal FK, Elganzoury AM, Fathalla MM, et al. Low-dose intra-articular autologous conditioned serum in treatment of primary knee osteoarthritis. Egyptian Rheumatology and Rehabilitation 2014;41:98–102.
31. Baltzer AW, Ostapczuk MS, Stosch D, et al. A new treatment for hip osteoarthritis: clinical evidence for the efficacy of autologous conditioned serum. Orthop Rev (Pavia) 2013;5:59–64.
32. Darabos N, Haspl M, Moser C, et al. Intraarticular application of autologous conditioned serum (ACS) reduces bone tunnel widening after ACL reconstructive

surgery in a randomized controlled trial. Knee Surg Sports Traumatol Arthrosc 2011;19(Suppl 1):S36–46.

33. Becker C, Heidersdorf S, Drewlo S, et al. Efficacy of epidural perineural injections with autologous conditioned serum for lumbar radicular compression: an investigator-initiated, prospective, double-blind, reference-controlled study. Spine (Phila Pa 1976) 2007;32:1803–8.

34. Goni VG, Singh Jhala S, Gopinathan NR, et al. Efficacy of epidural perineural injection of autologous conditioned serum in unilateral cervical radiculopathy: a pilot study. Spine (Phila Pa 1976) 2015;40:E915–21.

35. Wright-Carpenter T, Opolon P, Appell HJ, et al. Treatment of muscle injuries by local administration of autologous conditioned serum: animal experiments using a muscle contusion model. Int J Sports Med 2004;25:582–7.

36. Heisterbach PE, Todorov A, Fluckiger R, et al. Effect of BMP-12, TGF-beta1 and autologous conditioned serum on growth factor expression in Achilles tendon healing. Knee Surg Sports Traumatol Arthrosc 2012;20:1907–14.

37. Majewski M, Ochsner PE, Liu F, et al. Accelerated healing of the rat achilles tendon in response to autologous conditioned serum. Am J Sports Med 2009; 37:2117–25.

38. Geburek F, Lietzau M, Beineke A, et al. Effect of a single injection of autologous conditioned serum (ACS) on tendon healing in equine naturally occurring tendinopathies. Stem Cell Res Ther 2015;6:126.

39. Hauri S, Hauri M. Autologous conditioned serum generated with the IRAP device. A new therapy for dogs? [abstract]. 35th Annual World Small Animal Veterinary Association Congress. Switzerland (Geneva), June 2-5, 2010.

40. Frisbie DD, Kawcak CE, Werpy NM, et al. Clinical, biochemical, and histologic effects of intra-articular administration of autologous conditioned serum in horses with experimentally induced osteoarthritis. Am J Vet Res 2007;68:290–6.

41. Weinberger T. Clinical experience with ACS/Orthokine/IRAP in horses. Equine Sports Med 2008;3:1–5.

42. Jöstingmeier U, Reinecke J, Hertsch B. Comparison of intraarticuar injection of autologous conditioned serum (ACS, irap) vs sodium hyaluronate and corticosteroid in front limb coffin joint derived lameness [abstract]. Australian Equine Veterinarian 2010;29:75.

43. Österdahl J. Evaluation of autologous conditioned serum. Swedish Uni Agricultural Sci 2008;67:1–16.

44. Zhang W, Robertson J, Jones AC, et al. The placebo effect and its determinants in osteoarthritis: meta-analysis of randomised controlled trials. Ann Rheum Dis 2008;67:1716–23.

45. Meheux CJ, McCulloch PC, Lintner DM, et al. Efficacy of intra-articular platelet-rich plasma injections in knee osteoarthritis: a systematic review. Arthroscopy 2016;32:495–505.

46. Cavallo C, Filardo G, Mariani E, et al. Comparison of platelet-rich plasma formulations for cartilage healing: an in vitro study. J Bone Joint Surg Am 2014;96: 423–9.

47. Smith PA. Intra-articular autologous conditioned plasma injections provide safe and efficacious treatment for knee osteoarthritis: an FDA-sanctioned, randomized, double-BLIND, placebo-controlled clinical trial. Am J Sports Med 2016; 44(4):884–91.

48. King W, van der Weegen W, Van Drumpt R, et al. White blood cell concentration correlates with increased concentrations of IL-1ra and improvement in WOMAC

pain scores in an open-label safety study of autologous protein solution. J Exp Orthop 2016;3:9.

49. Sanchez M, Anitua E, Delgado D, et al. Ultrasound-guided plasma rich in growth factors injections and scaffolds hasten motor nerve functional recovery in an ovine model of nerve crush injury. J Tissue Eng Regen Med 2015. [Epub ahead of print].

50. Gouze JN, Gouze E, Palmer GD, et al. A comparative study of the inhibitory effects of interleukin-1 receptor antagonist following administration as a recombinant protein or by gene transfer. Arthritis Res Ther 2003;5:R301-9.

51. Terada S, Ota S, Kobayashi M, et al. Use of an antifibrotic agent improves the effect of platelet-rich plasma on muscle healing after injury. J Bone Joint Surg Am 2013;95:980-8.

52. Evans CH. Platelet-rich plasma a la carte: commentary on an article by Satoshi Terada, MD, et al.: "use of an antifibrotic agent improves the effect of platelet-rich plasma on muscle healing after injury". J Bone Joint Surg Am 2013;95: e801-2.

α₂-Macroglobulin

Autologous Protease Inhibition Technology

Jason M. Cuéllar, MD, PhD[a], Vanessa Gabrovsky Cuéllar, MD[b],
Gaetano J. Scuderi, MD[c],*

KEYWORDS

- α₂-macroglobulin (A2M) • Inflammation • Anti-inflammatory • Cytokines • Arthritis
- Osteoarthritis • Discogenic back pain • Autologous

KEY POINTS

- A2M has emerged as a potential treatment of cartilage-based pathology and inflammatory arthritis because of its ability to bait and trap inflammatory mediators.
- A2M has been successfully applied to musculoskeletal pathology to decrease pain and modulate cartilage degeneration.
- Autologous A2M can be concentrated from plasma using a unique filtration process.
- New recombinant formulations of A2M can even more precisely target molecular pathways of intra-articular and extra-articular and intervertebral disk disease.

INTRODUCTION

Musculoskeletal conditions causing pain are ubiquitous, making up a large percentage of physician visits each year. Etiology and treatment range widely, and it is not necessarily appropriate to discuss the application of a particular treatment of all aspects of musculoskeletal pain. Musculoskeletal pathology, however, can be generally divided into the following categories:

1. Intra-articular joint pain
2. Extra-articular pain
3. Spinal intervertebral (discogenic) pain

Intra-articular joint pain is most commonly attributed to idiopathic osteoarthritis (OA), posttraumatic OA (PTOA), and other systemic inflammatory arthropathies,

---

[a] Department of Orthopaedic Surgery, Cedars-Sinai Medical Center, 8700 Beverly Boulevard, Los Angeles, CA 90048, USA; [b] 450 North Roxbury Boulevard, Suite 602, Beverly Hills, CA 90210, USA; [c] 210 Jupiter Lakes Boulevard, Suite 3102, Jupiter, FL 33458, USA
* Corresponding author.
E-mail address: scuderimd@aol.com

Phys Med Rehabil Clin N Am 27 (2016) 909–918
http://dx.doi.org/10.1016/j.pmr.2016.06.008
1047-9651/16/© 2016 Elsevier Inc. All rights reserved.

such as rheumatoid arthritis (RA). In recent decades the development of tumor necrosis factor α (TNF-α) inhibitors have been a significant clinical impact on the treatment of RA, providing many patients with significant pain relief and disease progression modification. Unfortunately, no such treatment has been adopted for OA or PTOA. OA is a common problem affecting a large proportion of the population and can affect many joints, including but not limited to the spine, knee, shoulder, hip, fingers, and ankle. It is characterized by progressive cartilage degeneration and loss. Current treatment of OA is limited to physical therapy in attempts to improve joint stabilization, weight loss to reduce joint reactive forces, systemic anti-inflammatory medications (ie, nonsteroidal anti-inflammatory drugs [NSAIDS]) and intra-articular injections of substances, such as steroids or so-called joint lubricants like hyaluronic acid. Physical therapy often has limited benefit, especially as disease progresses, and patients often have difficulty losing weight if physical activity is painful. Systemic NSAIDS can have serious side effects, including gastrointestinal bleeding, and have recently been implicated in cardiac side effects, thus limiting their use. Intra-articular injections of steroids have been demonstrated to have no additional benefit compared with an exercise program alone in a randomized controlled trial[1] and may double the infection rate after total knee or hip replacement.[2] Furthermore, multiple studies have recently brought into question the efficacy of hyaluronic acid injections, leading the American Academy of Orthopaedic Surgeons (AAOS) to withdraw their recommendation of its clinical use.[3] Perhaps most importantly, none of these potential therapies can successfully prevent cartilage degeneration and osteoarthritis.

Distinct from cartilage pathology and osteoarthritis, extra-articular joint pain most commonly involves inflammation of tendons inserting at or near a joint. The most common examples of such enthesopathies are Achilles tendonitis, subacromial bursitis of the rotator cuff, and lateral epicondylitis of the elbow (tennis elbow). These often resolve with activity modification or with a short course of NSAIDS. Persistent enthesopathies can be difficult to treat, however, and have led to many attempts to treat with various types of platelet-rich plasma injections. Several studies have failed to demonstrate a significant benefit, however, with the possible exception of Achilles tendonitis,[4] although this too has been called into question in randomized studies.[5]

Spinal intervertebral discogenic pain is possibly the most controversial musculoskeletal pain etiology — invoking some physicians to question even its existence as a pain generator, whereas others advocate invasive surgical procedures, such as spinal fusion or total disk replacement surgery. The authors believe that discogenic pain does exist but that determining with certainty which particular disk(s) is(are) the source of back pain can be challenging. Nonsurgical treatments for this clinical entity have been limited until recently.[6] There is growing evidence that discogenic pain may be an inflammatory process, without any discrete mechanical pathology.[7] In contrast, spinal radiculopathic pain is caused by compression and/or inflammation of a spinal exiting nerve root, usually by a herniated intervertebral disc. Although this clinical entity most often resolves without surgical treatment approximately 80% to 90% of the time, the remaining cases can be treated successfully by surgical decompression.[8] This pathophysiology of radiculopathic pain should be differentiated from spinal intervertebral discogenic pain, because they are 2 distinct clinical problems.

In the setting of advanced cartilage disease and osteoarthritis, there is little that can be offered patients short of joint replacement. Even in early stages of disease, however, historically there have not been disease-modifying agents that are clinically effective. Discogenic back pain and enthesopathies present a similar challenge, because there has not been any clear effective clinical intervention to mediate the course of disease or symptoms. The concept of biologic rather than surgical treatment of musculoskeletal pathologies has led to the emergence of regenerative interventional therapies. With respect to cartilage degeneration in particular, another goal of emerging biologic therapies is to prevent the onset or progression of arthritides.

Osteoarthritis, for example, is mediated by numerous biomechanical and biochemical processes involved in its pathophysiology. Inflammatory cytokines have been demonstrated to increase production of metalloproteases that degrade cartilage, and the catabolic cartilage products further stimulate production of additional proinflammatory cytokines.[9-13] Recently, increased attention is given to inhibiting metalloproteases involved in cartilage catabolism, with the intention of modulating cartilage breakdown and preventing the cascade of inflammatory mediators involved in disease progression.

α₂-Macroglobulin (A2M) has emerged as a unique potential treatment of cartilage-based pathology and inflammatory arthritides. This article describes the unique method by which A2M can not only inhibit the associated inflammatory cascade but also disrupt the catabolic process of cartilage degeneration. Autologous concentrated A2M from plasma is currently in use by some providers to successfully treat various painful arthritides, including mild to moderate OA, PTOA, enthesopathies. and spinal discogenic back pain.

α₂-MACROGLOBULIN MODULATES THE INFLAMMATORY CASCADE AND CARTILAGE DEGRADATION

Two important biochemical networks that contribute to OA pathology include proinflammatory cytokines and matrix metalloproteinases (MMPs).[7] A2M is a major plasma glycoprotein best known for its ability to inhibit a broad spectrum of serine, threonine, and metalloproteases by a unique bait and trap method (**Fig. 1**).

A2M uses a 39–amino acid bait region that, when cleaved by a protease, induces a large irreversible conformational change that physically traps the protease within a steric cage. As part of the entrapment, the protease forms a covalent bond with A2M, exposing a receptor recognition site, triggering the endocytosis and eventual

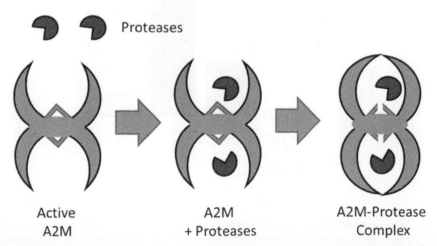

Proteases

| Active A2M | A2M + Proteases | A2M-Protease Complex |

Fig. 1. Pictorial representation of the mechanism by which A2M traps proteases. Each dimer traps a single protease. After the second trapped protease, the molecule then undergoes active transport for its elimination.

clearance of the A2M-protease complex. A2M has also been demonstrated to bind proinflammatory cytokines, such as TNF-α and IL-1β, and reduces the cytokine-induced up-regulation of collagenases in chondrocytes (**Fig. 2**).

Inflammation is an early stage in many painful pathologies, in particular OA, and is mediated primarily by TNF-α, interleukin (IL)-1β, and IL-6 but also involves several other cytokines and chemokines.[11] Along with their roles in mediating the inflammation, TNF-α and IL-1β down-regulate the production of extracellular matrix proteins in chondrocytes[14–16] and induce the up-regulation of MMPs, including those that degrade collagen, such as MMP-1, MMP-3, and MMP-13.[7–9] ADAMTS-4 (a disintegrin and metalloproteinase with thrombospondin motifs) is also up-regulated or activated by IL-1β; however, this is not the case for ADAMTS-5.[17–19] Transgenic mouse models with a modified ADAMTS-5 gene have attenuated OA pathology, suggesting that inhibitors of ADAMTS-5 should be included in any therapy that targets proteases.

The degradative products of cartilage catabolism can in turn stimulate production of inflammatory proteases, in addition to cytokines, which further contributes to increases in inflammatory proteases, specifically elastase and cathepsins.[20] Fragments of fibronectin and collagen are reported to stimulate the production of inflammatory cytokines, chemokines, and MMPs.[21,22] Consequently, the fragments of extracellular matrix proteins, and other degradative products in OA, produced by catabolic proteases might contribute to the inflammatory response that stimulates further protease

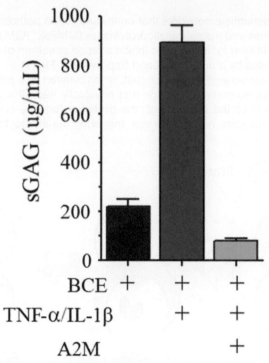

Fig. 2. A2M is chondroprotective against inflammatory cytokines. Treatment of bovine cartilage explants (*blue column*) with proinflammatory cytokines TNF-α and IL-1β (*red column*) induce chondrocytes within the cartilage to produce or activate proteases resulting in increased production of sulfated glycosaminoglycan (sGAG). Treatment with purified human A2M (*green column*) potently inhibited cartilage catabolism. BCE, bovine cartilage explant.

production. Moreover, proteases that cleave aggrecan to release the G3 domain (MMP-2, MMP-7, MMP-9, and MMP-13) are responsible for the formation of the fibronectin-aggrecan complex (FAC).[23]

Fibronectin (an extracellular matrix protein) and its fragments can stimulate cytokine production and activation of MMPs.[22] Aggrecan (a proteoglycan component of articular cartilage) undergoes extensive degeneration during aging and triggers signaling cascades, which augment joint and cartilage damage.[24] This cartilage degradation product, the FAC, has been shown to be associated with joint pathology as well as predict response to lumbar epidural steroid injection in patients with radiculopathy intervertebral disc herniation.[25,26]

A therapeutic agent that prevents the formation of the G3 domain of aggrecan reduces the FAC G3 domain and accordingly may be an efficacious treatment in painful pathophysiology. Because the production of G3 domain of aggrecan is catalyzed by different known classes of proteases, a common inhibitor of all of these proteases may represent an ideal therapeutic agent. This again suggests the potential and proposed mechanism of efficacy of A2M as a multipurpose protease inhibitor and anti-inflammatory mediator.

It has been shown ex vivo that A2M decreases cartilage catabolism, inhibiting the protease activity of ADAMTS-5, metalloproteinases, and other known mediators of the pathologic cartilage catabolism process[27] (see **Fig. 2**). Therefore, the inhibition of ADAMTS-5 and other metalloproteinases and mediators is the probable mechanism of action of A2M as an anticatabolic agent (**Fig. 3**).

Genetically engineered A2M variants with superior inhibition of ADAMTS-5 and other proteinases could further result in enhanced chondroprotection.

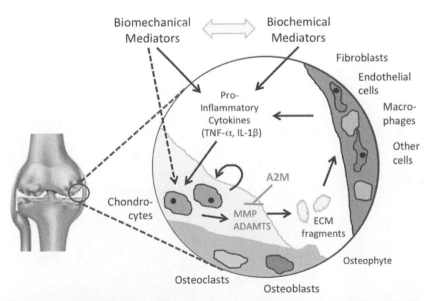

Fig. 3. Schematic of the inflammatory cascade, which occurs in OA — cartilage breakdown leads to extracellular matrix (ECM) breakdown products, such as FAC, which then stimulate the release of inflammatory cytokines, leading to a vicious cycle of further cartilage breakdown (positive feedback loop).

CLINICAL APPLICATION OF α_2-MACROGLOBULIN

A method of A2M concentration from autologous blood has recently been developed (Autologous Platelet Integrated Concentration [APIC]–Cell-Free [Cytonics, West Palm Beach, Florida]) and is currently undergoing a Food and Drug Administration clinical trial for the treatment of mild to moderate knee OA (**Fig. 4**).

A similar autologous formulation of A2M is achieved by APIC protein-rich plasma (Cytonics), which is approved by the Food and Drug Administration and has been used for various musculoskeletal conditions. The system uses a unique filtration step using a tangential flow filter (**Fig. 5**).

The concentration process is an office-based procedure that takes approximately 40 minutes and involves simple venipuncture and blood withdrawal for processing using tabletop centrifugation and ultrafiltration. The procedural steps are briefly as follows (see manufacturer guidelines for details):

1. Fill syringes provided with anticoagulant (acid citrate dextrose solution A [ACD-A]), 7 mL each.
2. Perform venipuncture on patient using standard precautions and fill each syringe with 45 mL blood.
3. Connect a blunt plastic cannula to each of the blood-filled syringes.
4. With cap secured, invert each syringe several times to achieve adequate mixing of blood and anticoagulant.
5. Remove the cap from the blunt plastic cannula and insert the cannula into the septum of the first APIC centrifuge tube.
6. Dispense 45 mL of anticoagulated blood from each syringe into the centrifuge tube. Note: do not invert or tilt the centrifuge tube because fluid may leak from the septum.
7. Load centrifuge tubes into the APIC centrifuge, using balanced technique, then close and lock the centrifuge lid.
8. Select the appropriate cycle and press "START."

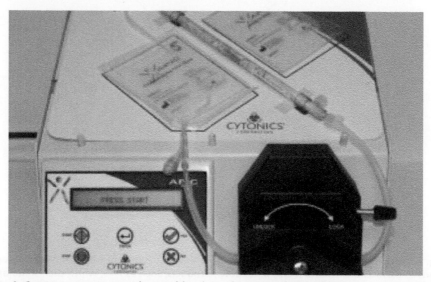

Fig. 4. System to process autologous blood, producing a solution that has approximately 6 times A2M concentration from blood.

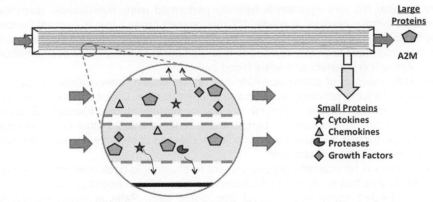

Fig. 5. Tangential flow filtration technology enables concentration of certain large proteins, such as A2M, whereas other smaller proteins, such as inflammatory cytokines, are diluted.

9. The spin cycle is complete after 4 minutes; carefully remove each centrifuge tube.
10. Connect the 60-mL syringe to the plasma collection needle.
11. Insert the plasma collection needle into the first centrifuge tube to a level 1 cm above the buffy coat.
12. Slowly collect 15 mL of plasma into the syringe, maintaining the position of the needle tip 1 cm above the buffy coat. Do not disturb the surface of the buffy coat. Repeat with other tubes.
13. Secure the syringe contents during transfer to the Concentration Kit.
14. Place the Concentration Kit onto the pump platform and press "Enter" on the pump keypad.
15. Remove the plasma collection needle from the syringe containing 45 mL of plasma and immediately connect the syringe to the blue port of the concentration bag.
16. Inject the plasma into the concentration bag and press "Enter" on the pump keypad.
17. Disconnect and discard the empty 60-mL syringe.
18. Load the tube into the pump head, lock the pump head lever, and press "START" on the pump keypad.
19. The process is complete in 20 minutes and will read "APIC Ready."
20. Immediately after the cycle completion, engage the white clamp on the waste bag tubing to prevent dilution.
21. Connect a syringe to the blue port of APIC Concentration Bag and draw the concentrated plasma into the syringe.
22. Disconnect the syringe containing the concentrated plasma.
23. Mix the concentrated plasma with autograft or allograft bone if indicated.
24. Apply concentrated A2M to appropriate clinical site.

There are several distinct clinical applications of autologous solutions rich in A2M, which have shown promising results to date. This includes treatment of intra-articular and extra-articular joint pain as well as spinal discogenic pain.[22,24] Mild to moderate OA of the knee, hip, and shoulder have been successfully treated with intra-articular injection of approximately 2 mL to 4 mL of A2M-rich concentrated plasma via APIC, with many patients experiencing pain relief for 6 months or more. Standard injection techniques familiar to orthopedists, rheumatologists, and physiatrists are used, such as the suprapatellar or anterolateral injection portal of the knee.

Intra-articular hip joint injection is typically performed using fluoroscopic guidance to ensure proper location. A phase 1/2 randomized control trial is currently under way to test the ability of a cell-free version of A2M-rich concentrate for the treatment of mild to moderate knee OA. The cell-free version contains similar A2M concentration while eliminating platelets and white blood cells.

Similarly, injection of autologous A2M-rich concentrate has been applied to painful extra-articular joint pathology, such as subacromial bursitis, lateral epicondylitiss, and Achilles tendonitis, with excellent clinical results in small studies (Gaetano Scuderi, 2016, personal communication). Large clinical trials of these pathologies have not yet been performed because these conditions are less commonly encountered than OA of the knee, hip, and shoulder.

When there is an inflammatory component to discogenic back pain, as evidenced by patients who test positive for FAC within the disc, A2M concentrate has also successfully treated spinal intervertebral discogenic pain. Patients report significant reduction in pain (4.9 mean improvement in Visual Analog Scale) and improved Oswestry Disability Index (ODI) scores (37-point mean ODI reduction) at the end of a 6-month study period.[28]

FUTURE DIRECTIONS

The early clinical success of A2M supplementation to a variety of musculoskeletal conditions is encouraging. Larger, prospective clinical trials are anticipated that may further support these preliminary results. The application of A2M is distinct from other autologous treatments, because its development is firmly grounded in a proposed mechanism of action based on understanding of cartilage pathology and inflammatory pain. Based on this science, the next step is to attempt to further improve on wild-type A2M mechanism, to perhaps more specifically address or augment its role in the pathophysiology at the site of disease. Genetic modifications of A2M are already under way, and several candidates demonstrate superior ability to modulate cartilage degeneration, for instance, compared with the wild type. Early evidence using reverse transcriptase–polymerase chain reaction shows up-regulation of collagen type 2 and aggrecan, precursors for cartilage regeneration. In some instances, these modifications specifically target metalloproteases known to be involved in OA and the development of joint pain. Further clinical characterization of these modified variants is anticipated, along with the ability to specifically target known pathologic mechanisms of disease progression. The development of a recombinant variant for clinical use will further enhance the clinical success of A2M in the treatment of musculoskeletal disease.

REFERENCES

1. Henriksen M, Christensen R, Klokker L, et al. Evaluation of the benefit of corticosteroid injection before exercise therapy in patients with osteoarthritis of the knee: a randomized clinical trial. JAMA Intern Med 2015;175(6):923–30.
2. Xing D, Yang Y, Ma X, et al. Dose intraarticular steroid injection increase the rate of infection in subsequent arthroplasty: grading the evidence through a meta-analysis. J Orthop Surg Res 2014;9:107.
3. Treatment of Osteoarthritis of the Knee, 2nd ed., AAOS, Recommendation 9. Available at: www.AAOS.org.
4. Guelfi M, Pantalone A, Vanni D, et al. Long-term beneficial effects of platelet-rich plasma for non-insertional Achilles tendinopathy. Foot Ankle Surg 2015;21(3): 178–81.

5. de Vos RJ, Weir A, van Schie HT, et al. Platelet-rich plasma injection for chronic Achilles tendinopathy: a randomized controlled trial. JAMA 2010;303(2):144–9.
6. Lu Y, Guzman JZ, Purmessur D, et al. Nonoperative management of discogenic back pain: a systematic review. Spine (Phila Pa 1976) 2014;39(16):1314–24.
7. Ohtori S, Inoue G, Miyagi M, et al. Pathomechanisms of discogenic low back pain in humans and animal models. Spine J 2015;15(6):1347–55.
8. Saal JA, Saal JS. Nonoperative treatment of herniated lumbar intervertebral disc with radiculopathy: an outcome study. Spine (Phila Pa 1976) 1989;14:431–7.
9. Tetlow LC, Adlam DJ, Woolley DE. Matrix metalloproteinase and proinflammatory cytokine production by chondrocytes of human osteoarthritic cartilage: associations with degenerative changes. Arthritis Rheum 2001;44(3):585–94.
10. Mengshol JA, Vincenti MP, Coon CI, et al. Interleukin-1 induction of collagenase 3 (matrix metalloproteinase 13) gene expression in chondrocytes requires p38, c-Jun N-terminal kinase, and nuclear factor kappaB: differential regulation of collagenase 1 and collagenase 3. Arthritis Rheum 2000;43(4):801–11.
11. Lefebvre V, Peeters-Joris C, Vaes G. Modulation by interleukin 1 and tumor necrosis factor alpha of production of collagenase, tissue inhibitor of metalloproteinases and collagen types in differentiated and dedifferentiated articular chondrocytes. Biochim Biophys Acta 1990;1052(3):366–78.
12. Reboul P, Pelletier JP, Tardif G, et al. The new collagenase, collagenase-3, is expressed and synthesized by human chondrocytes but not by synoviocytes. A role in osteoarthritis. J Clin Invest 1996;97(9):2011–9.
13. Kapoor M, Martel-Pelletier J, Lajeunesse D, et al. Role of proinflammatory cytokines in the pathophysiology of osteoarthritis. Nat Rev Rheumatol 2011;7(1): 33–42.
14. Saklatvala J. Tumour necrosis factor alpha stimulates resorption and inhibits synthesis of proteoglycan in cartilage. Nature 1986;322(6079):547–9.
15. Goldring MB, Fukuo K, Birkhead JR, et al. Transcriptional suppression by interleukin-1 and interferon-gamma of type II collagen gene expression in human chondrocytes. J Cell Biochem 1994;54(1):85–99.
16. Stove J, Huch K, Günther KP, et al. Interleukin-1beta induces different gene expression of stromelysin, aggrecan and tumor-necrosis-factor-stimulated gene 6 in human osteoarthritic chondrocytes in vitro. Pathobiology 2000;68(3):144–9.
17. Glasson SS, Askew R, Sheppard B, et al. Deletion of active ADAMTS5 prevents cartilage degradation in a murine model of osteoarthritis. Nature 2005;434(7033): 644–8.
18. Rogerson FM, Chung YM, Deutscher ME, et al. Cytokine-induced increases in ADAMTS-4 messenger RNA expression do not lead to increased aggrecanase activity in ADAMTS-5-deficient mice. Arthritis Rheum 2010;62(11):3365–73.
19. Tortorella MD, Malfait AM, Deccico C, et al. The role of ADAM-TS4 (aggrecanase-1) and ADAM-TS5 (aggrecanase-2) in a model of cartilage degradation. Osteoarthr Cartil 2001;9(6):539–52.
20. Miller RE, Lu Y, Tortorella MD, et al. Genetically engineered mouse models reveal the importance of proteases as osteoarthritis drug targets. Curr Rheumatol Rep 2013;15(8):350.
21. Fichter M, Körner U, Schömburg J, et al. Collagen degradation products modulate matrix metalloproteinase expression in cultured articular chondrocytes. J Orthop Res 2006;24(1):63–70.
22. Homandberg GA, Wen C, Hui F. Cartilage damaging activities of fibronectin fragments derived from cartilage and synovial fluid. Osteoarthr Cartil 1998;6(4): 231–44.

23. Scuderi GJ, Woolf N, Dent K, et al. Identification of a complex between fibronectin and aggrecan G3 domain in synovial fluid of patients with painful meniscal pathology. Clin Biochem 2010;43:808–14.
24. Oshita H, Sandy JD, Suzuki K, et al. Mature bovine articular cartilage contains abundant aggrecan that is C-terminally truncated at Ala719-Ala720, a site which is readily cleaved by m-calpain. Biochem J 2004;382(Pt 1):253–9.
25. Scuderi GJ, Golish SR, Cook FF, et al. Identification of a novel fibronectin-aggrecan complex in the synovial fluid of knees with painful meniscal injury. J Bone Joint Surg Am 2011;93:336–40.
26. Scuderi GJ, Cuellar JM, Cuellar VG, et al. Epidural interferon gamma immunoreactivity: a biomarker for lumbar nerve root irritation. Spine (Phila Pa 1976) 2009; 34(21):2311–7.
27. Wang S, Wei X, Zhou J, et al. Identification of alpha2-macroglobulin as a master inhibitor of cartilage-degrading factors that attenuates the progression of post-traumatic osteoarthritis. Arthritis Rheumatol 2014;66(7):1843–53.
28. Scuderi GJ, Montesano PX, Cuellar J. Improving response to treatment for patients with DDD With the use of the fibronectin-aggrecan complex: Med Sci Sports Exerc 2016 May;48(5 Suppl 1):511–2.

Performing a Better Bone Marrow Aspiration

Mayo F. Friedlis, MD[a],*, Christopher J. Centeno, MD[b]

KEYWORDS

- Bone marrow aspiration • Bone marrow aspiration technique
- Bone marrow stem cells • Stem cells • Image-guided bone marrow aspiration

KEY POINTS

- Bone marrow aspiration (BMA) is the technique used to harvest stem cells for use in regenerative medicine.
- The use of ultrasound or fluoroscopy guidance represents an advance over traditional palpation-guided techniques. BMA combining anesthesia with guidance can improve patient comfort.
- Newer techniques for BMA allows for higher yields of stem cells.
- Patient preparation, equipment, anesthesia, use of guidance, and medical and other considerations for performing BMA are important.

INTRODUCTION

Patients often consider bone marrow aspiration (BMA) to be painful and difficult. Traditionally, BMAs were often performed using palpation-guided techniques that may work well in thin patients but were uncomfortable for most patients and difficult in heavier patients. Additionally, the authors' experience suggests that this procedure is often not performed in a way that maximizes yield. This article helps physicians understand how to obtain the highest possible stem cell yield while reducing patient discomfort.

BASIC SCIENCE OF STEM CELLS

The International Society for Cellular Therapy definition of a mesenchymal stem cell (MSC)[1] includes a cell line that

- Is plastic adherent
- Expresses CD105, CD73, and CD90 and lacks expression of CD45, CD34, CD14 or CD11b, CD79alpha or CD19, and HLA-DR surface molecules
- Must be capable of trilineage differentiation to osteoblasts, adipocytes, and chondroblasts in vitro

---

[a] Stem Cell Arts, 5550 Friendship Blvd, Chevy Chase, MD 20815, USA; [b] Centeno Schultz Clinic, 403 Summit Blvd, Suite 201, Broomfield, CO 80021, USA
* Corresponding author.
E-mail address: mfriedlis@gmail.com

Phys Med Rehabil Clin N Am 27 (2016) 919–939
http://dx.doi.org/10.1016/j.pmr.2016.06.009
1047-9651/16/© 2016 Elsevier Inc. All rights reserved.

Stem cells are part of the body's natural healing processes. They are responsible for repair of injured tissues in the body on an ongoing basis.[2] Hence, healing can be enhanced by injecting or surgically placing stem cells into damaged or injured areas.

A recent PubMed search for *mesenchymal stem cells* reveals more than 40,000 publications.[3] Some studies have shown that MSCs can heal cartilage, bone, ligament, and tendon.[4-7] Interventional orthopedics is the use of percutaneous techniques under imaging guidance to deliver MSCs and other orthobiologics to promote healing and avoid the need for surgery. There are early clinical data to suggest that, in the future, many orthopedic conditions that previously required surgical intervention may be treatable with guided placement of MSCs.

Later the authors provide an overview of the types of stem cells available in bone marrow (**Fig. 1**).

Mesenchymal Stem Cells

MSCs, also known as marrow stromal cells or colony-forming fibroblasts, are multipotent adult stem cells that have shown clinical potential as therapeutic agents in regenerative medicine.[8-13] They are derived from other mesodermal tissues. Experiments in the 1980s and 1990s demonstrated that local environmental factors cause MSCs to differentiate into different cell types. For example, culturing MSCs with ascorbic acid, inorganic phosphate, or dexamethasone causes them to differentiate into osteoblasts, whereas exposure to transforming growth factor beta causes them to differentiate into chondrocytes.[11] More recent research has revealed that MSCs are actually a heterogeneous population of similar cells rather than one distinct cell type.[14]

Hematopoietic Stem Cells

Hematopoietic stem cells (HSCs) are stem cells that are responsible for the production of blood; they are also secondarily involved in muscle repair.[15] In the body they are recruited from the bone marrow when local muscle satellite cells are unable to complete muscle repair.

Endothelial Progenitor Cells

Endothelial progenitor cells are recruited from bone marrow to facilitate vascular homeostasis and neovasculogenesis.[16] This cell type may be useful for reestablishing vascularity in chronically injured musculoskeletal tissues.

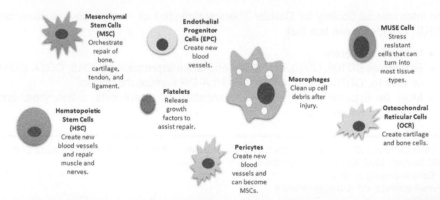

Fig. 1. The bone marrow contains many cells in addition to stem cells to help with orthopedic injuries. The focus of a BMA is to maximize MSC yield. MUSE, multilineage differentiating stress enduring. (*Courtesy of* Christopher J. Centeno, MD, Broomfield, Colorado.)

Pericytes

Pericytes reside around blood vessels and are recruited from the bone marrow for neovasculogenesis.[17] Some investigators have suggested that they can differentiate into MSCs when injuries occur.[18]

Osteochondral Reticular Cells

These stem cells are concentrated in the metaphysis of long bones but not in the perisinusoidal space. They can differentiate into osteoblasts, chondrocytes, and reticular marrow stromal cells.[19]

Multilineage Differentiating Stress-Enduring Cells

Multilineage differentiating stress-enduring cells can differentiate into endoderm, mesoderm, and ectoderm. They are activated by physical stress and act as a reserve cell source. They are also involved in regenerative homeostasis and tissue repair.[20]

Although bone marrow contains many types of stem and other cells to help orthopedic injuries, the focus of a BMA is to maximize MSC yield.

BASIC SCIENCE OF BONE MARROW AND BONE MARROW ASPIRATION

Drilling into the bone marrow is one of the oldest known medical procedures, with evidence dating back more than 7000 years.[21] The first attempts to obtain an actual bone marrow sample for diagnostic reasons were independently undertaken by Pianese (Italy) and Wolff (Germany) in 1903.[22] The modern Jamshidi needle (**Fig. 2**), first described in 1971,[23] is a commonly used tool for entering the bone marrow cavity.

SAFETY, INDICATIONS, CONTRAINDICATIONS, MEDICATIONS, AND PATIENT PREPARATION

BMA has been performed safely for more than 30 years. A large European Union registry including BMA and bone marrow biopsy shows a serious adverse event

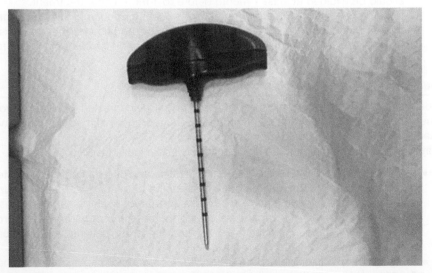

Fig. 2. A Jamshidi needle is one of several types of trocars that can be used in BMA. (*Courtesy of* Christopher J. Centeno, MD, Broomfield, Colorado.)

rate of 16 in 27,700 procedures. There was one fatality from pulmonary embolism. Pain at the draw site is the most common adverse event.[24]

Indications

BMA is indicated for treatment the following conditions:

- Osteoarthritis[25]
- Tears of ligaments or tendons[26,27]
- Avascular necrosis[5]

Contraindications

BMA is contraindicated in the following circumstances:

- There is significant anemia; check hematocrit (Hct) if unsure.
- There is local or systemic infection.
- There is active hematologic neoplasm, even if in treatment.
- There is anticoagulant treatment that cannot be stopped for the procedure.
- Patients are unable to be positioned for the procedure.
- There is immune compromise. Patients with immune compromise should not be treated.
- Cancer may be a contraindication. A recent study showed no increased risk of tumor growth when stem cells were used in conjunction with resection of bone cancer and graft placement[28]
- Rheumatoid disease: The authors have treated patients with rheumatoid disease provided they are not in an acute inflammatory phase. The effects of immunosuppressant or biological therapies for rheumatologic diseases on the efficacy of stem cell treatment are unknown.
- Medications: Some medications must be avoided:
  ○ Because of its antiinflammatory and antianabolic effects, prednisone is contraindicated for 4 to 6 weeks before treatment.[29]
  ○ Statins seem to have a very negative effect on stem cell proliferation and should be avoided at least 1 month before to 1 month after treatment.[30]
  ○ Nonsteroidal antiinflammatory medications seem to reduce platelet aggregation and function.[31] In the experience of one of the authors, they may also reduce MSC proliferation. They should be avoided for 1 week before and for 6 weeks after treatment.

Patient Selection, Body Size, and Positioning

Older patients may have fewer stem cells. They can still be harvested, but a larger volume of bone marrow will be needed to compensate. If properly stimulated, they have been shown to work adequately for tissue repair.[32]

Imaging and BMA can be more challenging in certain individuals:

- Body mass index (BMI): BMI, within limits, is not a predictive factor for knee osteoarthritis outcome[25] but may be more challenging to perform. Larger body size and habitus increase the amount of excess soft tissue to be penetrated; these cases will require longer trocars, which will increase the opportunity for error and pain. The standard trocar is 3.5 in, and for larger patients a 6-in trocar may be required.
- Imaging is more difficult in larger individuals. Fluoroscopic imaging may be beneficial for guidance in these individuals when compared with ultrasound. The ideal position for performing BMA at the posterior superior iliac crest (PSIS) is prone

because it allows for the proper imaging of the multiple draw sites[33] located in that area. If patients cannot assume this position easily, it is possible to cannulate the anterior superior iliac crest (ASIS). Such cases are best left for experienced practitioners, as the lateral anterior femoral cutaneous nerve is located here.
- Larger patients and those with respiratory problems may have increased difficulty with respiration in the prone position. The authors recommend that new practitioners gain experience before taking on more challenging cases or refer them to experienced practitioners.

How Much Bone Marrow Aspiration Can Be Safely Drawn?

These guidelines are based on the authors' experience and patient size:

- Small woman/child (90–105 lb): no more than 50 mL
- Average woman, small man, or a patient with lower Hct (105–150 Hct): 60 to 70 mL
- Larger man/woman (150–250 lb): up to 120 mL

General Bone Marrow Aspiration Volume Requirements for Different Joints

These guidelines are based on the authors' experience:

- Bilateral knee osteoarthritis (OA): 120 mL
- Unilateral knee OA: 60 to 90 mL
- Medium joint (elbow/transverse tarsal joint axis (TT) ankle): 60 mL
- Small joint/intervertebral disc (IVD): 40 to 60 mL
- Very small joint (finger/foot single): 30 mL one side

PREPARATION FOR BONE MARROW ASPIRATION
Types of Trocars and Differing Techniques

- The bone can be penetrated using either a hand trocar or a commercially available powered driver, such as the one shown in **Fig. 8C**. The choice of tool will depend on the patients' age and bone density and physician preference. Some physicians may prefer a hand trocar; others will prefer a powered driver.
- Bone hardness changes across the lifecycle and becomes softer with age. A greater effort will be required to penetrate the bone of younger individuals and athletes.
- Hand trocars are recommended for older patients (55 years or older) or those with osteoporosis; use of a driver could result in overpenetration.

Maximizing Mesenchymal Stem Cells
Yield

- To maximize MSC yield, the authors recommend targeting the posterior superior iliac spine (**Fig. 3**) because it contains more MSCs than other bone aspiration sites like the tibia.[33]
- As shown in **Fig. 4**, the ilium has a thick portion and a thin portion. The thickest part of the ilium is the target.
- Drawing small volumes (5–15 mL) from many sites increases MSC yield; drawing a large volume (more than 10–15 mL) from a single bone site reduces MSC yield.[34–36]
- MSCs reside in the subcortical areas; pericytes reside around blood vessels. Penetrating the bone marrow space probably dislodges cortical and perivascular pericytes (**Fig. 5**).

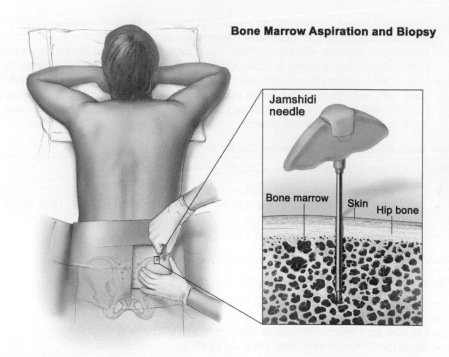

Bone Marrow Aspiration and Biopsy

Jamshidi needle

Bone marrow   Skin   Hip bone

Fig. 3. This image shows a patient lying prone on a table, prepped and draped for BMA from the posterior superior iliac spine. (*Courtesy of* Terese Winslow LLC, Alexandria, Virginia. 2016; with permission.)

- Drawing from more sites maximizes subcortical MSC yield and allows access to pericytes.
- There are other strategies for drawing stem cells. Some practitioners call for going deeper into the marrow and extracting cells at different depths through side port trocars, such as the one shown in **Fig. 6**.[37] There are no published data on the efficacy of this method with regard to improving MSC yield.
- Others practitioners suggest using the same entry position and manipulating the trocar to get different areas of the marrow. Again, no data exist on the relative efficacy of this technique over simply penetrating the cortex at multiple sites (**Fig. 7**).
- In the authors' experience and based on the peer-reviewed literature cited, using multiple small-volume (5–10 mL) draw sites produces the highest yield.
- MSCs reside in the subcortical areas; pericytes reside around blood vessels.[38] Drawing from more sites maximizes subcortical MSC yield and allows access to pericytes.

Equipment and Supplies

The following supplies are required for a 60-mL bone marrow draw (**Fig. 8**):

- 20 mL 0.5% ropivacaine, 27-gauge 0.5-in skin needle, 22-gauge 3.5-4.0 11/16-in needle
- Sterile, disposable, 11-gauge Jamshidi trocars, 2-gauge, or similar, power drill with bit
- Scalpel blade (if a drill is to be used)

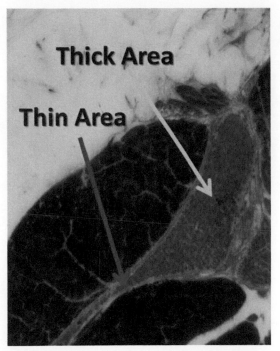

Fig. 4. Cross section of the iliac crest showing thick and thin areas. Penetrating the thin area of the pelvis increases the likelihood of passing through the marrow space. The thick area has a large marrow space with less risk of passing through the marrow-rich area and much higher likelihood of drawing whole marrow. (*Courtesy of* Christopher J. Centeno, MD, Broomfield, Colorado.)

- 5 mL syringe with 5000 IU of heparin in normal saline
- Two 30-mL syringes each preloaded with 30,000 IU of heparin (1000 IU of heparin for each milliliter)
- Steri-Strips (3M, St Paul, MN), gauze, tape

Guidance

- Using guidance, either fluoroscopy or ultrasound (US), allows greater precision with anesthesia and placement of the trocar.
- Guidance allows the ilium to be penetrated at predefined intervals to maximize MSC harvest.
- The authors think that using guidance for stem cell aspiration should be the standard of care; the authors discuss advantages and disadvantages of each type next.

Fluoroscopy

- In the authors' experience, fluoroscopy is easier to learn, and it facilitates exact placement of the trocar within the anesthetized area. Bony landmarks identified with the fluoroscope help with targeting specific sites.
- Fluoroscopy is more comfortable for patients, as there is less soft tissue to be penetrated (because of the steeper insertion vector) than with the US approach. Fluoroscopy also makes it easier to manipulate the trocar.

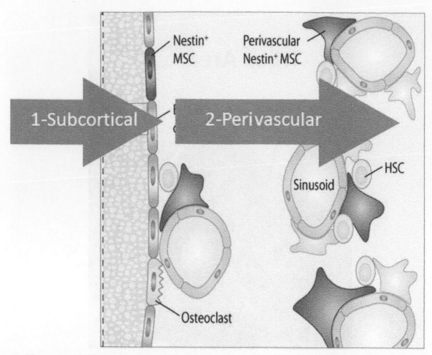

Fig. 5. There are 2 opportunities to dislodge marrow MSCs. (*Courtesy of* Christopher J. Centeno, MD, Broomfield, Colorado.)

Ultrasound

- US does not expose patients or the physician to radiation.
- US does not require a large procedural suite. US makes it more challenging to position the trocar within the anesthetized area and to achieve proper depth. Use of a skin marker can help.
- US will require a larger anesthetized area because the trocar will have to travel a longer distance through the soft tissue.

TECHNICAL CONSIDERATIONS
Patient Preparation

- Position patients prone with a pillow under the abdomen to minimize lordosis in the lumbar spine. Sterilely prep and drape the area over the PSIS (**Fig. 9**).
- For volumes of more than 30 mL of BMA, both left and right iliac crests must be prepped and draped.
- **Fig. 10** shows the target sites for BMA.

Anesthesia Notes

Anesthesia dramatically reduces patient discomfort. However, care must be taken in the selection of anesthetics because some are toxic to stem cells. Lidocaine and Marcaine are toxic and should not be used for BMA. Ropivacaine seems to be safe at lower concentrations.[39] Although local anesthesia is very effective at preventing discomfort from the bone marrow drilling procedure, some patients may experience pain when BMA is drawn out of the bone marrow cavity.

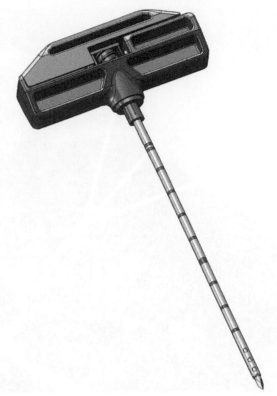

Fig. 6. BMA needle featuring side ports (only) manufactured by Marrow Cellutions. (*Courtesy of* Ranfac Corp, Avon, MA; with permission.)

Critical Importance of Clot Prevention

- Clots trap stem cells and make them unavailable for their intended use.
- If a commercial closed system is used for preparation, clot formation will not be evident to the operator.
- Heparin, administered through the trocar, is used to prevent clotting before the aspirate is drawn out. The amounts are listed later.
- Preload the syringe to be used for withdrawing the aspirate with heparin. The amounts and volumes for each of these are noted later.

BONE MARROW ASPIRATION STEP-BY-STEP
Positioning of Guidance

- With patients positioned on the table, prepped, and draped, position the guidance. Select (A) or (B):
  - (A) Fluoroscopy: Orient the beam of the x-ray 15° ipsilateral oblique. This placement will expand the view of the target sites allowing for an easier approach (**Fig. 11**).
  - (B) US: Identify the direction of the US head needed to perform the aspiration. A curved low-frequency probe is used (**Fig. 12**).
    - The target is the thick part of the ilium. On the US screen the thickest part of the ilium appears like a mountain of bone. Cannulate the thick part of this mountain (**Fig. 13**).

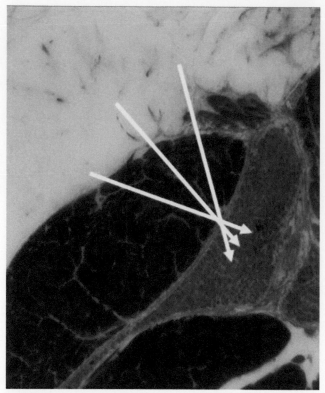

Fig. 7. The single-entry, multiple-direction draw technique. *Arrows*, orientation of the trocar. (*Courtesy of* Christopher J. Centeno, MD, Broomfield, Colorado.)

- Use sterile gel and gloves.
- Use a skin marking pen to mark all the different locations that will be needed to accomplish 3 to 5 aspirations (**Fig. 14**).

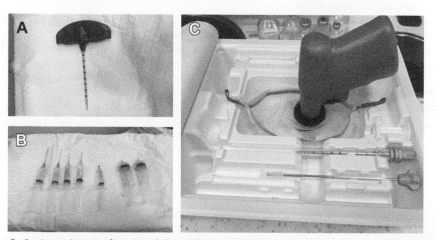

Fig. 8. Basic equipment for BMA: (*A*) Jamshidi needle, (*B*) syringes, and (*C*) Arrow OnControl Driver. (*Courtesy of* Teleflex Inc, Morrisville, NC; with permission.)

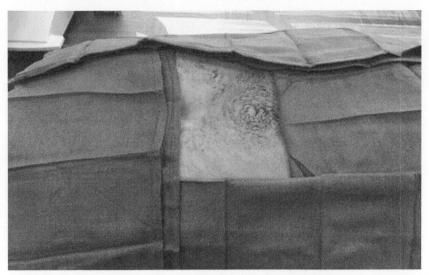

Fig. 9. A patient lying prone, prepped for BMA. (*Courtesy of* Christopher J. Centeno, MD, Broomfield, Colorado.)

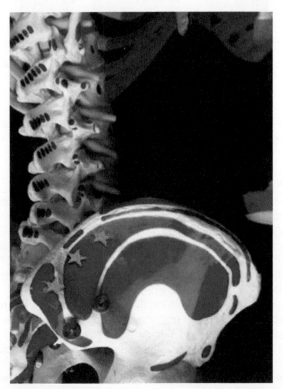

Fig. 10. Model of the ilium showing the target sites for BMA. (*Courtesy of* Christopher J. Centeno, MD, Broomfield, Colorado.)

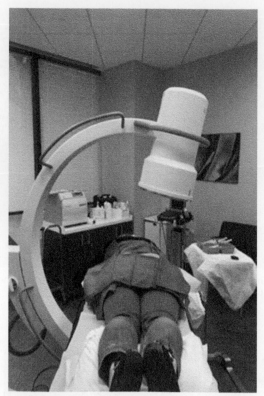

Fig. 11. The Ziehm Solo fluoroscope is at 15° ipsilateral to PSIS. (*Courtesy of* Ziehm Imaging, Inc, Orlando, FL; with permission.)

■ Start all aspirations from a point lateral on the ilium using a single skin puncture. Align the US head with these preset markings, for both anesthetization and penetration of the cortex (see **Fig. 14**).

Apply Anesthesia

- Identify a starting point that will allow access to 3 to 5 different sites on the ilium from one location (see **Fig. 14**).
- Anesthetize with a large skin weal, approximately 1 cm.
- Anesthetize each target using an appropriate length, with a 22- to 25-gauge needle.
- Identify the first target approximately 1 cm from the edge along the posterior surface of the ilium.
- Care should be taken not to perform this procedure too far laterally or inferior to the sacroiliac (SI) joint in order to protect the superior cluneal nerves and the superior gluteal nerve, artery and vein (NAV) bundle (**Fig. 15**).
- Care should be taken to penetrate the periosteum with anesthesia at each target site.
- Move the needle in a circular fashion to anesthetize an area about 2 cm in diameter. Use about 7 mL of anesthetic for this injection point and the tract leading up to it (**Fig. 16**).

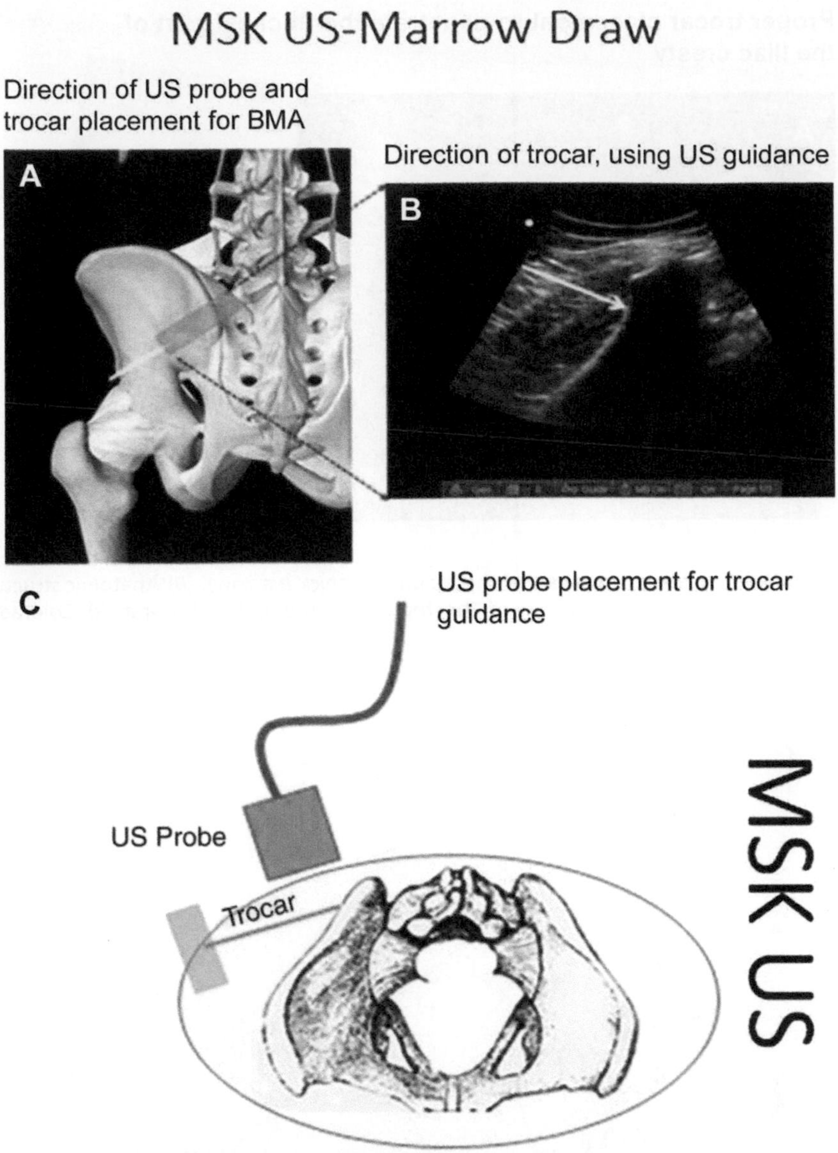
MSK US-Marrow Draw
Direction of US probe and trocar placement for BMA
A
Direction of trocar, using US guidance
B
C
US probe placement for trocar guidance
US Probe
Trocar
MSK US

Fig. 12. (*A*) US head orientation to the ilium, (*B*) the view on the US machine of the appropriate approach of anesthetizing needle or trocar, and (*C*) the relationship of the trocar and US head to the pelvis. MSK, musculoskeletal. *Arrows* show orientation of the trocar. (*Courtesy of* Christopher J. Centeno, MD, Broomfield, Colorado.)

- The second target (and any subsequent targets) will be about 2 cm from the first one, about 1 cm from the edge of the ilium. Anesthetize as before.

Penetrate the Bone

- Select either a hand trocar or a powered driver. Most cases can be done using a Jamshidi trocar, especially in patients 55 years or older, whose bones may be too

Proper trocar placement to penetrate the thickest part of the Iliac crestv

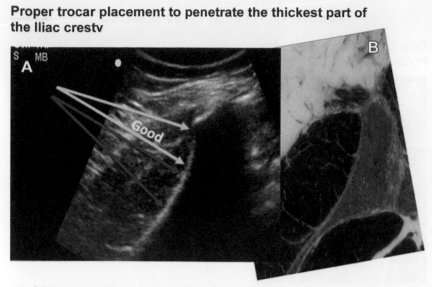

Fig. 13. (A) Cannulate the top part of the mountain (*thick marrow*). (B) Anatomic structure depicted on the US screen. (*Courtesy of* Christopher J. Centeno, MD, Broomfield, Colorado.)

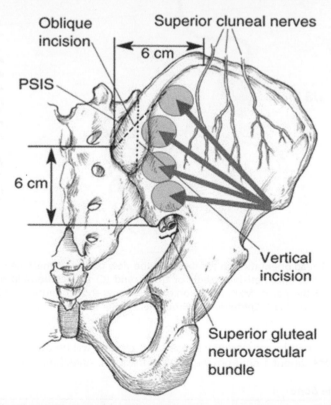

Fig. 14. Draw site targets. One skin site, multiple bone targets. (*Courtesy of* Christopher J. Centeno, MD, Broomfield, Colorado.)

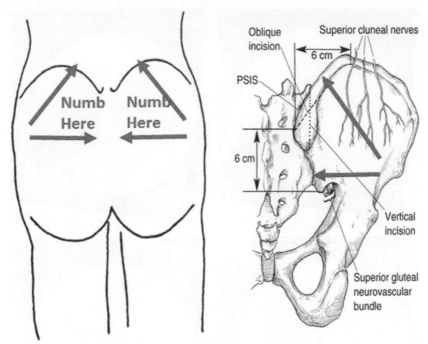

Fig. 15. Target site for anesthesia, relative to the SI joint, the gluteal nerves, and the superior gluteal NAV bundle. (*Courtesy of* Christopher J. Centeno, MD, Broomfield, Colorado.)

osteoporotic to make the drill safe. For younger patients and athletes, a driver will probably make the job much faster and easier.

- o A trocar can pierce the skin without a scalpel wound. A commercially available drill bit may not be as easy to introduce and will require a scalpel wound. **Fig. 17** shows the shape, size, and depth of the scalpel wound.
- **Fig. 17**A shows the size and shape of the scalpel wound, and **Fig. 17**B shows the necessary depth of penetration. The pelvis is spherical. The trocar/driver will be on the inside of the sphere pushing out. Drilling on a curved surface is challenging. If the trocar/driver slides slide down into nonanesthetized soft tissue or over the top of the ilium, patients will experience pain and possible complications.
- To prevent errors, approach the ilium perpendicular, or at a right angle, to the surface of the curvature. The exact angle will differ for each of the 3 to 5 penetrations to be performed, as each will be in a different part of the curve. It is a good idea to recheck the direction and make corrections, if needed.
- Tap the trocar with the hand to penetrate the skin. Then advance the trocar or drill through the anesthetized area, down to the bone.
- Patients should feel only the pressure of the trocar or driver but no pain. If patients experience pain, the trocar/driver may be outside the anesthetized area. Reposition the trocar to find the planned location or reapply anesthesia. Query patients to ensure there is no pain.
- To maintain control, advance the trocar with small oscillations of the hand, turning the handle back and forth while applying pressure, rather than rotating it completely. There will be a decrease in resistance when the cortex is penetrated and the marrow cavity is entered. This depth is the target depth. Patients may feel discomfort when this depth is reached.

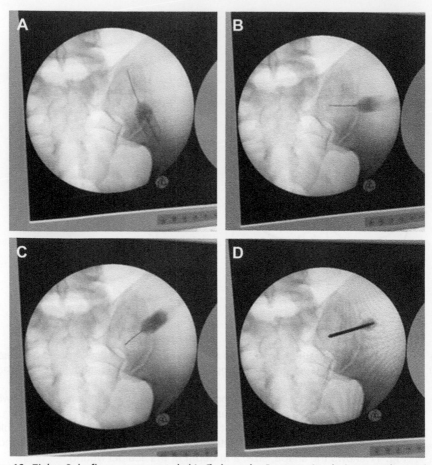

Fig. 16. Ziehm Solo fluoroscope panels (*A–C*) show the 3 target sites being anesthetized using fluoroscopic guidance. (*D*) The trocar placed at the same site that was anesthetized. (*Courtesy of* Ziehm Imaging, Inc, Orlando, FL; with permission.)

- When using a drill, operate it continuously rather than pulsing it. This continuous operation will make it easier to sense, both by the sound of the drill and the resistance, when the marrow cavity is entered.
- When the trocar/driver reaches the marrow cavity, it should be firmly stuck in the bone. If it is loose, continue drilling until the trocar/driver is solidly in the bone. In addition, most commercial trocars and drill bits have a 1-cm marking system that should also help determine how far the tip is advancing.
- For either method, you can tell if the trocar is solidly implanted in bone by performing a tap test. Take one finger and tap on the end of the trocar. If it feels solid, then it is firmly implanted in bone. If it is loose or moves, it needs to be further advanced.
- To prevent clots, remove the inner stylet. Inject approximately 0.3 to 0.5 mL of heparin in normal saline, 500 to 750 IU/mL, through the trocar and into the bone marrow.

Withdraw the Aspirate

- Attach one of the 30-mL syringes preloaded with 30,000 IU of heparin in normal saline (total volume 3–5 mL) and begin withdrawing bone marrow.

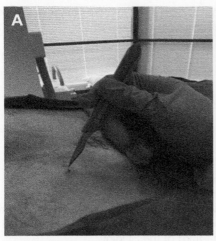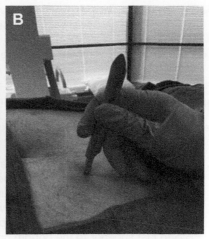

Fig. 17. (A) The size and shape of the scalpel wound. (B) The necessary depth of penetration.

Withdraw 5 to 15 mL from each site. If bone marrow does not flow easily, consider going deeper or redirecting altogether by selecting another site.

- As the BMA meets the heparin, note that the two will not mix. Quickly tap the syringe to force the heparin to mix with the BMA to reduce the chances of clotting.
- Caution: It is rare, but some patients will experience severe pain when marrow aspirate is withdrawn. The pain is brief but can be quite intense and unusual, sometimes mimicking a radiculopathy. It may be helpful to pulse the syringe, pulling gently but in a pulsewise fashion, to slowly extract the BMA out of the marrow cavity.
- Withdraw the trocar carefully by pulling it back, and while still in the tissue using the same skin site (ie, not withdrawing it from the skin) redirect it to the next target.
- After completing 3 sites, remove the 30 mL syringe and cap it. Keeping the syringe in continuous motion for the duration of the procedure may help prevent clotting.
- When all sites are completed and the trocar is withdrawn, put pressure over the wound to assure hemostasis.
- Approach the other side of the ilium in the same fashion.

Provide Aftercare

- Have patients lie on their back with knees bent for 5 minutes to place pressure over the entry wounds and promote hemostasis. Redress the wounds if necessary.
- The authors place a Tegaderm (3M, St Paul, MN) dressing on the wounds and ask patients to keep them dry until the next morning. After that, patients can shower and replace the dressing with a Band-Aid (Johnson & Johnson Consumer Inc, New Brunswick, NJ) and Neosporin (Johnson & Johnson Consumer Inc).
- Opioid medication may be appropriate for postprocedural pain.

Clinical Notes

- In the authors' experience, most patients will not feel the drilling and tolerate the procedure well.
- Some patients will feel discomfort when the trocar/driver reaches the bone cavity and when heparin is injected, so it is best to warn them.

- Some patients will feel pain when bone marrow is withdrawn. For those who feel it, it may be severe. However, it is brief and patient complaints are rare. Communication is key.
- Patients needing a repeat procedure can be scheduled 6 to 12 weeks following the first procedure.

QUICK REFERENCE FOR ULTRASOUND-GUIDED BONE MARROW ASPIRATION

The following guide is provided as a quick reference for use in the office or procedure room.

1. Check patients' Hct. It should be more than 30 to 38 (hemoglobin [Hgb]10.0–12.5). If it is lower, target volumes should be adjusted down.
2. Prep the low back and pelvis per your clinic protocol.
3. Use curved low-frequency US probe with sterile gel and gloves; map out the area to be numbed with a sterile surgical pen. This area should be from just lateral to PSIS to just superior to the bottom one-third of the SI joint.
4. Under active US guidance, use a long 25- or 22-gauge needle to numb the area from the skin, soft tissues, and periosteum along the planned BMA sites. Numb the entire area you have outlined with the surgical pen. This should be 10 to 20 mL of anesthetic per side.
5. Prepare medications: 5000 IU heparin in a 5-mL syringe with normal saline and as many 30-mL syringes with 30,000 IU heparin each as required for the planned harvest volume.
6. On the first side anesthetized, insert the trocar long under the US probe toward the top one-third of the mountain made up by the posterior aspect of the ilium. At the chosen BMA site, put constant forward pressure on the trocar and turn the handle back and forth until it breaks through the cortex.
7. Perform a tap test. Once the cortex is engaged and there is a slight loss of resistance, tap the end of the trocar side to side to ensure that it is firmly engaged in bone. If so, inject approximately 500 to 750 IU of heparin into the bone site.
8. Place the 30-mL syringe on the trocar and pull back on the plunger. *Flick the syringe as the first BMA enters the syringe to ensure that it mixes with the heparin.*
9. Draw 5 to 15 mL at this site and repeat for a total of 3 to 5 sites on the left and 3 to 5 sites on the right, depending on desired final volume.
10. The maximum safe volume depends on patient size. In a patient less than 105 lb, limit the withdrawal to 50 mL; in an average man, it should not be more than 90 to 120 mL; and in a large man, it should not be more than 120 to 150 mL.

QUICK REFERENCE FOR FLUOROSCOPE GUIDED BONE MARROW ASPIRATION

The following guide is provided as a quick reference for use in the office or procedure room.

11. Check patients' Hct. It should be more than 30 to 38 (Hgb 10.0–12.5). If it is lower, target volumes should be adjusted down.
    a. Prep the low back and pelvis per your clinic protocol.
    b. C-arm is anteroposterior with a 15° ipsilateral oblique on the PSIS.
    c. Under active fluoroscopic guidance, use a long 25- or 22-gauge needle to numb the area from the skin, soft tissues, and periosteum along the planned BMA target sites. Numb the entire target area. This area should require 10 to 20 mL of anesthetic per side.

   d. Draw medications: 5000 IU heparin in a 5-mL syringe with normal saline and as many 30-mL syringes with 30,000 IU heparin each as required for the desired final volume.

   e. Return to the side that was first numbed, and insert the trocar through the skin wheal that was used for anesthesia and advance so that it is positioned at the first chosen target. The trocar enters at approximately a 30° angle. Once a BMA target site is contacted, put constant forward pressure on the trocar and turn the handle back and forth until it breaks through cortex; note the slight loss of resistance.

   f. Perform a tap test. Once the cortex is engaged, tap on the end of the trocar side to side to ensure that it is firmly engaged in bone. If so, then inject approximately 500 to 750 IU of heparin into the bone site through the trocar.

   g. Place the 30-mL syringe on the trocar and pull the plunger back. Flick the syringe as the first BMA enters to ensure that it mixes with the heparin.

   h. Draw 5 to 15 mL at this site and repeat at 3 to 5 sites on the left and 3 to 5 sites on the right depending on desired final volume.

   i. The maximum safe volume depends on patient size. In a patient less than 105 lb, limit withdrawal to 50 mL; in an average male, it should not be more than 90 to 120 mL; and in a large male, it should not be more than 120 to 150 mL.

REFERENCES

1. Dominici M, Le Blanc K, Mueller I, et al. Minimal criteria for defining multipotent mesenchymal stromal cells. The International Society for Cellular Therapy position statement. Cytotherapy 2006;8(4):315–7.

2. Murphy MB, Moncivais K, Caplan AI. Mesenchymal stem cells: environmentally responsive therapeutics for regenerative medicine. Exp Mol Med 2013;45(11): e54.

3. Pubmed search for "mesenchymal stem cells". Available at: http://www.ncbi.nlm.nih.gov/pubmed/?term=mesenchymal+stem+cells. Accessed April 21, 2016.

4. Haleem AM, Singergy AAE, Sabry D, et al. The clinical use of human culture-expanded autologous bone marrow mesenchymal stem cells transplanted on platelet-rich fibrin glue in the treatment of articular cartilage defects: a pilot study and preliminary results. Cartilage 2010;1(4):253–61.

5. Hernigou P, Mathieu G, Poignard A, et al. Percutaneous autologous bone-marrow grafting for nonunions. J Bone Joint Surg Am 2006;88(1 Suppl 2):322–7.

6. Buda R, Vannini F, Cavallo M, et al. One-step arthroscopic technique for the treatment of osteochondral lesions of the knee with bone-marrow-derived cells: three years results. Musculoskelet Surg 2013;97(2):145–51.

7. Schnabel LV, Lynch ME, van der Meulen MCH, et al. Mesenchymal stem cells and insulin-like growth factor-I gene-enhanced mesenchymal stem cells improve structural aspects of healing in equine flexor digitorum superficialis tendons. J Orthop Res 2009;27(10):1392–8.

8. Friedenstein AJ, Gorskaja JF, Kulagina NN. Fibroblast precursors in normal and irradiated mouse hematopoietic organs. Exp Hematol 1976;4(5):267–74.

9. Foster T, Puskas B, Mandelbaum B. Platelet-rich plasma: from basic science to clinical applications. Am J Sports Med 2009;37:2259–72.

10. Kevy S, Jacobson M. Preparation of growth factors enriched autologous platelet gel. In: Proceedings of the 27th Annual Meeting of Service Biomaterials. St. Paul, MN, April, 2001.

11. Marx RE. Platelet-rich plasma: evidence to support its use. J Oral Maxillofac Surg 2004;62(4):489–96.

12. Pourcho A, Smith J, Wisniewski S, et al. Intraarticular platelet-rich plasma injection in the treatment of knee osteoarthritis: review and recommendations. Am J Phys Med Rehabil 2014;93:S108–21.
13. Al-Ajlouni J, Awidi A, Samara O, et al. Safety and efficacy of autologous intra-articular platelet lysates in early and intermediate knee osteoarthrosis in humans: a prospective open-label study. Clin J Sport Med 2015;25(6):524–8. Available at: http://journals.lww.com/cjsportsmed/Fulltext/2015/11000/Safety_and_Efficacy_of_Autologous_Intra_articular.10.aspx.
14. Sun Y, Feng Y, Zhang CQ, et al. The regenerative effect of platelet-rich plasma on healing in large osteochondral defects. Int Orthop 2010;34(4):589–97.
15. Otto A, Collins-Hooper H, Patel K. The origin, molecular regulation and therapeutic potential of myogenic stem cell populations. J Anat 2009;215(5):477–97.
16. Szmitko P, Wang C, Weisel R, et al. Biomarkers of vascular disease linking inflammation to endothelial activation. Circulation 2003;108:2041–8.
17. Lamagna C, Bergers G. The bone marrow constitutes a reservoir of pericyte progenitors. J Leukoc Biol 2006;80(4):677–81.
18. Caplan AI. All MSCs are pericytes? Cell Stem Cell 2008;3(3):229–30.
19. Worthley DL, Churchill M, Compton JT, et al. Gremlin 1 identifies a skeletal stem cell with bone, cartilage, and reticular stromal potential. Cell 2015;160(1–2):269–84.
20. Wakao S, Kitada M, Kuroda Y, et al. Multilineage-differentiating stress-enduring (Muse) cells are a primary source of induced pluripotent stem cells in human fibroblasts. Proc Natl Acad Sci U S A 2011;108(24):9875–80.
21. Parapia LA. Trepanning or trephines: a history of bone marrow biopsy. Br J Haematol 2007;139(1):14–9.
22. Rubinstein M. Aspiration of bone marrow from the iliac crest: comparison of iliac crest and sternal bone marrow studies. J Am Med Assoc 1948;137(15):1281–5.
23. Jamshidi K, Swaim WR. Bone marrow biopsy with unaltered architecture: a new biopsy device. J Lab Clin Med 1971;77(2):335–42.
24. Bosi A, Bartolozzi B. Safety of bone marrow stem cell donation: a review. Transplant Proc 2010;42(6):2192–4.
25. Centeno C, Pitts J, Al-Sayegh H, et al. Efficacy of autologous bone marrow concentrate for knee osteoarthritis with and without adipose graft. BioMed Res Int 2014;2014:1–9.
26. Centeno C, Pitts J, Al-Sayegh H, et al. Anterior cruciate ligament tears treated with percutaneous injection of autologous bone marrow nucleated cells: a case series. J Pain Res 2015;8:437–47.
27. Centeno C, Al-Sayegh H, Bashir J, et al. A prospective multi-site registry study of a specific protocol of autologous bone marrow concentrate for the treatment of shoulder rotator cuff tears and osteoarthritis. J Pain Res 2015;8:269–76.
28. Hernigou P, Flouzat Lachaniette CH, Delambre J, et al. Regenerative therapy with mesenchymal stem cells at the site of malignant primary bone tumour resection: what are the risks of early or late local recurrence? Int Orthop 2014;38(9):1825–35.
29. Wyles CC, Houdek MT, Wyles SP, et al. Differential cytotoxicity of corticosteroids on human mesenchymal stem cells. Clin Orthop Relat Res 2015;473(3):1155–64.
30. Izadpanah R, Schächtele DJ, Pfnür AB, et al. The impact of statins on biological characteristics of stem cells provides a novel explanation for their pleotropic beneficial and adverse clinical effects. Am J Physiol Cell Physiol 2015;309(8):C522–31.

31. Schippinger G, Pruller F, Divjak M, et al. Autologous platelet-rich plasma preparations: influence of nonsteroidal anti-Inflammatory drugs on platelet function. Orthop J Sports Med 2015;3(6). 2325967115588896. p. 3.
32. Beane OS, Fonseca VC, Cooper LL, et al. Impact of aging on the regenerative properties of bone marrow-, muscle-, and adipose-derived mesenchymal stem/stromal cells. PLoS One 2014;9(12):e115963.
33. Marx RE, Tursun R. A qualitative and quantitative analysis of autologous human multipotent adult stem cells derived from three anatomic areas by marrow aspiration: tibia, anterior ilium, and posterior ilium. Int J Oral Maxillofac Implants 2013;28(5):e290–4.
34. Batinić D, Marusić M, Pavletić Z, et al. Relationship between differing volumes of bone marrow aspirates and their cellular composition. Bone Marrow Transplant 1990;6(2):103–7.
35. Muschler GF, Boehm C, Easley K. Aspiration to obtain osteoblast progenitor cells from human bone marrow: the influence of aspiration volume. J Bone Joint Surg Am 1997;79(11):1699–709.
36. Fennema EM, Renard AJS, Leusink A, et al. The effect of bone marrow aspiration strategy on the yield and quality of human mesenchymal stem cells. Acta Orthop 2009;80(5):618–21.
37. Scarpone M, Kuebler D, Harrell C. Marrow Cellution Bone Marrow Aspiration System and Related Concentrations of Stem and Progenitor Cells.
38. Ehninger A, Trumpp A. The bone marrow stem cell niche grows up: mesenchymal stem cells and macrophages move in. J Exp Med 2011;208(3):421–8.
39. Rahnama R, Wang M, Dang AC, et al. Cytotoxicity of local anesthetics on human mesenchymal stem cells. J Bone Jt Surg 2013;95(2):132–7.

Regenerative Approaches to Tendon and Ligament Conditions

Michael N. Brown, DC, MD[a,b,*], Brian J. Shiple, DO[c],
Michael Scarpone, DO[d]

KEYWORDS

- Soft tissue injuries • Tendon and ligament injuries • Stem cell therapies
- Regenerative medicine

KEY POINTS

- Healing of soft tissue injuries and lesions are often incomplete leaving the patient with residual pain, joint dysfunction, and functional disabilities.
- There are multiple types of platelet preparations which need to be properly selected depending on phases of healing.
- Stem cells derived from multiple sources may help modulate tissue repair.
- Extracellular matrix proteins and scaffolding may help facilitate tissue remodeling by providing a mechanical and biological environment for cells to migrate into, align and proliferate.
- Growth factors modulate tissue repair.

INTRODUCTION

Soft tissue pathology caused by acute injury, cumulative stress, or the sequelae of biomechanical faults and degenerative changes represent a significant portion of the practice of physical medicine and rehabilitation and sports medicine physicians. For many years, nonoperative management choices included rest, physical therapy, splinting and orthosis, medications, and physical modalities that often left patients with few other options for management of soft tissue injury. Healing of soft tissue injuries and lesions is often incomplete, leaving the patient with residual pain, joint dysfunction, and functional disabilities. Patients and physicians who

[a] 1515, 116th Avenue NE, Suite #202, Bellevue, WA 98004, USA; [b] 10 Harris Court, Building A, Suite 1, Monterey, CA 93940, USA; [c] 1788 Wilmington Pike, Suite 2000, Glenn Mills, PA 19342, USA; [d] Trinity Sports Medicine & Performance Center, 3151 Johnson Road, Suite 2, Steubenville, OH 43952, USA
* Corresponding author. 1515, 116th Avenue NE, Suite #202, Bellevue, WA 98004.
E-mail address: drbr1@aol.com

Phys Med Rehabil Clin N Am 27 (2016) 941–984
http://dx.doi.org/10.1016/j.pmr.2016.07.003
1047-9651/16/© 2016 Elsevier Inc. All rights reserved.

pmr.theclinics.com

manage these conditions are left searching for treatment options and alternatives. Intratendinous injections of corticosteroid may reduce stiffness and pain but also reduce the physical forces required to injury the tendon in the future.[1–3] Injury to ligaments often results in joint effusion, altered movement, muscle weakness, reduced functional performance, and may result in significant loss of time out of play.[4]

Over the past 2 decades, technological advancements are emerging that use a "tissue engineering" approach to these conditions. Langer and Vacanti[5] first described 4 basic components required in tissue engineering: a structural scaffold, a cell source, biological modulators, and mechanical modulators. As various biologic and biocellular techniques have emerged, physicians have been trying to make the translational application to clinical practice where various treatment protocols are being developed. Unfortunately, the empirical experience with these techniques far exceeds the validation of these techniques in controlled studies.

The anterior cruciate ligament (ACL) is of particular importance, with some unique features that warrant discussion. Worldwide, young athletes experiencing anterior cruciate ligament injuries range from 17% to 61%.[6] In the United States, 350, 000 ACL reconstructive surgeries are performed annually.[7] The ACL is thought to have a poor healing capacity with a substantially higher rate of failure, which has led to a unanimous abandonment of suture repair and adoption of ACL reconstruction as the goal standard of care for ACL injuries, especially in younger athletes, whose primary goal is to return back to high-level sports activity.[4] Because the ACL is an intra-articular, extrasynovial ligament, ACL injury and the disruption of the synovial sheath do not allow a local hematoma formation to take place, which is crucial for the onset of the inflammatory response that would stimulate primary healing.[8] Despite ACL reconstruction, those athletes who successfully return back to play are at high risk for a second injury[9] and will have a less favorable outcome.[10] Importantly, ACL injuries are associated with long-term clinical sequelae despite ACL reconstruction, such as meniscus tears, chondral lesions, and the onset of posttraumatic osteoarthritis.[11–16] Recent technological advancements in tissue engineering and regenerative medicine have demonstrated promising use of novel biologic/tissue engineering techniques that include growth factors, stem cells, and the use of bio-scaffolding to improve ACL healing and repair.[17]

Primary disorders of tendons (tendinopathy), due to overuse or age-related degeneration, are common problems encountered in the day-to-day practice. Although there are no accurate figures specifically related to tendon disorders, studies from primary care show 16% of the general population suffer from rotator cuff shoulder pain and 21% in the elderly.[18,19] The incidence of rotator cuff pain is even more common in the sports community. It has been stated that injuries to tendons are involved in 30% to 50% of all sports injuries.[20] Rotator cuff disease is the most common upper extremity disability.[21] Due to hypocellularity and hypovascularity in tendinopathy, the natural ability of tendons to heal is extremely low.[22]

As biocellular techniques and tissue engineering protocols continue to emerge, we will need a more comprehensive classification system based on ultrasonography and clinical presentation to identify which type of tissue engineering strategy would be most appropriate for the category of tendinopathy. Developing both diagnostic and interventional skills using high-resolution ultrasonography will become increasingly important as regenerative medicine and tissue engineering techniques and protocols continue to emerge. Sensitivity figures of 0.98 are reported when using a 10-MHz or greater frequency ultrasound probe when detecting full-thickness rotator cuff tears.[23]

It is becoming more commonplace for non-radiologists to become experienced with ultrasonography who can develop similar high levels of accuracy when diagnosing partial-thickness tears as compared with musculoskeletal radiologists, which is statistically better, than general radiologists and sonographers.[24–32] Unfortunately, ultrasonography still remains user dependent[23] and will continue to place demands on practicing physicians to improve diagnostic ultrasonography skills. Once the proper skill level is achieved, it will help ensure appropriate assessment and categorization of ligament and tendon injuries in order select the appropriate intervention to improve outcomes. In addition, regenerative medicine and tissue engineering techniques currently being used remain, for the most part, empirical and will require validation through clinical trials. The purpose of this article was to discuss basic concepts and strategies using a tissue engineering approach to soft tissue injuries of tendons and ligaments.

TENDON INJURY AND PATHOPHYSIOLOGY

Tendinopathy can be described by specific location, which can play a role in determining the type of tendinopathy involved. Tendinopathy can be found within the main body of the tendon, its insertion site on bone (enthesis), and the structures around the tendon (peritenon).[33,34] These different forms of tendinopathy can coexist within the same tendon.

Histology-based studies of the rotator cuff tendon, as well as other tendon injuries, have demonstrated the absence of acute inflammatory cells.[35–40] Other studies are not in agreement with this and have found histologic evidence of inflammation.[41,42] A normal tendon is extensible, which participates in a stretch-recoil cycle.[43] However, in tendinopathic tendons extensibility is lost and becomes more rigid, which may complicate the control of joint position.[44] Alteration of extensibility affects the capacity to respond to tensile loads and plastic deformation of tendinopathic tendons can lead to micro-injury or complete tendon failure.[45] Several classification systems have been proposed based on histopathology.[46–49]

Various etiologic theories have been proposed in the literature that divide causes into extrinsic and intrinsic factors. Extrinsic factors would include impingement syndrome,[50] overuse,[51,52] or multifactorial causes.[53] Intrinsic factors include hypoperfusion theory,[54] degenerative,[55] degeneration-microtrauma,[56] apoptotic theory,[57] and extracellular matrix (ECM) modification.[58] Rotator cuff tendinopathy, resulting in a tear requiring surgical repair, is particularly problematic. Repaired tendon tissue rarely achieves functionality equal to that of the insertion site of the original tendon to bone and is not regenerated after repair. Instead, the injured tissue is replaced with a "reactive scar" rich in collagen type III rather than collagen type I, which is mechanically weaker than the original zone of calcified cartilage at the enthesis formed during embryogenesis.[59] Studies have demonstrated a high rate of failure of tendon healing following repair.[60–64] The high rate of failure to heal after rotator cuff repair has led to a surge of interest in the use of regenerative orthopedic medicine techniques to augment the tendon repair and healing process.[65–73]

Tendon healing is organized into distinct stages.[74] Following injury there is hemorrhage and clot formation with platelet degranulation with release of cytokines and growth factors heralding the inflammatory stage of tendon healing. At that time, neutrophils and macrophages enter the hematoma and begin phagocytosis of necrotic material and pieces of the ECM (3–7 days after tendon injury).[74] The proliferative phase is heralded by extrinsic cells from the peritenon, soft tissues, such as tendon sheath, fascia, periosteum, and subcutaneous tissues, but also intrinsic cells from the epitenon and endotenon migrate and proliferate at the injured site.[75,76] Vasoactive and chemotactic factors are released that promote angiogenesis and stimulation of teno-cyte proliferation and migration to the site of injury.[74] In this process, granulation tissue is formed by mainly type III collagen.[77] Initial collagen fibers are not initially parallel but still contribute to biomechanical strength. The amount of collagen progressively in-creases and in week 4, the fibroblasts from the endotenon proliferate. After 40 days, these intrinsic fibroblasts play a critical role in tendon healing and producing new collagen by recycling collagen.[78,79] The tendon tissues mature and the fibers become more fully oriented according to tensile forces. The proliferative phase lasts approximately 2 months and biomechanical and tensile strength is restored in the remodeling phase when collagen is aligned in the longitudinal axis and cross-linking is complete.[78] The newly remodeled tendon remains hypercellular and type III collagen is gradually replaced by type I collagen, which is more cross-linked to withstand ten-sile loads.[79] There are numerous growth factors and cytokines that modulate the various healing cascades during the tendon repair process (**Fig. 1**).

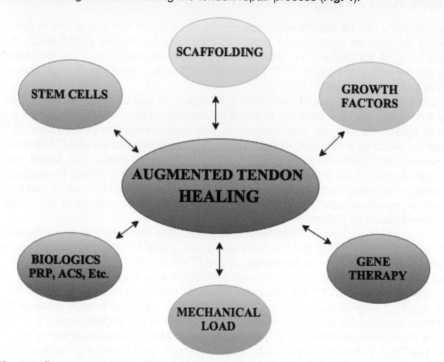

Fig. 1. Influence on augmented tendon healing.

Insertional tendinopathy represents another unique pathophysiologic state in tendons. Typically, the superficial tendon layer is healthy and the deep layer is where the enthes-opathy or insertional tendinosis exists. The superficial portion of the tendon is consis-tently under a greater strain than the deeper layer because the superficial portion is a further distance from the central axis of rotation of the joint. Insertional tendinopathy re-sults from the differential effects of mechanical stimulation. Some orthopedic re-searchers have proposed a "stress-shielded" model in which an incision of the superficial layer redistributes the load equally from the deep to superficial portions of the tendon, thus the re-stressing causes a recovery of the tendon's mechanical properties.[80]

The presence of different strain patterns within a tendon opens up the potential for altering mechanical loads provided in certain joint positions that are more likely to stress a specific area of the tendon commonly affected by tendinopathy. Understanding the sequential progression of loading strategies applied to a tendon post regenerative injection procedure may be an important component of the "regenerative medicine" paradigm that can apply a controlled stress or mechanical load that can progress during the different phases of healing to improve outcomes. Significant work will need to be done in the future to prove which specific movement patterns or rehabilitation protocols are more efficacious to improve tendon and ligamentous healing.

LIGAMENT INJURY AND PATHOPHYSIOLOGY

A normal ligament is primarily composed of type I collagen, which is responsible for the tissue strength and resilience. This collagen is densely packed and cross-linked, which accounts for the stability and strength of the ligament. Following injury similar to what has been described in tendon injury, healing fibroblasts during the proliferative phase synthesize type III collagen rather than type I, which is produced in a much smaller quantity during this phase of tissue healing.[81,82] During the healing process, the production of abnormal cross-linked collagen and smaller-diameter collagen fibers, as well as the reduction of tightly packed collagen fibers together produce a ligament with reduced stiffness and strength thereafter.[83–88] Studies of experimental medial collateral ligament (MCL) injuries have demonstrated the injured ligament exhibits greater stress relaxation. This makes the healing ligament less efficient in maintaining tensile loads than a normal ligament and it ends up with abnormal "creep properties." This pathophysiological processes allows the ligament to elongate more under tensile loads.[84,89] Following ligamentous injury and subsequent laxity of the joint leads ultimately to osteoarthritis of the joint.[90,91] Ligament injuries in athletes often lead to the inability of the injured athlete to participate at the preinjury level of activity, even after a decade from the date of injury.[92] In addition, a common sequelae of ligament injury is a reported early onset of posttraumatic osteoarthritis.[93]

Approximately two-thirds of patients with ACL injury are treated with ACL reconstruction. Although the objectives of undergoing ACL reconstruction surgery is to reestablish function and prevent subsequent damage to the articular cartilage and other soft tissues, there is mounting evidence that articular cartilage degeneration progresses despite surgery and/or different surgical technique.[15,94–96] The primary factor responsible for osteoarthritis progression after ligamentous injury is joint instability and the associated increased shear motion between the articular cartilage surfaces. ACL injury, in particular, the envelope of joint motion becomes greater producing a tibiofemoral offset increasing shear stress at the cartilage-bone interface.[90,97–99] This in turn may increase the external adduction moment and increase the load in the medial compartment, which accelerates arthritic progression.[90,100] The loss of function, stability, and performance leads to the onset of osteoarthritis progression. This has led us to search for methods of treatment that restore the properties of normal ligament function and prevention of posttraumatic osteoarthritis.[101–106]

THE USE OF DIAGNOSTIC AND INTERVENTIONAL ULTRASOUND

Diagnostic musculoskeletal ultrasonography is becoming a commonly used office-based procedure and diagnosing tendon and ligament injury and pathology.[107] This imaging modality is quickly becoming a critical diagnostic and interventional tool for physicians specializing in regenerative injection therapies. Precision diagnosis is a critical component of therapeutic intervention and it is important for physicians deploying biocellular interventions, tissue growth factors, ECM and scaffolding, and other interventions within a ligament or tendon. Diagnostically, ultrasound has particular value in demonstrating the pathophysiologic state of a tendon or ligament. Modern diagnostic ultrasonography, especially with high-resolution capacity, can display the entire physiologic spectrum of pathologic states in soft tissue, such as ligaments and tendons in all phases of healing.[108] The pathophysiologic state of the tissues is translated into detectable echodensity and echogenic changes easily detected by high-resolution ultrasonography.[109] In addition, diagnostic ultrasound also has proven value to be able to perform dynamic examination of the integrity of ligaments and soft tissues during motion testing.[109] We have discussed previously the change in "stiffness" of tendinopathic tendons. Tissue elastography provides a means for the modern ultrasonographer to identify changes in "tissue stiffness," identifying areas of focused tendinopathic changes within the tendon or specific tissue that may escape detection during a static 2-dimensional (2D) examination of gray-scale differences. The use of shear-wave elastography and the more recent development of strain elastography and 3D elastography in assessing tendon pathology is still being defined. This new technology shows promise further evaluating tendon and soft tissue pathology and may become a means to monitor outcome of regenerative interventions in the future.[110,111] The higher the resolution and processing power the more definition and resolution is achieved in evaluating fibrocartilage structures in the knee, such as the meniscus. The meniscus fibrocartilage is composed of densely packed collagen fibers interposed with chondrocytes. This cellular architecture is responsible for the homogeneous hyperechoic appearance seen on ultrasonography. Although ultrasound cannot penetrate deep into the joint proper to directly visualize the entire meniscus structure, there are multiple ultrasonography findings that would suggest underlying cartilage injury.[112] Para meniscal cysts can be easily identified and are frequently seen as a hypoechoic and occasionally anechoic structure adjacent to the meniscus.[113] Our empirical experience has involved the use of ultrasound to evaluate the meniscotibial, meniscal capsular ligament attachments, peripheral tears in the meniscus, and dynamic examination of the ligamentous attachments of the meniscus to evaluate meniscus extrusion and instability with valgus and varus stress maneuvers. These various findings provide a classification scheme for different interventions based on pathophysiology and clinical findings.

Many articles have been published defining the criteria for partial and full-thickness tears of the rotator cuff. The sensitivity and specificity of diagnostic ultrasound in rotator cuff pathology is also well established, as well as the pitfalls associated with use of ultrasound in this regard.[114–116] Although ultrasonography has demonstrated that sensitivity can be as high as 100% for full-thickness tears similar to MRI, ultrasound has a lower sensitivity for diagnosing partial-thickness tears.[116] It is the process of stratification of ligamentous and tendon pathology by clinical examination and ultrasonography that provides a basis for therapeutic intervention using regenerative injection procedures. The use of ultrasonography and stratifying or classifying specific tendon pathology or ligamentous pathology requires a significant skill level and is still user dependent.

STRATEGIES FOR REGENERATIVE INJECTION THERAPIES AND AUGMENTED TENDON AND LIGAMENT HEALING

There have been an increasing number of physicians in various disciplines turning to the use of platelet-rich plasma (PRP) or other cell-based injections for soft tissue injuries or degenerative pathology within tendons and ligaments. The authors having spent many years performing such interventions and are beginning to deemphasize the importance of stem cells or specific cellular intervention and emphasize the importance of a "tissue engineering" approach to tendon and ligamentous pathology. This approach is multifactorial, as noted in **Fig. 1**. A tissue engineering approach requires the physician to match a precision diagnosis with the biocellular intervention. This requires not only the selection of the specific cell type and source that is most appropriate for a specific tissue pathology or injury, but the selection of appropriate adjuvant growth factors and ECM proteins to more effectively augment healing. Physicians using a tissue engineering approach should be readily aware of when and when not to use specific biocellular intervention based on a given pathologic state in the tissue. They can then select specific adjuvant ECM proteins, bioactive scaffolding, cellular preparations and growth factors to enhance healing and promote cell differentiation to a targeted tissue. It is also critically important that the regenerative orthopedic medicine practitioner develop a keen understanding of physical rehabilitative medicine principles that should be used after their intervention. Specific gradual soft tissue loading strategies following an intervention can have a profound effect on tissue healing.[20,117] Physical medicine and rehabilitation principles also require an understanding of the use of orthotics, bracing, and splinting and physical modalities that may be beneficial for short-term recovery from an intervention before and/or after the procedure.

PLATELET-RICH PLASMA AND AUTOLOGOUS PLATELET PRODUCTS

PRP is the most commonly used autologous source of a variety of growth factors used in regenerative orthopedic procedures in an attempt to augment tendon and ligament healing. Both plasma and platelets are rich sources of bioactive proteins, including growth factors, ECM proteins, and other signaling molecules.[118] Platelets contain granules: α, δ, and λ. Alpha (α) granules play a pivotal role in platelet function. There are approximately 50 to 80 α granules per formed platelet and contain more than 30 proteins, including platelet-derived growth factor (PDGF), transforming growth factor (TGF-β, β1 and β2 isomers), platelet factor 4 (PF4), interleukin-1 (IL-1), platelet-derived angiogenesis factor (PDAF), vascular endothelial growth factor (VEGF), epidermal growth factor (EGF), platelet-derived endothelial growth factor (PDEGF), epithelial cell growth factor (ECGF), and insulinlike growth factor (IGF).[118] The properties of PRP are based on the production and release of these factors when the platelets are activated.[119] Dense granules within platelets contain neuromodulators and inflammatory modulators, such as histamine and serotonin. By exposure to collagen, thrombin, or calcium, platelets release growth factors and cytokines.[118]

PRP has been used for years as a source of growth factors to augment soft tissue healing, but this has not been without problems. Physicians using high-resolution ultrasound and PRP injections to evaluate and treat tendinopathic tendons and tendon can attest to the fact that tendons are difficult to heal and tendons can fail to heal with a single intervention. It is commonplace that patients need to be reevaluated to determine if there has been interval resolution of tendinopathy or healing of a tear. Careful documentation under ultrasound examination may demonstrate the need for either multiple interventions or a change in strategy to augment tendon healing. We remain cognizant of the fact that in some studies a single PRP injection compared with placebo controls has found no significant difference between the study and control groups.[120] Similar results were reported by Rodeo and colleagues.[121] Despite some negative studies, there continues to be evidence to support the use of platelet products in clinical practice. For example, surgical repaired flexor tendon injuries in the forelimb of horses demonstrated a higher failure strength with greater elastic modulus 24 weeks postoperatively after being treated with PRP compared with the control group with only saline injection. Histologically, the PRP group demonstrated better collagen organization and increased metabolic activity.[122] It was noted in this study, that the PRP group demonstrated better collagen organization and increased metabolic activity.[122]

Inconsistency reported in various studies could prove that there is not a clear dose-response relationship using PRP. High PRP concentration may support wound healing, yet some investigators think that overdosing PRP can lead to poorly differentiated scar tissue by overstimulating cells and the release of growth factors in such a high concentration may have negative effects causing increased inflammation.[123] Another natural source for a variety of growth factors, including anti-inflammatory cytokines, would be autologous conditioned serum (ACS), which contains anti-inflammatory cytokines or interleukins (IL-4, IL-10, IL-13) and IL-1 receptor antagonist in addition to growth factors basic fibroblast growth factor (bFGF), hepatocyte growth factor (HGF), and TGFb.[124] It was noted that there was a positive effect of ACS in Achilles tendon healing with accelerated organization of repaired tissue, increased collagen mRNA, increased collagen deposition reflected by tendon thickness, and increased mechanical strength.[124] Despite this, the repaired tendon remained biomechanically inferior to native tendon controls.[124]

No doubt, growth factors play an important role in the healing course of tendon tissue. Clinicians using growth factors as an attempt to augment tendon or ligament healing face a number of problems, such as which specific growth factors could be used as standalone therapy or what combinations of growth factors should be used appropriately for a given clinical presentation. This has not been established in various research protocols. In addition, the short duration of action of many growth factors limits the potential long-term effects using injection therapy, especially in lieu of the fact that healing tendons can take months or years to heal. The next conceivable step in research protocols would be to establish a specific protocol or model by using a combination of growth factors, biocompatible scaffolds, and specific biocellular intervention. In vitro studies have demonstrated that the addition of PRP to human tenocytes resulted in cell proliferation, collagen deposition, and improved gene expression for matrix-degrading enzymes and endogenous growth factors.[125] We can also stimulate tendon healing by a well-ordered angioneogenesis.[126] These investigators highlight the importance of understanding the timing of an administration of growth factors and their dosage for designing effective growth factor therapy.[78] It is of critical importance that we continue to perfect specific protocols and to create selection criteria for interventions for the future of regenerative musculoskeletal medicine.

In clinical practice, physicians specialized in diagnostic and interventional ultrasound in musculoskeletal (MSK) medicine have the capacity to repeat evaluations and monitor clinical outcomes. By repeated clinical evaluation and ultrasonography, examination can make appropriate changes to the treatment regimen as necessary, which may include repeat interventions to improve clinical outcomes. This is difficult to duplicate in research protocols and therefore empirical experience and utilization of regenerative procedures continue to outpace research evidence for the use of various biocellular and biologic intervention.

Plate-Rich Plasma Classification and Terminology

Because there are many protocols for preparing PRP and the products of these preparation methods differ in both cellular and molecular composition, it is becoming increasingly important for physicians to classify the type of PRP or platelet preparation that is being used for a specific intervention. Several classification systems exist,[118,127–129] but more importantly regardless of the classification system used, it is critically important to select the appropriate platelet preparation for the pathophysiology or condition being selected to treat. The initial classification was published in 2006 by Mishra.[130] Mishra and colleagues[127] proposed a new classification system. This classification system included identifying type A PRP with platelet concentrations less than 5 times blood concentration and type B PRP with platelet concentrations 5 times normal blood concentration. Simply speaking, PRP categories were noted as pure PRP (P-PRP) and leukocyte-rich PRP (L-PRP). This classification was later noted to be insufficient because different PRP centrifuge devices create platelet products with different platelet cell counts and leukocyte counts, which has potential repercussions on the biologic effect and clinical outcomes. Not long after Mishra's classification system was published, Dohan and colleagues[118] published their classification system. However, this was really aimed at the surgical community and divided PRP and platelet-rich fibrin products that at the time were more important in creating surgical grafts to be used in the surgical application of tissue repair in the operative setting. Then the platelet activation white blood cell (PAW) classification system was published by DeLong in 2012 leading to 32 PRP categories.[118] This system requires a platelet concentration range reflecting a close proximity to the actual platelet quantity, the activation mode in the presence of white cells, and so forth.[118] With the advent of the "Double-Spin Suspension" method of creating a pure PRP, we now have a PRP product that is high in platelet concentration with few to no red blood cells (RBCs) and an elevated or baseline leukocyte count with a significantly reduced neutrophil count. This is in contrast to the P-PRP, which has a low platelet count of 1 to 3 times concentration and no leukocytes or RBCs. Most of the research to date has included L-PRP versus P-PRP. To date there has not been a peer-reviewed human study featuring a double-spin suspension method pure PRP yet. However, this method has gained popularity in clinical practice and the investigators have extensive experience using this method as their go-to product with good clinical experience, anecdotal to date. One of the investigators participated in a new PRP classification article published in the spring of 2015 that took into account all known factors that may be important to differentiate when studying the PRP literature and more importantly when designing future PRP research studies. In this latest classification article, the investigators pointed out it is not enough to report the concentration of the PRP used to treat a subject as "times × baseline platelet count" because a 5 times baseline platelet count in a subject with a baseline platelet count of 160,000 is much different from a subject with a baseline platelet count of 340,000 platelets per microliter. Therefore, the new recommendation for classifying a platelet treatment when evaluating an article or designing the next PRP study is to adopt the PLRA system. "P" stands for platelet concentration as expressed in platelets per microliter and the volume of PRP delivered to the target should be recorded as well. That way, an actual dose of platelets can be determined and compared between similar studies. Next the presence or absence of "L" for leukocytes should be recorded and if leukocytes are present the concentration of neutrophils should be recorded as well. The next symbol is "R" for RBCs should be recorded as present or not, and finally "A" for activation should be recorded if the sample was exogenously activated or not.

Without the research details regarding the biochemical features and qualities of the double-spin suspension method of the newest pure PRP system available, we can make some observations of the well-studied L-PRP versus the P-PRP systems available to date. L-PRP can be detrimental to healing of injured tendons because it induces catabolic and inflammatory effects on tendon cells and may prolong the effects of healing tendons. On the other hand, when considering P-PRP may not have the desired effect on acutely injured tendons and may result in the formation of excessive scar due to the potential of P-PRP eliciting a cellular anabolic effect.[129] L-PRP elicits more extensive catabolic response in differentiated tenocytes and induces a higher level of inflammatory response. L-PRP induces the expression of type III collagen, which as we have already discussed involves early granulation tissue formation. P-PRP elicits the expression of type I collagen, which is more desired in mature ligament and tendon tissue.[129] Thus, the utilization of L-PRP may be deleterious to chronically injured tendons or chronic degenerative tendinosis, but may be beneficial during the acute phase of healing. P-PRP may be more appropriate for induction of type I collagen in the proliferative phase or remodeling phase of healing.[129] Because L-PRP induces inflammatory responses and differentiated tenocytes, using L-PRP to treat already-inflamed tendinopathic tendons may only exacerbate the tendon disorder by prolonging the inflammatory phase and thereby impairing the healing process.[129] It may be more appropriate to use P-PRP to augment the repair of tendinopathic tendons because of its anabolic properties and low inflammatory effects.[129] Because of the anabolic effect of P-PRP, its use in acutely injured tendons may elicit fibrosis or scar formation because of induction of tenocyte stem/progenitor cells to produce too much collagen at the injury site.[129] Thus, one needs to exercise caution in using P-PRP in acutely injured tendons. Gene expression of IL-1 beta, IL-6, and TNF-alpha is upregulated by L-PRP; thus, induction of catabolic effects on tendon cells could be detrimental to effects on injured tendons and impair healing.[131,132] Because P-PRP elicits anabolic effects, its probably best suited use would be in late-stage healing, thus enabling it to augment and accelerate tendon healing. The effects of leukocyte-rich versus leukocyte-poor and its effect on the side occurring cascade may explain, in part, the variable outcomes of PRP treatment in clinical trials.

PLATELET LYSATES AND PLATELET RELEASATES USE IN AUGMENTED TENDON AND LIGAMENT HEALING
Platelet Lysate

A platelet lysate involves the preparation of a platelet concentrate in which platelets are centrifuged into a pellet and exposed to freezing temperatures, thereby lysing the platelet cell membrane, releasing platelet growth factors from the alpha granule and reconstituting in plasma. The plasma is then filtered and a growth factor–rich plasma is created. This has been widely used in cell cultures, especially mesenchymal stem cell (MSC) cultures, as a replacement for fetal bovine serum. The authors discontinued the use of lysates when it was discovered the number of unaffected platelets by the cryolysis was a variable percentage even with triple freeze thaw cycles. We empirically appreciated platelet releasates affected 100% of the platelet population as verified with our own laboratory-based platelet counters and thus the release of much more growth factors. This will need to be documented in further studies.

Platelet Releasates

A platelet releasate involves the production of a platelet concentrate or PRP. Platelets are then activated with thrombin, calcium chloride, or collagen. Platelet lysates and releasates have been used for years for their growth-promoting effects in cell cultures.[133] Releasates are used for the alpha-granule–derived growth factors, such as PDGF, TGF-beta, IGF, VEGF, FGF-2/b, and EFG.[134,135] A platelet releasate was investigated with regard to its effect on TSC (tenocyte stem and progenitor cells). This involved activating platelets with calcium chloride rather than thrombin. It was noted that the platelet releasate promoted TSC proliferation and differentiation into active tenocytes as well an increase in collagen production.[132]

THE USE OF STEM CELLS IN LIGAMENT AND TENDON INJURY

In 1994, adult MSCs were discovered to play an active role in connective tissue repair.[136] Since that time, multiple sources of stem cells have been identified and studied, including tenocyte-derived stem cells,[137] adipose-derived stem cells,[138] amniotic-derived cells,[139] dermal fibroblasts,[140] and bone marrow–derived MSCs.[141] The theoretic basis for current clinical application of stem cells is to use these cells as a reservoir for musculoskeletal tissue repair. The most common clinical sources of stem cells are from bone marrow aspiration or from lipoaspirates. These cells delivered to a precise location, typically with ultrasonography, rely on local growth factor signaling or the addition of exogenous factors to drive the stem cells to differentiate into the target cell line.[141,142] Most adult bone marrow consists of blood cells in various stages of differentiation. These components can be divided into plasma, RBCs, platelets, and nucleated cells. The adult stem cell fraction is present in the nucleated cells of the marrow.[143] Bone marrow concentrate (BMC) is produced by density gradient centrifugation of bone marrow usually aspirated from the iliac crest. However, actual stem cell numbers from bone marrow are less than 0.01% or 1/100,000 nucleated cells. Its major function is to deliver MSCs to the injury site. Like PRP, BMAC is also rich in platelets and therefore growth factors.[144] With the ease of marrow blood aspiration it can be readily accessed by surgeons intraoperatively or within the clinical setting in a timely fashion. Because of the ease of bone marrow aspirate techniques, there has been clinical utility and various strategies used to influence the cells down a tenogenic line, including the application of growth factors.[145] Some investigators feel there is mounting evidence to show that bone marrow stem cells (BMSCs) used with specific protocols to differentiate into a tenogenic line can produce tendon tissue when exposed to the appropriate environmental cues.[67] There is evidence that bone marrow–derived MSCs only act as a signaling cell to the local tissue niche and do not affect tissue healing by differentiating into a specific cell lineage but rather induce healing by a cell-signaling mechanism that affects the local resident stem cells in the niche and do not differentiate into the repaired tissue.[146]

An intriguing study was published by Hernigou and colleagues,[65] in which they followed 90 patients following rotator cuff repair. Forty-five patients received bone marrow aspirate concentrate injections with rotator cuff repair intraoperatively and 45 patients received rotator cuff surgical repair only. These patients were followed for 10 years with ultrasound and MRI. At 6 months' follow-up, the study group that received the combined BMC and surgery were 100% healed versus 67% of the control group. At 10-year follow-up, the study group that received the combined BMC and surgery demonstrated that 87% of the study group maintained an intact tendon versus 44% of the control.[65] Several other studies have also demonstrated the ability of MSCs to improve healing of tendons or ligaments.[147–150] Despite these positive findings, there are studies that have failed to show the application of bone marrow–derived, culture-expanded MSCs to augment the healing process of rotator cuff tendon tears despite evidence that they are present and metabolically active.[66] Laboratory studies of injured tendons in rats demonstrated the addition of MSCs to a rotator cuff injury model did not improve the structure, composition, or strength of the healing tendon attachment site.[66]

Adipose tissue–derived stem cells (ASCs) have shown promise in animal models of tendon repair.[151] Like bone marrow, adipose tissue is also derived from embryonic germ layer mesoderm. Adipose tissues contain a relatively large number of undifferentiated cells, which include stem cells and progenitor cells capable of producing tissues arising from embryonic mesoderm, such as cartilage, ligament, tendon, muscle, and bone.[152] ASCs have been shown to have an increased angiogenic capacity compared with bone marrow.[153] Despite the excellent availability of MSCs in adipose tissue, isolating the cells from adipose stroma (stromal vascular fraction), typically requires a process of enzymatic digestion. This process has come under scrutiny of the Food and Drug Administration (FDA) and at present is considered a violation of the "more than minimal manipulation" rule set forth by the FDA. It is anticipated that multiple techniques will emerge that will satisfy FDA regulations and yet provide physicians with a safe means to extract MSCs from adipose tissue in sufficient numbers to have clinical utility in a same-day surgery setting.

ASCs have been of significant interest in musculoskeletal orthopedic application. Some researchers have questioned the utility of ASCs in ligament tissue engineering and were unable to demonstrate expression of ligament markers with ASC placation.[154] ASCs have been shown to be as effective as other MSCs by their multipotency and proliferation capacity. It is believed that ASCs present an ideal cell source for experimental and clinical research on tendon engineering.[155] Experimental studies of tendon repair have shown ASCs to exhibit a significant increase in tendon cell strength, direct differentiation toward tenocytes and endothelial cells, and an increase in angiogenic growth factors. These findings suggest that ASCs may have a positive effect on primary tendon repair and may be useful for future cell-based therapy,[151] although most existing clinical information to date has been generated using culture-expanded marrow-derived MSCs. There is information to suggest that MSCs from fat, placenta, umbilical cord, and muscle have similar, but not identical functional potential.[156–158] Despite this, the question of which exogenously supplied MSC source might be optimal for a given clinical situation has not yet been established.[146] In addition, researchers still need to sort out which biocellular intervention and tissue engineering strategy is most efficacious. It will also be necessary to define and characterize tendinopathy and tendon tears, and which of these lesions is the most amenable to a specific cellular medicine intervention protocol.

THE USE OF EXTRACELLULAR MATRIX PROTEINS AND TISSUE SCAFFOLDING

The use of ECM proteins and scaffolding to augment tendon and ligament healing is becoming an important strategy in tissue repair.[5,59] In tendon injury and repair for example, the bone-to-tendon interface after healing has little resemblance to the native tendon fibro-osseous insertion site; instead, the normal 4 distinct zones of the tendon insertion are joined by a layer of fibrovascular scar tissue composed of predominately type III collagen.[159] This tissue is significantly weaker than the original insertion and contributes to the substantial number of failures through both natural and surgical repair.[160] Therefore, a scaffold is one particular strategy that may provide a suitable mechanical and biological environment for cells to migrate into and provide a bridge between the tendon and bone or the tendon defect to facilitate the alignment of cellular proliferation and collagen deposition.[161] There are many scaffold-based and biological approaches that have been investigated in an effort to improve tendon and ligament healing and provide mechanical integrity. This would include natural and synthetic matrices for cell and tissue in-growth.[162] One of the problematic issues using allogeneic ECMs is induction of inflammatory responses in the host.[163] Therefore, it is important to select the proper ECM or scaffolding strategy for the type of target tissue, phase of healing, and extent of injury. Fibrin gel, for example, offers a few advantages in these situations because of the properties of fibrin, such as controllable degradation rates, that can match tissue regeneration, good biocompatibility, adhesive properties, and nontoxic degradation byproducts.[164] Fibrin gel self-assembles into a scaffold by mimicking the last step of blood clotting to support cell, proliferation, differentiation, and tissue regeneration.[164] It can also be used as a cell carrier to protect cells from the forces produced during preparation and delivery processes.[164] Fibrin gel also provides high cell-seeding efficiency and uniform cell distribution.[165] The degradation rate of fibrin gel can be regulated with aprotinin and tranexamic acid (trans-4-aminomethyl-cyclohexane-1- carboxylic acid) to precisely match tissue regeneration.[166]

Decellularized adipose tissue (DAT) as a bioactive matrix within a hydrogel is also being explored as a scaffold and means of regenerative cell delivery within an ECM matrix. An injectable composite scaffold incorporating DAT as a bioactive matrix within a hydrogel phase capable of in situ polymerization would be advantageous for ASC delivery in the filling of small or irregular soft tissue defects.[167] Nonoperative musculoskeletal practitioners are beginning to become more interested in injectable scaffolding to fill tissue defects with combination with platelet, stem cell, and other biocellular interventions.

There is significant work being done with regard to implantable bio-scaffolds that are either now approved for operative tendon and ligament repair or being used in animal models to evaluate their potential use.[168] In the near future, implantable scaffolding membranes will be available using minimally invasive techniques that will be placed under ultrasound guidance. Amnionic membranes in vivo and in vitro studies are beginning to demonstrate that the biochemical properties of amniotic membranes can help reduce inflammation and enhance soft tissue healing.[169]

Hyaluronic acid (HA) is demonstrating increased cell viability and proliferation, in a dose-dependent manner. Importantly, HA also stimulates the synthesis of type I collagen without an increase in type III collagen.[170] Because of tenocyte apoptosis and decreased collagen synthesis, there is an increased risk of tendon rupture.[46] HA in different concentrations can have a modulation effect on cell migration,[171] adhesion,[172] and proliferation.[173]

Another novel ECM that has become available for use in orthopedic regenerative injection procedures is a flowable tissue matrix allograft derived from human placental connective tissue.[174] The human placenta is a rich source of biological tissue and the ECM components contain collagens (types I, III, IV, V, and VI), fibronectin, nidogen, laminin, proteoglycans, and hyaluronan, as well as growth factors.[175] Another important advantage to placental tissue sources of ECM proteins is that they are nonimmunogenic, which elicits little to no immune response.[176] We present several case examples in this article in which this novel tissue matrix was used to treat ligament and tendon pathology.

IMPLANTABLE COLLAGEN MATRIX FOR TENDON HEALING

The composition of collagen is altered in injured tendons as well as upregulation of proinflammatory cytokines, which ultimately effects the tensile strength of the healing tendon and thus perpetuating potential future failure.[59] Implanting a collagen matrix graft can initiate the healing cascade, which can facilitate tendon healing and alter the cytokine environment in which the matrix graft is placed. Orthopedic literature has demonstrated that healing of the rotator cuff following rotator cuff repair is problematic.[60–64] Implantation of bio-scaffolding is currently being explored as an important component of the biologic approach to successful rotator cuff tendon repair.[59] It has been proposed that the use of a bio-inductive purified bovine collagen implant can be applied over the bursal surface of a partial rotator cuff tear using arthroscopic deployment (**Fig. 2**).[177] The application of a collagen tissue matrix graft applies a small amount of tension along the tendon, which functions as a bioreactor rather than a full tendon anchor. Mild tension applied by the tissue graft causes induction of tissue healing.[177] The membrane composed primarily of collagen and implanted under arthroscopic technique initiates bleeding and therefore the activation of platelets in the clotting cascade secondary to exposure of the bare collagen within the implant. The resulting clot encompasses the implanted membrane activating a cytokine cascade that is thought to promote healing.[177] Orthopedic researchers reviewing data from sheep tendon models and computer remodeling help demonstrate that new tissue reduces peak strain at the partial tear site and may help with the balance of biologic activity and the biomechanical aspect of healing tendons.[178] They demonstrated when using the collagen matrix graft that in clinical trials of 24 partial rotator cuff tears that the implant consistently induced new tendon tissue in all 24 subjects. Healing was verified by serial MRI demonstrating new tissue that was well integrated within the host tissue and progressive tissue maturation.[179]

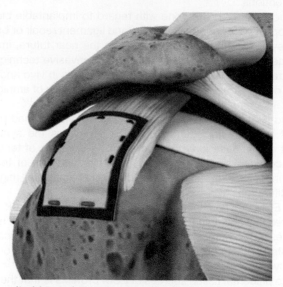

Fig. 2. Rotation medical bio-inductive implant (bovine patch) for RC tendon repair. (*Courtesy of* Rotation Medical, Plymouth, MN; with permission.)

THE USE OF TISSUE GROWTH FACTORS IN AUGMENTED TENDON AND LIGAMENT HEALING

The tendon healing process is a complex orchestration of cellular biology that is heavily influenced by numerous secreted molecules.[180] **Table 1** on the right is a brief summary of just a few of the growth factors and biocellular processes that are involved in the phases of healing a tendon and ligament. We provide only a cursory review of growth factors that influence tendon and ligament healing that are currently under investigation as a potential means to augment the healing cascade.

Table 1
Summary of a few of the growth factors and biocelluar processes that are involved in the phases of healing a tendon and ligament

Inflammatory	Proliferative	Remodeling
Platelets	Cellularity and matrix production	Cellularity and matrix production
Neutrophils		
Monocytes	Collagen type III	Collagen type III ↓
Erythrocytes	Activation of local tendon stem/progenitor cells	Collagen type I ↑
Circulation-derived mesenchymal stem cells		
IL-6, -1β	bFGF	BMP 12, 13, 14
bFGF	BMP 12, 13, 14	IGF-1
IGF-1	IGF-1	TGFβ
PDGF	PDGF	
TGFβ	TGFβ	
VEGF	VEGF	

Abbreviations: bFGF, basic fibroblast growth factor; BMP, bone morphogenetic protein; IGF, insulinlike growth factor; IL, interleukin; PDGF, platelet-derived growth factor; VEGF, vascular endothelial growth factor.

Transforming Growth Factor β_1

Transforming growth factor beta 1, for example, is likely to be involved in the mechanism of scar tissue formation in the presence of recruited macrophages in the inflammatory phase of healing.[160] However, its application to injured tendons, although yielding increased tissue proliferation, did not contribute to increasing tendon strength.[159]

Bone Morphogenic Protein-12

Bone morphogenic protein (BMP) 12 and 14 are expressed in active fibroblasts and are present throughout the healing process of bone-to-tendon insertion.[181] BMP-12 induces the formation of tendon and ligament like tissue and is involved in the differentiation of stem cells to tenocytes.[182]

Bone Morphogenic Protein-14

BMP-14 plays a role in tendon collagen organization. It has been shown when introduced into rat Achilles tendon to induce ECM synthesis and cellular proliferation and increase expression of ECM and cell adhesion–related genes.[183]

Other Bone Morphogenic Proteins

BMP-2 and BMP-7 were shown to induce collagen production when added to cultured tenocytelike cells derived from samples of human rotator cuff (RC) tendons.[67] For these reasons, the ability of BMPs to augment RC repair is currently under investigation. Studies in sheep and rat models have shown BMP therapy alone is beneficial for RC repair.[121]

Insulinlike Growth Factor-1

Insulin growth factor-1 (IGF-1) is an anabolic polypeptide that directly affects all major cell types involved in soft tissue healing. IGF-1 not only affects muscle cells but also tenoblasts, ligament fibroblast, and other fibroblastic cell types and also induces angiogenesis required for wound healing.[184] The singular loss of IGF-1 can have drastic effects on wound cell proliferation, decreased collagen, and hydroxyproline concentrations. No other growth factor is known to singularly affect positive wound-healing parameters to the same degree as IGF-1.[184] IGF-1 stimulates protein synthesis and cell proliferation while decreasing swelling and has been observed in the healing of the bone-to-tendon junction.[185]

Basic Fibroblast Growth Factor

Basic fibroblast growth factor (bFGF) increases proliferation and expression of collagen type III and can facilitate BMSC proliferation and differentiation into tenocytes.[186] bFGF has been shown to be a potent stimulator of angiogenesis, cellular migration, and proliferation in both in vivo and in vitro studies.[187]

Platelet-Derived Growth Factor

PDGF-b has been proposed to be a critical cytokine in the repair of tendons and ligaments. PDGF-b has been shown to promote chemotaxis, cell proliferation, ECM production, surface integrin expression, and revascularization in fibroblasts.[69] In a sheep RC repair model, scaffolds infused with PDGF-b demonstrated improved histologic scores and ultimate load-to-failure compared with repairs using empty scaffolds alone.[69]

Vascular Endothelial Growth Factor

The potent angiogenic effect of VEGF has been well documented. This may be important because impaired blood supply in tendons leads to apoptosis in tendons.[69] VEGF activity rises after the inflammatory phase. VEGF in RC repair has been shown to improve tensile strength in animal tendon healing models with VEGF augmentation.[188]

OTHER NOVEL INTERVENTIONS TO AID IN TENDON HEALING

Tenex FAST (Focused Aspiration of Scar Tissue), now called Tenex Health TX Procedure, became available in 2011 when the FDA approved a unique needle ultrasonic tenotomy for the treatment of tendinopathies.[189–191] This device has a probe in which the tip vibrates at ultrasonic rates and can emulsify tissue in front of the tip and simultaneously irrigates the emulsified tissue through an outflow suction feature.[189,190] This technology was adopted from a previous fundoplication procedure used to remove cataracts from the eye.[190] Nirschl[192] described his surgical findings in tendinopathy cases and described "angiofibrotic hyperplasia" with disrupted collagen fibers, increased cellularity, and neovascularization in tendinopathic tendons. The authors' personal experience has been that in certain cases of tendinopathy, this unique ultrasound-guided tenotomy procedure can be helpful in debridement of the angiofibrotic scar at the enthesis of tendinopathic tendons before using a regenerative injection procedure or placement of a percutaneous ECM graft. This technique was used and described in some of the case examples described below.

CASE STUDIES: REGENERATIVE INJECTION THERAPIES AND MINIMAL INVASIVE PROCEDURES FOR AUGMENTATION OF TENDON AND LIGAMENT HEALING

Clinical outcomes of 6 patients presenting with symptomatic tendinopathy refractory to conservative treatment (nonsteroidal inflammatory drugs [NSAIDs], physical therapy (PT), immobilization, and other modalities) underwent the Tenex procedure followed by a flowable placental tissue amniotic membrane graft injected under ultrasound guidance. These flowable injectable placental amniotic membrane grafts contain both placental tissues and fluids. We refer to these products in the following cases as amniotic membrane grafts or autologous matrix graft (AMG)s.

Providing a biocompatible ECM scaffold that can help facilitate proper tissue remodeling and repair may be able to overcome the inherent limitations of normal tendon and ligament repair. Although there are a variety of ECM scaffolds available for therapeutic use,[193] ECMs derived from placental tissues have many unique qualities that make them a promising option for treating these soft tissue injuries. In addition to providing a collagen-based matrix, placental tissue has both anti-inflammatory and immunosuppressive properties. In addition, placental tissues contain a wide range growth factors, many of which are known to aid in the healing and regeneration of musculoskeletal tissues.

MATERIALS AND METHODS

During 2015, 4 patients presented with tendon or ligament injuries that were refractory to conservative treatment. The injuries included 1 case of Achilles tendinosis, 1 partial RC tendon tear, 1 case of mild scarring of the ulnar collateral ligament, and 1 case of lateral epicondyle tendinosis. All 4 patients were men and ranged in age from 22 to 62 years old.

TREATMENT

All treatments were performed in an outpatient setting. In each case, the defective tendon or ligament was debrided under ultrasound guidance. Following debridement, 0.5 mL of an AMG diluted in 1.5 mL normal saline solution (NSS) was injected under ultrasound guidance into the site of injury.

FOLLOW-UP

The patients were followed up with statistically validated functional questionnaires and ultrasound imaging at 3 weeks, 3 months, and 6 or 9 months.

RESULTS

There was significant improvement of symptoms and statistically validated functional scores in all posttesting scores compared with pretesting scores.

SUMMARY

The use of placental tissue to treat tendon and ligament damage was associated with improved subjective reports and statistically validated functional scores with reduced pain and structural improvement on ultrasound imaging in a diverse group of cases.

CASE EXAMPLE 1: ACHILLES–PLACENTAL MATRIX
History

A 45-year-old man presented to the outpatient sports medicine clinic reporting burning and pinching pain in the back of the left ankle provoked by activity and persisting into the night. He ranked his pain at 6 (of 10) and his VISA-A questionnaire score was 6 (of 100). The pain had persisted despite conservative treatment involving a CAM boot and physical therapy for 6 weeks.

Examination

When examined, the Achilles tendon exhibited mild swelling without redness but was severely tender medial and lateral to the tendon. Four to 5 cm proximal to the insertion, the tendon was thickened. His ankle demonstrated normal pulse, sensation, range of motion, strength, and ligament stability and he tested negative for Tinel sign. Radiographs revealed minimal osteophyte formation at the Achilles insertion with neither subtalar nor tibiotalar arthrosis. Diagnostic 2D and 3D ultrasound with Doppler was used to identify the following complications: neovascularity, retrocalcaneal bursa fluid, mild enthesophyte changes at the insertion, and partial interstitial tearing of the tendon at the site of the significantly thickened area. **Fig. 3** demonstrates preinjection ultrasound findings on left Achilles tendon demonstrating neovascularization, interstitial tearing and tendon thickening on initial examination and resolution of neovascularization and improved fibular pattern organization 16 weeks postinjection.

Treatment

The Tenex procedure was performed under local anesthesia. The proximal area of the damaged tendon and the distal aspect of the tendon at the calcaneus were tenotomized and debrided. After the Tenex treatment, 0.5 mL PX50 with 1.5 mL of NSS was injected into the proximal tendinotic area of the Achilles tendon under ultrasound guidance. After the procedure, the patient received a CAM boot and a prescription of oxycodone/acetaminophen (5 mg/325 mg #25 as needed).

Follow-Up

Three weeks after the procedure, the patient reported feeling better; his VISA-A questionnaire improved from 6 to 61 (of 100), and his pain dropped from 6 to 1 (of 10). Despite mild tenderness and swelling, he reported increased tolerance to activities of daily living. On examination, the thickened area of the Achilles tendon was resolving and flattening. He received physical therapy for the following 4 weeks, including friction massage, range of motion, and eccentric strengthening. On completion of physical therapy (7 weeks after the procedure), he reported his pain at 0 to 1 and the swelling and tenderness had completely resolved. The burning pain was absent but

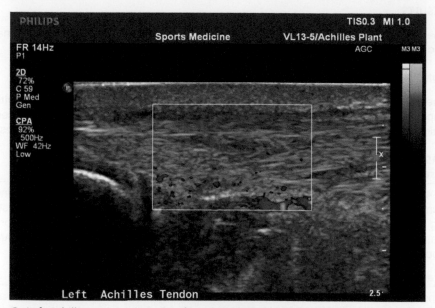

Fig. 3. Left Achilles preinjection view demonstrating neovascularity and visualizing tendon thickening and hyperechoicity (interstitial tearing).

intermittently returned when the ankle was fatigued. The thickened area of the tendon continued to resolve since the last examination. The patient participated in activity as tolerated for the following 4 weeks. At the 12-week follow-up, the patient reported no pain, 100% tolerance for activities of daily living, and 95 of 100 on his VISA-A questionnaire. Initial ultrasound findings demonstrated interstitial tearing of Achilles tendon (**Fig. 4**). Postprocedure ultrasound demonstrated improved fibular pattern reorganization 16 weeks postprocedure (**Fig. 5**).

At the 1-year follow-up, the VISA-A questionnaire score had improved to 99 (of 100). **Table 2** reviews clinical course of this case.

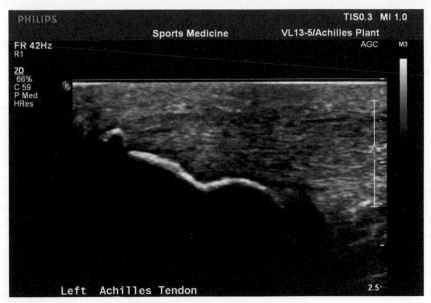

Fig. 4. Left Achilles preinjection visualizing interstitial tearing.

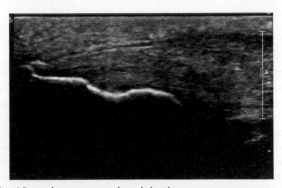

Fig. 5. Left Achilles 16 weeks postprocedure injection.

Table 2 Case 1				
Initial Results	**3 wk**	**12 wk**	**1 y**	**16 mo**
6	1	0	0	0
Severe tenderness Constant burning Night pain Limp	Very little pain No burning No night pain Normal gait	Very little tenderness No burning Normal gait	No tenderness No burning	No tenderness No burning Some stiffness on waking
Decreased tolerance	Increased tolerance	Within normal limits	Within normal limits	Within normal limits
6/100	61/100	95/100	95/100	95/100
Thickened tendon Neovascularity Interstitial tearing	Thickened tendon resolving and flattening	Some tendon thickening with resolving of neovascularity	No pictures	Tendon thickening with improved linear fiber patterns and less neovascularity

CASE EXAMPLE 2: SHOULDER (CALCIFIC ROTATOR CUFF)
History

A 62-year-old man presented with left shoulder pain (4 of 10) with any overhead exercise. Pain was reported to reduce his activity level by 75%. He reported no mechanism of injury. At his surgical consult, the physician recommended conservative care but the patient did not respond. At the completion of conservative care, his shoulder quick dash results were 31.8% disability (68.75% for sports).

Examination and Imaging

The shoulder had no redness, swelling, deformity, or ecchymosis, but an MRI revealed a partial tear of the RC and mild calcific tendinopathy. The patient exhibited normal pulses, sensation, range of motion, and strength in both shoulders. However, his left supraspinatus tendon was tender and his left shoulder tested positive for impingement sign and Hawkins sign. Radiographs showed some inferior spurring of the acromioclavicular joint and arthrosis of the acromioclavicular joint and the inferior aspect of the glenohumeral joint. Ultrasound examination demonstrated partial RC tear and some calcification (**Fig. 6**). Ultrasound elastography demonstrated corresponding tendon tissue softening secondary to tendinopathy (**Fig. 7**).

Treatment

To provide access to the RC for the Tenex device, an 18-gauge needle was inserted to reach the tendon (**Fig. 8**) of the supraspinatus and infraspinatus as an introducer and a number 11 scalpel blade opened the skin through a small stab incision. Under ultrasonic guidance, the Tenex device was used to aspirate and debride the calcification around the partial tear of the RC. Immediately after the Tenex procedure, 0.5 mL of an AMG was mixed with 1.5 mL of NSS and was injected into the proximal tendinotic area of the Achilles tendon under ultrasound guidance. After the procedure, the patient received a prescription for Hydrocodone (7.5 mg/325 mg #25 1 every 6 hours as needed for pain).

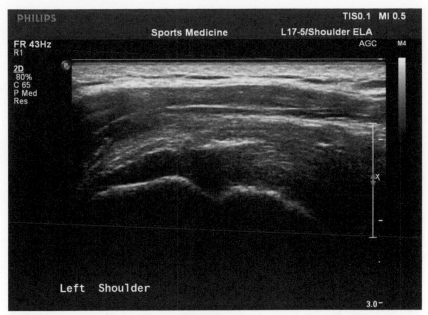

Fig. 6. Left shoulder preinjection noting partial tear and residual calcification.

Follow-Up

At the 6-week follow-up, the patient reported the pain intensity remained 5/5 on a 0–10 pain scale, but the frequency decreased from constant to intermittent. The quick dash shoulder assessment improved to 2.3% disability (18.75% for sports). The

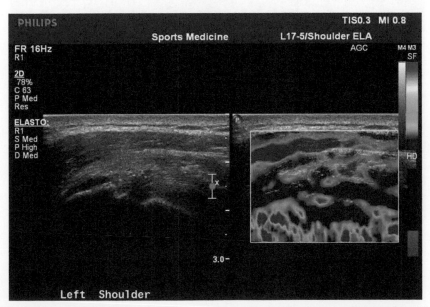

Fig. 7. Left shoulder preinjection with partial tear noted with corresponding tendon tissue softening on elastographic image.

962

962   Brown et al

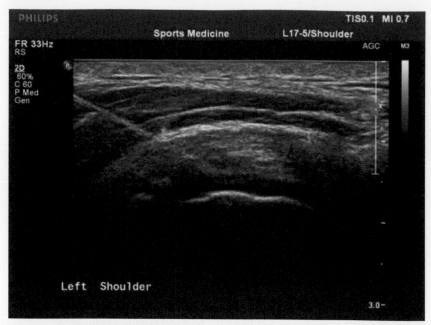

Fig. 8. Supraspinatus tendon injection.

supraspinatus was mildly tender. He was positive for the Kennedy-Hawkins sign, yet reported improved strength and ability to work out and lift. Ultrasonic investigation revealed a partial tear still present at the supraspinatus-infraspinatus junction with previous placental tissue graft apparent in the tendon (**Fig. 9**). There was a small

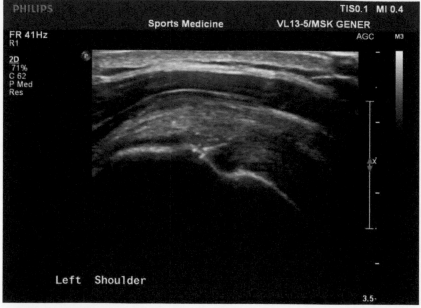

Fig. 9. Left shoulder 6 weeks postinjection noting tendon thickening and partial tear but less prominent.

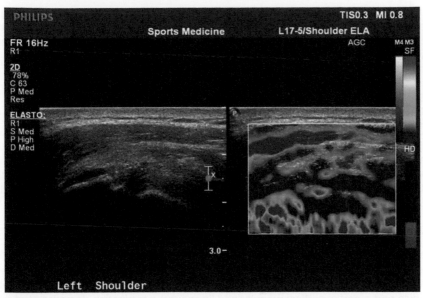

Fig. 10. Left shoulder 6 weeks after noting partial tear and improved elastographic changes (tissue hardening).

hyperechoic area with residual calcification. Ultrasound tissue elastography demonstrated partial tear improving and interval improvement in tissue stiffness (**Fig. 10**). He was then given physical therapy, including the following modalities: scapular lift, strengthening, and anterior capsular stretching. At approximately 12 weeks, he had significant improvement. He had pain only with bench press and some weight-lifting

Table 3 Case 2			
	Initial Results	**6 wk**	**9 mo**
Pain level	4 Constant	4 Intermittent	0
Subjective report	Tenderness Pain with overhead activity	Mild tenderness Improved strength No night pain	No complaints
ADLs	Self-reported as decreased 75%	Self-reported as decreased 50% but able to return to lifting	No limitations
Disability	Quick Dash: 38.1% Quick Dash Sports: 68.75% Positive Hawkins sign	Quick Dash: 2.3% Quick Dash Sports: 18.75%	Quick Dash: 0% Quick Dash Sports: 0%
Ultrasound and MRI findings	(MRI) Calcification of rotator cuff Partial tear of rotator cuff	(Ultrasound) Partial tear still visible.	No image available

Abbreviation: ADLs, activities of daily living.

maneuvers. A second AMG injection treatment was given 9 months after the original treatment into the supraspinatus and infraspinatus tendons. Within 4 weeks after the second AMG injection, his quick dash shoulder assessment showed 0% disability and 0% sports disability. **Table 3** reviews the clinical course of this case.

CASE EXAMPLE 3: RIGHT MEDIAL ELBOW PAIN IN A COLLEGE PITCHER: SECOND-DEGREE ULNAR COLLATERAL LIGAMENT SPRAIN
History

A 22-year-old male college pitcher presented with right elbow pain that was achy and tight at rest and sharp with activity. His pain level was reported as a 6 (of 10), which he reported to reduce his activity level by 70%. In addition, he was unable to throw the ball without significant pain. His quick dash score indicated a 28.3% disability (81.25% for sports).

Examination

The patient presented with decreased range of motion in the joint, as he lacked 2° of extension. On examination, the ulnar nerve was somewhat prominent and a diagnostic ultrasound revealed a mild tear of the ulnar collateral ligament (UCL) at the medial epicondyle and a partial cortical irregularity. Ultrasound examination demonstrated over collateral ligament partial tear with cortical irregularity (**Fig. 11**).

Treatment

Under local anesthesia, 0.5 mL of the AMG was combined with 1.5 mL NSS and injected into the defective area of the UCL under ultrasound guidance. After the procedure, the elbow was immobilized and the patient received a prescription for oxycodone/acetaminophen (5 mg/325 mg #25 as needed). In addition to the AMG placental tissue treatment, the athlete underwent a multidisciplinary rehabilitation protocol that involved physical therapy, sports chiropractor, and a performance coach. Sixteen weeks later at the completion of the season the athlete underwent a second AMG injection and continued with a multidisciplinary rehabilitation protocol.

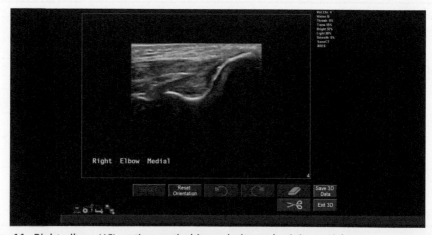

Fig. 11. Right elbow UCL noting cortical irregularity and origin partial tear.

Follow-Up

After 3 weeks, the quick dash assessment improved to 18.8% disability (75.1% for sports). A mild tear was still visible under ultrasound and he reported only a 40% reduction in daily activity (an improvement from the 70% reported before treatment). At the 6-week follow-up, the patient reported minimal pain and had been able to resume pitching. The quick dash assessment improved to 11.37% disability (31.25% for sports) and he reported only a 28% reduction in daily activity. Ultrasound examination demonstrated hypoechoic areas with collagen content from placental injection still visualized and interval healing (**Fig. 12**). At 12 weeks postprocedure, his quick dash assessment had improved to 6% disability (6.75% for sports) and he reported very little discomfort when pitching. **Table 4** reviews the clinical course in this case. Ultrasound examination at 12 weeks demonstrated UCL seen with more organized fibers and residual cortical changes in hypoechogenicity (**Fig. 13**).

Ultrasonography examination at 16 weeks demonstrated restoration of linear pattern and resolving partial tear of UCL origin (**Fig. 14**).

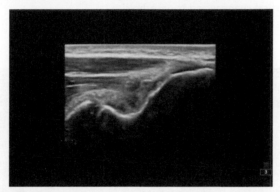

Fig. 12. Right elbow 6 weeks postinjection noting hypoechoic areas with collagen content from placental injection still visualized.

Table 4 Case 3				
	Initial Results	**6 wk**	**12 wk**	**16 wk**
Pain level	6	1	0	0
Subjective report	Achy and tight at rest Sharp pain with activity	Minimal Pain but able to start pitching	Very mild stiffness when pitching	No pain
ADLs	Self-reported elbow evaluation as decreased 70%	Self-reported elbow evaluation as decreased 28%	Self-reported elbow evaluation as decreased 14%	No problems with ADLs
Disability	Quick Dash: 28.33% Quick Dash Sports: 81.25%	Quick Dash: 11.37% Quick Dash Sports: 31.25%	Quick Dash: 6% Quick Dash Sports: 6.75%	Quick Dash-0% Quick Dash Sports: 0%
Ultrasound and MRI findings	Mild tear of UCL Partial cortical irregularity	Mild tear of UCL visible	Residual hypoechoic area at origin at UCL	Beginning resolution of hypoechoic area at origin at UCL

Abbreviations: ADLs, activities of daily living; UCL, ulnar collateral ligament.

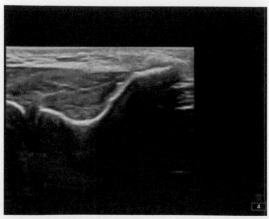

Fig. 13. Right elbow 12 weeks postinjection noting UCL is seen with more organized fibers with still origin cortical changes and hyperechoicity.

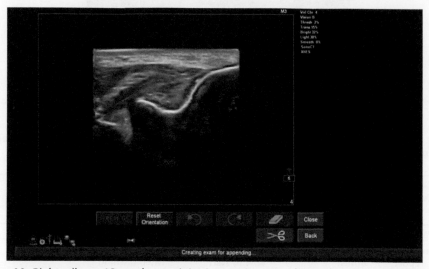

Fig. 14. Right elbow 16 weeks postinjection noting nice linear ligament pattern and resolving partial tear at ligament origin.

CASE 4: A CASE OF CHRONIC LATERAL ELBOW PAIN
History

A 45-year-old nurse who presented with 6 months of chronic lateral elbow pain in the right upper extremity. She had failed all conservative treatment, including rest, bracing, physical therapy, NSAIDs, and steroid injections. Surgery was offered.

Examination

The patient presented with tenderness to palpation over the anterior and lateral flat surface of the right humeral capitulum. Middle finger extension against resistance elicited pain at the lateral epicondyle. Placing elbow at 20° flexion with pronated varus stress test was positive for +1 laxity and severe pain. Tenderness to palpation was also noted over posterior lateral epicondyle. Initial ultrasound examination demonstrated defect in the ECRB (extensor carpi radialis, brevis) and radial collateral ligament (**Figs. 15** and **16**).

Elastography of Radial Collateral Ligament Defect Before Treatment

Pretreatment shear elastography demonstrated increased stiffness of tissue at attachment site noted in red (**Fig. 17**).

Assessment

A hypoechoic defect was observed by diagnostic ultrasound indicating tear of the origin of the ECRB and radial collateral ligament (RCL), lateral collateral ligament (LCL), and tendinosis of the extensor carpi radialis longus (ECRL).

Treatment

A sequence of 4 PRP injections of ×6 concentration, RBC 0, neutrophil poor, leukocyte rich, inactivated, was injected into the defects at the origin of the ECRB, ECRL, RCL, and LCL under ultrasound guidance in long axis and short axis views with a 25-gauge × 1.5-inch needle; 1 to 2 mL total dose was injected per treatment to the targets. Treatments were administered every 2 months to allow adequate recovery and healing time.

Outcome

Patient was asymptomatic with interval resolution of hypoechoic defect and tear in the RCL and ECRB. There was restoration of RCL and LCL ligament tension and instability by elastography and physical examination respectively. Repeat ultrasonography examination demonstrated interval healing of common extensor and RCL (**Figs. 18** and **19**).

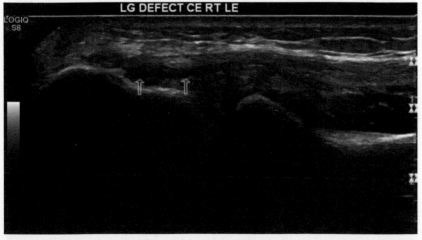

Fig. 15. Large defect in right left upper extremity (elbow). *Arrow* indicates long defect in common extensor tendon (right).

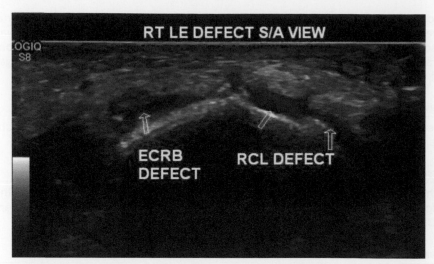

Fig. 16. ECRB and RCL defect at elbow. *Arrows* ECRB (extensor carpi radialis brevis) defect and RCL (radial collateral ligament) defect.

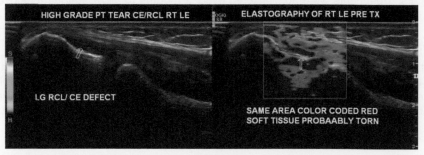

Fig. 17. RCL defect elastography. *Arrow* indicates large radial collateral ligament and common extensor tendon defect.

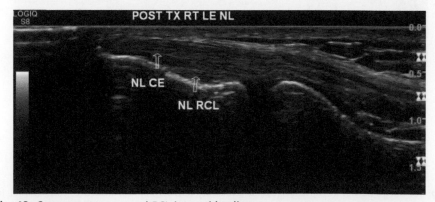

Fig. 18. Common extensor and RCL interval healing.

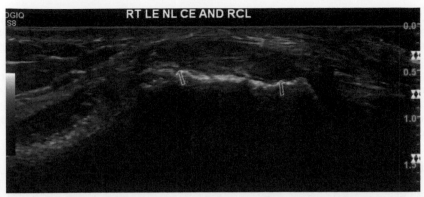

Fig. 19. Demonstrates extensor tendon and RCL interval healing.

Table 5 Case 4			
	Initial Results	**4 wk**	**1 y**
Pain level	8–9	0–1	0
Subjective report	Severe tenderness Night pain Difficulty gripping objects	No night pain Grip and strength improvement	No pain Grip strength improved
Disability	Patient-reported elbow pain questionnaire 92/100	Patient-reported elbow pain questionnaire 3/100	Patient-reported elbow pain questionnaire 0/100
Ultrasound and examination findings	Elastographic softening of extensor tendon and lateral epicondylar tendinosis		

CASE EXAMPLE 5: WORSENING LATERAL ELBOW PAIN
History

For 10 years, a 47-year-old male patient suffered consistent and worsening elbow pain (8 or 9 of 10) that interfered with his activities of daily living and persisted at night. Conservative treatments that included stretches, strengthening, and NSAIDs failed to alleviate symptoms. The patient rated elbow evaluation was 92% disability (of 100). His grip was weakened, such that he was continually dropping items.

Examination

He had tenderness in the later epicondyle of the humerus and pain that inhibited wrist and middle finger extension. Ultrasound evaluation revealed elastographic softening of the extensor tendons and lateral epicondylar tendinosis. Initial ultrasound elastography demonstrated decreased tensile strength (**Fig. 20**). Doppler ultrasound demonstrated neovascularization (**Fig. 21**).

Treatment

Tenex treatment was performed under local anesthesia for 120 seconds. The extensor tendons were tenotomized and debrided at the origin of the lateral epicondyle of the humerus. Immediately after Tenex treatment, 0.5 mL AMG was diluted in 1.5 mL NSS and injected into the Tenex-treated area of the tendon under ultrasound guidance (**Fig. 22**).

Follow-Up

After 4 weeks, the patient's pain decreased to 1 or 0 (of 10) with no night pain since 1 week after the procedure. The patient evaluated his elbow at 3% disability (of 100). His strength steadily improved, so that at 3 weeks he was able to perform activities of daily living, and at 4 weeks he returned to light weight lifting. **Table 5** reviews the clinical course in this case. One year posttreatment ultrasonography examination demonstrated decreased thickening of tendon with some mild hypoechogenicity despite patient being asymptomatic (**Fig. 23**). One year after injection treatment tissue elastography demonstrated interval resolution of tendon softening secondary to tendinopathy (**Fig. 24**).

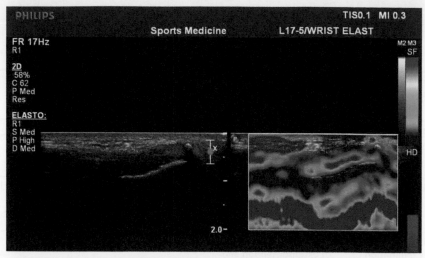

Fig. 20. Right elbow demonstrating decreased tensile strength.

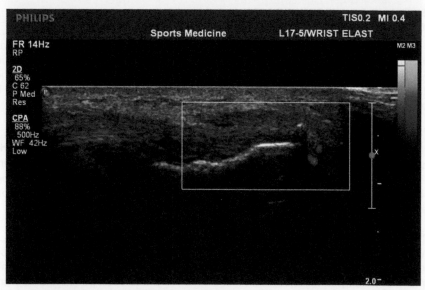

Fig. 21. Right elbow demonstrating neovascularity.

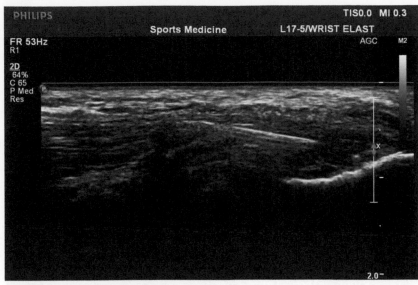

Fig. 22. Right elbow placental cell injection.

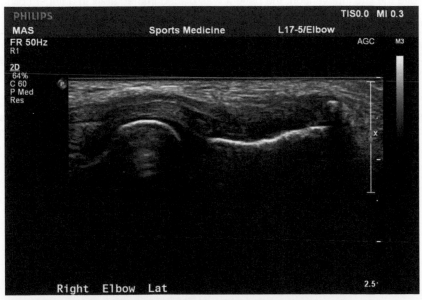

Fig. 23. Right elbow 1 year after procedure noting decreased thickening of tendon with some mild hyperechoicity that is reported as asymptomatic.

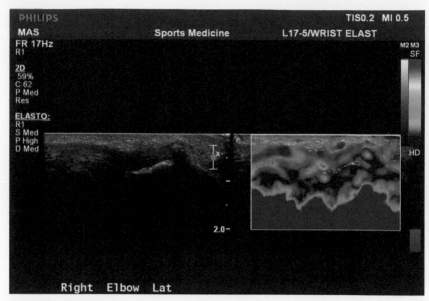

Fig. 24. Right elbow 1 year postinjection noting resolution of tendon softening.

CASE EXAMPLE 6: MALLET FINGER
History

A 65-year-old man presented with an 8-week history of mallet finger deformity right hand 3rd distal interphalangeal (DIP). The patient was warned that the therapeutic window for a reasonable outcome had passed and the patient may not respond to intervention. The patient was offered hand surgical consult and the patient declined. Despite the late intervention, the patient was placed immediately in a finger splint.

Examination and Imaging

Physical examination demonstrated mallet finger injury (**Fig. 25**).

Diagnostic ultrasound demonstrated a ruptured and retracted dorsal extensor tendon (**Fig. 26**).

Treatment

After demonstration of near approximation of tendon attachment with passive extension, he was offered a trial of PRP injection followed by dorsal extension splint in hyperextension for 6 weeks (**Fig. 27**). The volume of pure PRP injected into the tendon

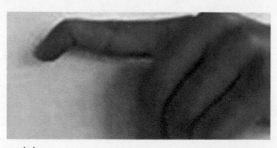

Fig. 25. Mallet finger injury.

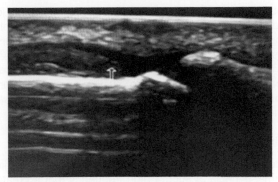

Fig. 26. Extensor tendon avulsion third DIP right.

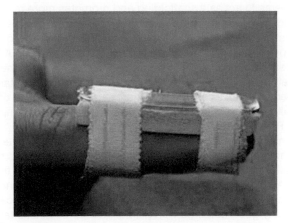

Fig. 27. Mallet finger splint.

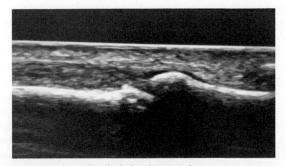

Fig. 28. Extensor tendon avulsion healed third DIP right.

defect was 0.2 mL to fill the gap and the 0.3 mL was seen filling the joint. The patient was seen for and delivered a second PRP injection on 6-week follow-up for mild persistent pain on palpation. Ultrasound demonstrated good interval healing and extensor tendon strength was normal to examiner resistance.

After 10 weeks in a continuous hyperextension dorsal splint program (see **Fig. 27**), the patient was pain free and had 5/5 strength with a normal DIP joint and no mallet deformity. Postprocedure ultrasonography examination demonstrated extensor tendon avulsion healed (**Fig. 28**).

CLINICAL CASE DISCUSSION

Tenex is a procedure that uses a dual cannula system with normal saline irrigation that oscillates the internal cannula at such a high frequency that it creates an ultrasonic sound wave that cuts and debrides necrotic tendon tissue, small calcific bone spurs, and calcific densities in tendons and then aspirates the diseased tissue through a hand-held probe guided by ultrasound guidance. The procedure potentially creates a void in the tendon structure after treatment. The tendon will heal without further intervention within 12 to 24 weeks. The addition of placental ECM containing collagen and growth factors seems to act as a scaffolding and promotes more rapid healing of the resultant intratendinous wound. The growth factors may also help decrease pain and regulate inflammation. The addition of the placental ECM appears to decrease postprocedure pain, promote more rapid healing, and improve function. A larger randomized controlled research study would be needed to truly validate the effects of this combination treatment. Two cases of ECRB tears with concomitant tears of the RCL are presented. The initial case demonstrates interval resolution of tendon defect appreciated on ultrasonography as well as physical findings and symptoms following a sequence of 4 PRP injections.

In the case of mallet finger, the combination of splinting and 2 sequential PRP injections resulted in normal healing of the tendon despite a full-thickness tear and retraction. In consideration of the previously discussed negative studies on the effect of PRP injections in the Achilles tendon and the RC, our empirical experience continues to demonstrate cases like this and thus calls for further studies. Empirically, the authors have had reasonably good outcome with partial and full-thickness tendon tears and high-grade partial avulsions. Clearly the clinical decisions made with regard to treatment intervention are important. The type of PRP, cell counts, amount, deployment techniques, and the decision of whether or not to use an ECM graft to augment healing is of significant importance.

SUMMARY

Interventional regenerative orthopedic medicine techniques have emerged that are directed to injuries of ligaments and tendons as well as degenerative states of these tissues. The utilization of high-resolution ultrasound has provided a means for specialty physicians practicing in the musculoskeletal system to perform examinations with a high level of precision that aims to document and classify specific tendon and ligament pathology. Using high-resolution ultrasound guidance in conjunction with "tissue engineering" principles that include the use of biocellular, scaffolding, growth factor, and rehabilitative medicine principles are beginning to demonstrate a means to augment ligament and tendon healing to tissues that historically do not heal well and are prone to chronicity. Patient suffering from ligamentous and joint instability as well as chronic tendon injury and tendinopathy are beginning to seek alternatives to conventional orthopedic methods of management. The surgical approach to ligament and tendon repair is reported to have high failure rates and less than ideal outcomes and thus there is an increasing interest in both intraoperative and nonoperative interventions using biocellular interventions and tissue engineering principles to augment healing and improve clinical outcomes. Research studies highlighting biocellular techniques are producing mixed results where some interventions demonstrate no significant difference to a control group, whereas others are demonstrating promise of these interventions. Physicians practicing regenerative medicine principles can conduct repeat evaluations and repeat diagnostic imaging, such as high-resolution ultrasound, to document changes in soft tissues or the lack thereof and make alterations in protocols to encourage higher levels of soft tissue healing and improved clinical outcomes. This process of the "practice of medicine" is difficult to evaluate in controlled studies and will need to be carefully incorporated in future research protocols that will be validated through clinical outcomes based research.

REFERENCES

1. Phelps D, Sonstegard D, Matthews L. Corticosteroid injection effects on the biomechanical properties of rabbit patellar tendons. Clin Orthop 1974;100: 345–8.
2. Wood T, Cooke P, Goodship A. The effect of anabolic steroids on the mechanical properties and crimp morphology of the rat tendon. Am J Sports Med 1988;16: 153–8.
3. Noyes F, Grood E, Nussbaum N, et al. Effect of intraarticular corticosteroids on ligaments properties: a biomechanical and histological study in rhesus knees. Clin Orthop 1977;123:197–209.
4. Hewett TE, Di Stasi SL, Myer GD. Current concepts for injury prevention in athletes after anterior cruciate ligament reconstruction. Am J Sports Med 2013;41: 216–24.
5. Langer R, Vacanti J. Tissue engineering. Science 1993;260:920–6.
6. Louw Q, Manilall J, Grimmer K. Epidemiology of knee injuries among adolescents: a systematic review. Br J Sports Med 2008;42:2–10.
7. Hing E, Cherry D, Woodwell D. National Ambulatory Medical Care Survey: 2004 summary. Adv Data 2006;374:1–33.
8. Leong N, Petrigliano F, McAllister D. Current tissue engineering strategies in anterior cruciate ligament reconstruction. J Biomed Mater Res A 2014;102: 1614–24.
9. Shelbourne KD, Gray T, Haro M. Incidence of subsequent injury to either knee within 5 years after anterior cruciate ligament reconstruction with patellar tendon autograft. Am J Sports Med 2009;37:246–51.
10. Spindler K, Huston L, Wright R, et al. The prognosis and predictors of sports function and activity at minimum 6 years after anterior cruciate ligament reconstruction: a population cohort study. Am J Sports Med 2011;39:348–59.
11. Levine J, Kiapour A, Quatman C, et al. Clinically relevant injury patterns after an anterior cruciate ligament injury provide insight into injury mechanisms. Am J Sports Med 2013;41:385–95.
12. Chu C, Beynnon B, Buckwalter J, et al. Closing the gap between bench and bedside research for early arthritis therapies (EARTH): report from the AOSSM/NIH U-13 Post-Joint Injury Osteoarthritis Conference II. Am J Sports Med 2011;39:1569–78.

13. Lohmander L, Ostenberg A, Englund M, et al. High prevalence of knee osteoarthritis, pain, and functional limitations in female soccer players twelve years after anterior cruciate ligament injury. Arthritis Rheum 2004;50:3145–52.
14. Nebelung W, Wuschech H. Thirty-five years of follow-up of anterior cruciate ligament-deficient knees in high-level athletes. Arthroscopy 2005;21:696–702.
15. von Porat A, Roos E, Roos H. High prevalence of osteoarthritis 14 years after an anterior cruciate ligament tear in male soccer players: a study of radiographic and patient relevant outcomes. Ann Rheum Dis 2004;63:269–73.
16. Quatman CE, Kiapour A, Myer GD, et al. Cartilage pressure distributions provide a footprint to define female anterior cruciate ligament injury mechanisms. Am J Sports Med 2011;39(8):1706–13.
17. Kiapour A, Murray M. Basic science of anterior cruciate ligament injury and repair. Bone Joint Res 2014;3:20–31.
18. Urwin M, Symmons D, Allison T, et al. Estimating the burden of musculoskeletal disorders in the community: the comparative prevalence of symptoms at different anatomical sites, and the relation to social deprivation. Ann Rheum Dis 1998;57:649–55.
19. Chard M, Hazleman R, Hazleman B, et al. Shoulder disorders in the elderly: a community survey. Arthritis Rheum 1991;34:766–9.
20. Kannus P. Tendons—a source of major concern in competitive and recreational athletes. Scand J Med Sci Sports 1997;7:53–4.
21. Gomoll A, Katz J, Warner J, et al. Rotator cuff disorders: recognition and management among patients with shoulder pain. Arthritis Rheum 2004;50:3751–61.
22. Benjamin M, Ralphs J. Tendons and ligaments—an overview. Histol Histopathol 1997;12:1135–44.
23. Hinsley H, Nicholls A, Daines M, et al. Classification of rotator cuff tendinopathy using high definition ultrasound. Muscles Ligaments Tendons J 2014;4(3): 391–7.
24. Ottenheijm R, Jansen M, Staal J, et al. Accuracy of diagnostic ultrasound in patients with suspected subacromial disorders: a systematic review and meta-analysis. Arch Phys Med Rehabil 2010;91(10):1616–25.
25. Smith T, Back T, Toms A, et al. Diagnostic accuracy of ultrasound for rotator cuff tears in adults: a systematic review and meta-analysis. Clin Radiol 2011;66(11): 1036–48.
26. Teefey S, Hasan S, Middleton W, et al. Ultrasonography of the rotator cuff. A comparison of ultrasonographic and arthroscopic findings in one hundred consecutive cases. J Bone Joint Surg Am 2000;82(4):498–504.
27. Teefey S, Middleton W, Payne W, et al. Detection and measurement of rotator cuff tears with sonography: analysis of diagnostic errors. AJR Am J Roentgenol 2005;184(6):1768–73.
28. Middleton W, Teefey S, Yamaguchi K. Sonography of the rotator cuff: analysis of interobserver variability. Am J Roentgenol 2004;183(5):1465–8.
29. Iannotti J, Ciccone J, Buss D, et al. Accuracy of office-based ultrasonography of the shoulder for the diagnosis of rotator cuff tears. J Bone Joint Surg Am 2005; 87(6):1305–11.
30. Moosmayer S, Smith HJ. Diagnostic ultrasound of the shoulder—a method for experts only? Results from an orthopedic surgeon with relative inexpensive compared to operative findings. Acta Orthop 2005;76(4):503–8.
31. Jeyam M, Funk L, Harris J. Are shoulder surgeons any good at diagnosing rotator cuff tears using ultrasound? A comparative analysis of surgeon vs radiologist. Int J Shoulder Surg 2008;2(1):4–6.

32. Al-Shawi A, Badge R, Bunker T. The detection of full thickness rotator cuff tears using ultrasound. J Bone Joint Surg [Br] 2008;90-B(7):889–92.
33. Kader D, Saxena A, Movin T, et al. Achilles tendinopathy: some aspects of basic science and clinical management. Br J Sports Med 2002;36:239–49.
34. Maffulli N, Kader D. Tendinopathy of tendo Achillis. J Bone Joint Surg Br 2002; 84:1–8.
35. Hashimoto T, Nobuhara K, Hamada T. Pathologic evidence of degeneration as a primary cause of rotator cuff tear. Clin Orthop Relat Res 2003;415:111–20.
36. Nirschl R. Rotator cuff tendinitis: basic concepts of pathoetiology. Instr Course Lect 1989;38:439–45.
37. Khan K, Cook J. The painful nonruptured tendon: clinical aspects. Clin Sports Med 2003;22:711–25.
38. Ishii H, Brunet J, Welsh R, et al. "Bursal reactions" in rotator cuff tearing, the impingement syndrome, and calcifying tendonitis. J Shoulder Elbow Surg 1997;6:131–6.
39. Astrom M, Rausing A. Chronic Achilles tendinopathy: a survey of surgical and histopathological findings. Clin Orthop 1995;316:151–64.
40. Regan W, Wold L, Coonrad R, et al. Mircroscopic histopathology of chronic refractory lateral epicondylitis. Am J Sports Med 1992;20:746–9.
41. Cetti R, Junge J, Vyberg M. Spontaneous rupture of the Achilles tendon is preceded by widespread and bilateral tendon damage and ipsilateral inflammation: a clinical and histopathologic study of 60 patients. Acta Orthop Scand 2003;74:78–84.
42. Matthews T, Hand G, Rees J, et al. Pathology of the torn rotator cuff tendon. Reduction in potential for repair as tear size increases. J Bone Joint Surg Br 2006;88:489–95.
43. Maganaris C, Narici M, Almekinders L, et al. Biomechanics and pathophysiology of overuse tendon injuries ideas on insertional tendinopathy. Sports Med 2004;34(14):1005–17.
44. Rack P, Ross H. The tendon of flexor pollicis longus: its effects on the muscular control of force and position at the human thumb. J Physiol 1984;351:99–110.
45. Woo SL. Mechanical properties of tendons and ligaments I: quasi-static and non-linear viscoelastic properties. Biorheology 1982;19:385–96.
46. Giai Via A, De Cupis M, Spoliti M, et al. Clinical and biological aspects of rotator cuff tears. Muscles Ligaments Tendons J 2013;3(2):70–9.
47. Cook J, Feller J, Bonar S, et al. Abnormal tenocyte morphology is more prevalent than collagen disruption in asymptomatic athletes' patellar tendons. J Orthop Res 2004;22:334–8.
48. Movin T, Gad A, Reinholt F, et al. Tendon pathology in longstanding achillodynia. Biopsy findings in 40 patients. Acta Orthop Scand 1997;68:170–5.
49. Riley G, Goddard M, Hazleman B. Histopathological assessment and pathological significance of matrix degeneration in supraspinatus tendons. Rheumatology 2001;40:229–30.
50. Neer C 2nd. Anterior acromioplasty for the chronic impingement syndrome in the shoulder: a preliminary report. J Bone Joint Surg Am 1972;5:441–50.
51. Codman E, Akerson I. The pathology associated with rupture of the supraspinatus tendon. Ann Surg 1931;93:348–59.
52. McMaster W, Troup T. A survey of interfering shoulder pain in United States competitive swimmers. Am J Sports Med 1993;21:67–70.
53. Wendelboe A, Hegmann K, Gren L, et al. Associations between body-mass index and surgery for rotator cuff tendinitis. J Bone Joint Surg Am 2004;86:743–7.

54. Lohr J, Uhthoff H. The microvascular pattern of the supraspinatus tendon. Cl. Orthop 1990;254:35–8.
55. Sano H, Ishii H, Trudel G, et al. Histologic evidence of degeneration at the insertion of 3 rotator cuff tendons: a comparative study with human cadaveric shoulders. J Shoulder Elbow Surg 1999;8:574–9.
56. Yadav H, Nho S, Romeo A, et al. Rotator cuff tears: pathology and repair. Knee Surg Sports Traumatol Arthrosc 2009;17:409–21.
57. Yuan J, Murrell G, Wei A, et al. Apoptosis in rotator cuff tendinopathy. J Orthop Res 2002;20:1372–9.
58. Riley G, Curry V, DeGroot J, et al. Matrix metalloproteinase activities and their relationship with collagen remodelling in tendon pathology. Matrix Biol 2002; 21(2):185–95.
59. Kovacevic D, Rodeo S. Biological augmentation of rotator cuff tendon repair. Clin Orthop Relat Res 2008;466:622–33.
60. Boileau P, Brassart N, Watkinson D, et al. Arthroscopic repair of full-thickness tears of the supraspinatus: does the tendon really heal? J Bone Joint Surg Am 2005;87:1229–40.
61. Galatz L, Ball C, Teefey S, et al. The outcome and repair integrity of completely arthroscopically repaired large and massive rotator cuff tears. J Bone Joint Surg Am 2004;86:219–24.
62. Gazielly D, Gleyze P, Montagnon C. Functional and anatomical results after rotator cuff repair. Clin Orthop Relat Res 1994;304:43–53.
63. Gerber C, Fuchs B, Hodler J. The results of repair of massive tears of the rotator cuff. J Bone Joint Surg Am 2000;82:505–15.
64. Harryman D, Mack L, Wang K, et al. Repairs of the rotator cuff: correlation of functional results with integrity of the cuff. J Bone Joint Surg Am 1991;73:982–9.
65. Hernigou P, Flouzat Lachaniette C, Delambre J, et al. Biologic augmentation of rotator cuff repair with mesenchymal stem cells during arthroscopy improves healing and prevents further tears: a case-controlled study. Int Orthop 2014; 38(9):1811–8.
66. Gulotta L, Kovacevic D, Ehteshami J, et al. Application of bone marrow-derived mesenchymal stem cells in a rotator cuff repair model. Am J Sports Med 2009; 37(11):2126–33.
67. Isaac C, Gharaibeh B, Witt M, et al. Biologic approaches to enhance rotator cuff healing after injury. J Shoulder Elbow Surg 2012;21:181–90.
68. Taniguchi N, Suenaga N, Oizumi N, et al. Bone marrow stimulation at the footprint of arthroscopic surface-holding repair advances cuff repair integrity. J Shoulder Elbow Surg 2015;24:860–6.
69. Bedi A, Maak T, Walsh C, et al. Cytokines in rotator cuff degeneration and repair. J Shoulder Elbow Surg 2012;21:218–27.
70. Mazzocca A, McCarthy M, Chowaniec D, et al. Rapid isolation of human stem cells (connective tissue progenitor cells) from the proximal humerus during arthroscopic rotator cuff surgery. Am J Sports Med 2010;38(7):1438–47.
71. Mazzocca AD, McCarthy MB, Chowaniec D, et al. Bone marrow-derived mesenchymal stem cells obtained during arthroscopic rotator cuff repair surgery show potential for tendon cell differentiation after treatment with insulin. Arthroscopy 2011;27(11):1459–71.
72. Ellera Gomes J, da Silva R, Silla L, et al. Conventional rotator cuff repair complemented by the aid of mononuclear autologous stem cells. Knee Surg Sports Traumatol Arthrosc 2012;20(2):373–7.

73. Tornero-Esteban P, Hoyas J, Villafuertes E, et al. Efficacy of supraspinatus tendon repair using mesenchymal stem cells along with a collagen I scaffold. J Orthop Surg Res 2015;10:124.
74. Sharma P, Maffulli N. Biology of tendon injury: healing, modeling and remodeling. J Musculoskelet Neuronal Interact 2006;6(2):181–90.
75. Hogan MV, Bagayoko N, James R, et al. Tissue engineering solutions for tendon repair. J Am Acad Orthop Surg 2011;19:134–42.
76. Majewski M, Schaeren S, Kohlhaas U, et al. Postoperative rehabilitation after percutaneous Achilles tendon repair: early functional therapy versus cast immobilization. Disabil Rehabil 2008;30:1726–32.
77. Müller SA, Todorov A, Heisterbach PE, et al. Tendon healing: an overview of physiology, biology, and pathology of tendon healing and systematic review of state of the art in tendon bioengineering. Knee Surg Sports Traumatol Arthrosc 2015;23(7):2097–105.
78. Oliva F, Via A, Maffulli N. Role of growth factors in rotator cuff healing. Sports Med Arthrosc 2011;19:218–26.
79. Ingraham J, Weber R, Childs E. Intrinsic tendon healing requires the recycling of tendon collagen fibril segments. J Hand Surg Eur Vol 2011;36:154–5.
80. Rumian AP, Draper ER, Wallace AL, et al. The influence of the mechanical environment on remodelling of the patellar tendon. J Bone Joint Surg Br 2009;91: 557–64.
81. Hsu S, Liang R, Woo S. Functional tissue engineering of ligament healing. Sports Med Arthrosc Rehabil Ther Technol 2010;2:2–10.
82. Liu S, Yang R, al-Shaikh R, et al. Collagen in tendon, ligament, and bone healing: a current review. Clin Orthop Relat Res 1995;318:265–78.
83. Shrive N, Chimich D, Marchuk L, et al. Soft-tissue "flaws" are associated with material properties of the healing rabbit medial collateral ligament. J Orthop Res 1995;13:923–9.
84. Frank C, Shrive N, Hiraoka H, et al. Optimization of the biology of soft tissue repair. J Sci Med Sport 1999;2(3):190–210.
85. Plaas A, Wong-Palms S, Koob T, et al. Proteoglycan metabolism during repair of the ruptured medial collateral ligament in skeletally mature rabbits. Arch Biochem Biophys 2000;374:35–41.
86. Frank C, McDonald D, Wilson J, et al. Rabbit medial collateral ligament scar weakness is associated with decreased collagen pyridinoline crosslink density. J Orthop Res 1995;13:157–65.
87. Frank C, McDonald D, Shrive N. Collagen fibril diameters in the rabbit medial collateral ligament scar: a longer term assessment. Connect Tissue Res 1997; 36:261–9.
88. Woo S, Abramowitch S, Kilger R, et al. Biomechanics of knee ligaments: injury, healing, and repair. J Biomech 2006;39:1–20.
89. Thornton G, Leask G, Shrive N, et al. Early medial collateral ligament scars have inferior creep behavior. J Orthop Res 2000;18:238–46.
90. Fleming B, Hulstyn M, Oksendahl HL, et al. Ligament injury, reconstruction, and osteoarthritis. Curr Opin Orthop 2005;16(5):354–62.
91. Koh J, Dietz J. Osteoarthritis in other joints (hip, elbow, foot, toes, wrist) after sports injuries. Clin Sports Med 2005;24:57–70.
92. Frank C. Ligament structure, physiology and function. J Musculoskelet Neuronal Interact 2004;4(2):199–201.
93. Øiestad B, Engebretsen L, Storheim K, et al. Knee osteoarthritis after anterior cruciate ligament injury. Am J Sports Med 2009;37(7):1434–43.

94. Almekinders L, Pandarinath R, Rahusen F. Knee stability following anterior cruciate ligament rupture and surgery. The contribution of irreducible tibial subluxation. J Bone Joint Surg Am 2004;86:983–7.

95. Asano H, Muneta T, Ikeda H, et al. Arthroscopic evaluation of the articular cartilage after anterior cruciate ligament reconstruction: a short-term prospective study of 105 patients. Arthroscopy 2004;20:474–81.

96. Beynnon B, Uh B, Fleming B, et al. Rehabilitation following anterior cruciate ligament reconstruction: a prospective, randomized, double-blind comparison of accelerated versus nonaccelerated rehabilitation. Am J Sports Med 2005;33:347–59.

97. Andriacchi T, Mundermann A, Smith R, et al. A framework for the in vivo pathomechanics of osteoarthritis at the knee. Ann Biomed Eng 2004;33:447–57.

98. Andriacchi T, Dyrby C. Interactions between kinematics and loading during walking for the normal and ACL deficient knee. J Biomech 2005;38:293–8.

99. Carter D, Beaupre G, Wong M, et al. The mechanobiology of articular cartilage development and degeneration. Clin Orthop 2004;427:S69–77.

100. Hill C, Seo G, Gale D, et al. Cruciate ligament integrity in osteoarthritis of the knee. Arthritis Rheum 2005;52:794–9.

101. Vaishya R, Agarwal A, Ingole S, et al. Current trends in anterior cruciate ligament reconstruction: a review. Cureus 2015;7(11):e378.

102. Nau M, Teuschl A. Regeneration of the anterior cruciate ligament: current strategies in tissue engineering. World J Orthop 2015;6(1):127–36.

103. Mautner K, Blazuk J. Where do injectable stem cell treatments apply in treatment of muscle, tendon, and ligament injuries? PM R 2015;7(4 Suppl):S33–40.

104. Hao Z, Wang S, Zhang X, et al. Stem cell therapy: a promising biological strategy for tendon-bone healing after anterior cruciate ligament reconstruction. Cell Prolif 2016;49(2):154–62.

105. Hanhan S, Ejzenberg A, Goren K, et al. Skeletal ligament healing using the recombinant human amelogenin protein. J Cell Mol Med 2016;20(5):815–24.

106. Gantenbein B, Gadhari N, Chan S, et al. Mesenchymal stem cells and collagen patches for anterior cruciate ligament repair. World J Stem Cells 2015;7(2):521–34.

107. Lento P, Primack S. Advances and utility of diagnostic ultrasound in musculoskeletal medicine. Curr Rev Musculoskelet Med 2008;1(1):24–31.

108. Lutz HT, Buscarini E, editors. WHO manual of diagnostic ultrasound, vol. 1, 2nd edition. Geneva (Switzerland): WHO Press; 2011. p. 12.

109. Mei-Dan O, Kots E, Barchilon V, et al. A dynamic ultrasound examination for the diagnosis of ankle syndesmotic injury in professional athletes. Am J Sports Med 2009;37(5):1009–16.

110. Gennisson J, Deffieux T, Fink T, et al. Ultrasound elastography: principles and techniques. Diagn Interv Imaging 2013;94:487–95.

111. Taljanovic MS, Melville D, Klauser A, et al. Advances in lower extremity ultrasound. Curr Radiol Rep 2015;3:19.

112. Akatsu Y, Yamaguchi S, Mukoyama S. Accuracy of high-resolution ultrasound in the detection of meniscal tears and determination of the visible area of menisci. J Bone Joint Surg Am 2015;97(10):799–806.

113. van Holsebeeck M. Sonography of large synovial joints. In: van Holsebeeck MT, editor. Musculoskeletal ultrasound. 2nd edition. St Louis: Mosby; 2001. p. 235–76.

114. Plasznik R. Sonography of the shoulder. In: van Holsebeeck MT, editor. Musculoskeletal ultrasound. 2nd edition. St Louis: Mosby; 2001. p. 463–513.

115. Rutten M, Jager G, Blickman J. From the RSNA refresher courses: US of the rotator cuff: pitfalls, limitations, and artifacts. Radiographics 2006;26(2):589–604.

6. Dinnes J, Loveman E, McIntyre L, et al. The effectiveness of diagnostic tests for the assessment of shoulder pain due to soft tissue disorders: a systematic review. Health Technol Assess 2003;7:1–166.

117. Davidson CJ, Ganion LR, Gehlsen GM, et al. Rat tendon morphologic and functional changes resulting from soft tissue mobilization. Med Sci Sports Exerc 1997;29:313–9.

118. Dohan Ehrenfest D, Rasmusson L, Albrektsson T. Classification of platelet concentrates: from pure platelet-rich plasma (P-PRP) to leucocyte- and platelet-rich fibrin (L-PRF). Trends Biotechnol 2009;27:158–67.

119. Dhillon M, Behera P, Patel S, et al. Orthobiologics and platelet rich plasma. Indian J Orthop 2014;48(1):1–9.

120. de Vos R, Weir A, van Shie H, et al. Platelet-rich plasma injection for chronic achilles teninopathy: a randomized controlled trial. JAMA 2010;303:144–9.

121. Rodeo S, Potter H, Kawamura S, et al. Biologic augmentation of rotator cuff tendon-healing with use of a mixture of osteoinductive growth factors. J Bone Joint Surg Am 2007;89:2485–97.

122. Bosch G, Van Shie H, de Groot M, et al. Effects of platelet-rich plasma on the quality of repair of mechanically induced core lesions in equine superficial digital flexor tendons: a placebo-controlled experimental study. J Orthop Res 2010; 28:211–7.

123. Serhan C, Savill J. Resolution of inflammation: the beginning programs the end. Nat Immunol 2005;6:1191–7.

124. Majewski M, Ochsner PE, Liu F, et al. Accelerated healing of the rat Achilles tendon in response to autologous conditioned serum. Am J Sports Med 2009; 37:2117–25.

125. de Mos M, van der Windt A, Jahr H, et al. Can platelet-rich plasma enhanced tendon repair? A cell culture study. Am J Sports Med 2008;36:1171–8.

126. Mishra A, Woodall J Jr, Vieira A. Treatment of tendon and muscle using platelet-rich plasma. Clin Sports Med 2009;28:113–25.

127. Mishra A, Harmon K, Woodall J, et al. Sports medicine applications of platelet rich plasma. Curr Pharm Biotechnol 2012;13:1185–95.

128. DeLong J, Russell R, Mazzocca A. Platelet-rich plasma: the PAW classification system. Arthroscopy 2012;28:998–1009.

129. Zhou Y, Zhang J, Wu H, et al. The differential effects of leukocyte-containing and pure platelet-rich plasma (PRP) on tendon stem/progenitor cells - implications of PRP application for the clinical treatment of tendon injuries. Stem Cell Res Ther 2015;6:173.

130. Mishra A, Pavelko T. Treatment of chronic elbow tendinosis with buffered platelet-rich plasma. Am J Sports Med 2006;34(11):1774–8.

131. Cavallo C, Filardo G, Mariani E, et al. Comparison of platelet-rich plasma formulations for cartilage healing: an in vitro study. J Bone Joint Surg Am 2014;96: 423–9.

132. Zhang J, Wang J. Platelet-rich plasma releasate promotes differentiation of tendon stem cells into active tenocytes. Am J Sports Med 2010;38:2477–86.

133. Eastment C, Sirbasku D. Human platelet lysate contains growth factor activities for established cell lines derived from various tissues of several species. In Vitro 1980;16:694–705.

134. Rendu F, Brohard-Bohn B. The platelet release reaction: granules' constituents, secretion and functions. Platelets 2001;12:261–73.

135. Maynard D, Heijnen H, Horne M, et al. Proteomic analysis of platelet alpha granules using mass spectrometry. J Thromb Haemost 2007;5:1945–55.

136. Bruder S, Fink D, Caplan A. Mesenchymal stem cells in bone development, bone repair, and skeletal regeneration therapy. J Cell Biochem 1994;56:283–94.
137. Pauly S, Klatte F, Strobel C, et al. Characterization of tendon cell cultures of the human rotator cuff. Eur Cell Mater 2010;20:84–97.
138. Strioga M, Viswanathan S, Darinskas A, et al. Same or not the same? Comparison of adipose tissue-derived versus bone marrow-derived mesenchymal stem and stromal cells. Stem Cells Dev 2012;21(14):2724–52.
139. Cananzi M, Atala A, De Coppi P. Stem cells derived from amniotic fluid: new potentials in regenerative medicine. Reprod Biomed Online 2009;18(Suppl 1): 17–27.
140. van Eijk F, Saris D, Riesle J, et al. Tissue engineering of ligaments: a comparison of bone marrow stromal cells, anterior cruciate ligament, and skin fibroblasts as cell source. Tissue Eng 2004;10:893–903.
141. Bianco P, Robey P, Simmons P. Mesenchymal stem cells: revisiting history, concepts, and assays. Cell Stem Cell 2008;2:313–9.
142. Chamberlain G, Fox J, Ashton B, et al. Concise review: mesenchymal stem cells: their phenotype, differentiation capacity, immunological features, and potential for homing. Stem Cells 2007;25:2739–49.
143. Kryger G, Chong A, Costa M, et al. A comparison of tenocytes and mesenchymal stem cells for use in flexor tendon tissue engineering. J Hand Surg Am 2007;32:597–605.
144. Smyth NA, Murawski CD, Haleem AM, et al. Establishing proof of concept: platelet-rich plasma and bone marrow aspirate concentrate may improve cartilage repair following surgical treatment for osteochondral lesions of the talus. World J Orthop 2012;3(7):101–8.
145. Lee J, Zhou Z, Taub P, et al. BMP-12 treatment of adult mesenchymal stem cells in vitro augments tendon-like tissue formation and defect repair in vivo. PLoS One 2011;6:e17531.
146. Caplan A, Correa D. The MSC: an injury drugstore. Cell Stem Cell 2011;9(1): 11–5.
147. Chong A, Ang A, Goh J, et al. Bone marrow-derived mesenchymal stem cells influence early tendon-healing in a rabbit Achilles tendon model. J Bone Joint Surg Am 2007;89(1):74–81.
148. Lim J, Hui J, Li L, et al. Enhancement of tendon graft osteointegration using mesenchymal stem cells in a rabbit model of anterior cruciate ligament reconstruction. Arthroscopy 2004;20(9):899–910.
149. Ouyang H, Goh J, Lee E. Use of bone marrow stromal cells for tendon graft-to-bone healing: histological and immunohistochemical studies in a rabbit model. Am J Sports Med 2004;32(2):321–7.
150. Ouyang H, Goh J, Lee E. Viability of allogeneic bone marrow stromal cells following local delivery into patella tendon in rabbit model. Cell Transplant 2004;13(6):649–57.
151. Uysal A, Mizuno H. Differentiation of adipose-derived stem cells for tendon repair. Methods Mol Biol 2011;702:443–51.
152. Zuk P, Zhu M, Ashjian P, et al. Human adipose tissue is a source of multipotent stem cells. Mol Biol Cell 2002;13:4279–95.
153. Casteilla L, Planat-Benard V, Laharrague P, et al. Adipose-derived stromal cells: their identity and uses in clinical trials, an update. World J Stem Cells 2011;3: 25–33.
154. Eagan M, Zuk P, Zhao K, et al. The suitability of human adipose-derived stem cells for the engineering of ligament tissue. J Tissue Eng Regen Med 2012;6:702–9.

155. Uysal A, Mizuno H. Tendon regeneration and repair with adipose derived stem cells. Curr Stem Cell Res Ther 2010;5(2):161–7.
156. Guilak F, Estes B, Diekman B, et al. Nicolas Andry award: multipotent adult stem cells from adipose tissue for musculoskeletal tissue engineering. Clin Orthop Relat Res 2010;468:2530–40.
157. Moretti P, Hatlapatka T, Marten D, et al. Mesenchymal stromal cells derived from human umbilical cord tissues: primitive cells with potential for clinical and tissue engineering applications. Adv Biochem Eng Biotechnol 2010;123:29–54.
158. Hass R, Kasper C, Böhm S, et al. Different populations and sources of human mesenchymal stem cells (MSC): a comparison of adult and neonatal tissue-derived MSC. Cell Commun Signal 2011;9:12.
159. Galatz L, Sandell L, Rothermich S, et al. Characteristics of the rat supraspinatus tendon during tendon-to-bone healing after acute injury. J Orthop Res 2006;24: 541–50.
160. Cheung EV, Silverio L, Sperling JW. Strategies in biologic augmentation of rotator cuff repair a review. Clin Orthop Relat Res 2010;468:1476–84.
161. Adams J, Zobitz M, Reach JJ, et al. Rotator cuff repair using an acellular dermal matrix graft: an in vivo study in a canine model. Arthroscopy 2006;22:700–9.
162. Hee C, Dines J, Dines D, et al. Augmentation of a rotator cuff suture repair using rhPDGF-BB and a type I bovine collagen matrix in an ovine model. Am J Sports Med 2011;39:1630.
163. Gilbert T, Freund J, Badylak S. Quantification of DNA in biologic scaffold materials. J Surg Res 2009;152:135–9.
164. Li Y, Meng H, Liu Y, et al. Fibrin gel as an injectable biodegradable scaffold and cell carrier for tissue engineering. ScientificWorldJournal 2015;2015:685690.
165. Swartz D, Russell J, Andreadis S. Engineering of fibrin-based functional and implantable small-diameter blood vessels. Am J Physiol Heart Circ Physiol 2005;288(3):H1451–60.
166. Jockenhoevel S, Flanagan T. "Cardiovascular tissue engineering based on fibrin-gel-scaffolds," in tissue engineering for tissue and organ regeneration. Chapter 3. In: Eberli D, editor. InTech; 2011.
167. Brown C, Yan J, Han T, et al. Effect of decellularized adipose tissue particle size and cell density on adipose-derived stem cell proliferation and adipogenic differentiation in composite methacrylated chondroitin sulphate hydrogels. Biomed Mater 2015;10:045010.
168. Longo U, Lamberti A, Maffulli N, et al. Tendon augmentation grafts: a systematic review. Br Med Bull 2010;94:165–88.
169. Niknejad H, Peirovi H, Jorjani M, et al. Properties of the amniotic cell membrane for potential use in tissue engineering. Eur Cell Mater 2008;15:88–99.
170. Osti L, Berardocco M, di Giacomo V, et al. Hyaluronic acid increases tendon derived cell viability and collagen type I expression in vitro: comparative study of four different hyaluronic acid preparations by molecular weight. BMC Musculoskelet Disord 2015;16:284.
171. Chen W, Grant M, Schor A, et al. Differences between adult and fetal fibroblasts in the regulation of hyaluronate synthesis: correlation with migratory activity. J Cell Sci 1989;94(Pt 3):577–84.
172. Klein E, Asculai S, Ben-Ari G. Effects of hyaluronic acid on fibroblast behavior in peritoneal injury. J Surg Res 1996;61(2):473–6.
173. Wiig M, Abrahamsson S, Lundborg G. Effects of hyaluronan on cell proliferation and collagen synthesis: a study of rabbit flexor tendons in vitro. J Hand Surg Am 1996;21(4):599–604.

174. Lullove E. A flowable placental tissue matrix allograft in lower extremity injuries: a pilot study. Cureus 2015;7(6):e275.
175. Saw V, Minassian D, Dart J, et al. Amniotic membrane tissue user group (AM-TUG): amniotic membrane transplantation for ocular disease: a review of the first 233 cases from the UK user group. Br J Ophthalmol 2007;91:1042–7.
176. Kubo M, Sonoda Y, Muramatsu R, et al. Immunogenicity of human amniotic membrane in experimental xenotransplantation. Invest Ophthalmol Vis Sci 2001;42:1539–46.
177. Ryu R, Ryu J, Abrams J, et al. Arthroscopic implantation of a bio-inductive collagen scaffold for treatment of an articular-sided partial rotator cuff tear. Arthrosc Tech 2015;4(5):e483–5.
178. Arnoczky S, Lavagnino M, Egerbacher M. The mechanobiological aetiopathogenesis of tendinopathy: is it the over-stimulation or the under-stimulation of tendon cells? Int J Exp Pathol 2007;88:21.
179. Bokor D, Sonnabend D, Deady L, et al. Preliminary investigation of a biological augmentation of rotator cuff repairs using a collagen implant: a 2-year MRI follow-up. Muscles Ligaments Tendons J 2015;5(3):144–50.
180. Evans C. Cytokines and the role they play in the healing of ligaments and tendons. Sports Med 1999;28:71–6.
181. Seeherman H, Archambault J, Rodeo S, et al. rhBMP-12 accelerates healing of rotator cuff repairs in a sheep model. J Bone Joint Surg Am 2008;90:2206–19.
182. Majewski M, Betz O, Ochsner PE, et al. Ex vivo adenoviral transfer of bone morphogenetic protein 12 (BMP-12) cDNA improves Achilles tendon healing in a rat model. Gene Ther 2008;15(16):1139–46.
183. Keller T, Hogan MV, Kesturu G, et al. Growth/differentiation factor-5 modulates the synthesis and expression of extracellular matrix and cell-adhesion related molecules of rat Achilles tendon fibroblasts. Connect Tissue Res 2011;52(4): 353–64.
184. Anderson D, Campbell P, Guanche C. The use of biological agents to accelerate recovery from rotator cuff repair: path to clinical application. Oper Tech Sports Med 2002;10(2):58–63.
185. Dahlgren L, Mohammed H, Nixon A. Temporal expression of growth factors and matrix molecules in healing tendon lesions. J Orthop Res 2005;23:84–92.
186. Yang G, Rothrauff B, Tuan R. Tendon and ligament regeneration and repair: clinical relevance and developmental paradigm. Birth Defects Res C Embryo Today 2013;99(3):203–22.
187. Folkman J, Klagsbrun M. Angiogenic factors. Science 1987;235(4787):442–7.
188. Zhang F, Liu H, Stile F, et al. Effect of vascular endothelial growth factor on rat Achilles tendon healing. Plast Reconstr Surg 2003;112:1613–9.
189. Koh J, Mohan P, Howe T, et al. Fasciotomy and surgical tenotomy for recalcitrant lateral elbow tendinopathy: early clinical experience with a novel device for minimally invasive percutaneous microresection. Am J Sports Med 2012;41:636–44.
190. Barnes D, Beckley J, Smith J. Percutaneous ultrasonic tenotomy for chronic elbow tendinosis: a prospective study. J Shoulder Elbow Surg 2015;24:67–73.
191. Pourcho A, Hall M. Percutaneous ultrasonic fasciotomy for refractory plantar fasciopathy after failure of a partial endoscopic release procedure. PM R 2015; 7(11):1194–7.
192. Nirschl R. Elbow tendinosis/Tennis elbow. Clin Sports Med 1992;11:851–70.
193. Badylak SF, Freytes DO, Gilbert TW. Extracellular matrix as a biological scaffold material: structure and function. Acta Biomater 2009;5(1):1–13.

Orthobiologics and Knee Osteoarthritis

A Recent Literature Review, Treatment Algorithm, and Pathophysiology Discussion

David M. Crane, MD[a,b,c,*], Kristin S. Oliver, MD, MPH[a,b,c,d],
Matthew C. Bayes, MD[a,c]

KEYWORDS

- Knee osteoarthritis • Fat lipoaspirate • Orthobiologics • Tissue engineering
- Meniscus • Extrusion • Stem cell depletion model • Multinodal pathophysiology

KEY POINTS

- There has been a tremendous growth in the regenerative medicine health care space since the beginning of platelet-rich plasma use in 1987.
- Tissue engineering is becoming a reality; however, difficult decisions such as how to best optimize care and treatment plans to treat knee osteoarthritis remain.
- In these early days of orthobiologics, we are seeing a pattern of studies emerge that seem to support the safety of these products.
- The literature seems to support orthobiologics in the treatment of knee osteoarthritis for 1 year or longer, depending on the age of the patient and disease severity.
- The current array of orthobiologic treatments and combinations will be a barrier of entry for many providers and patients.

INTRODUCTION

This article provides the reader with information in several areas regarding the use of orthobiologics in the treatment of knee osteoarthritis (OA).[1] These goals are (1) to provide a recent, brief literature review of the current options in orthobiologics as they pertain to the clinical treatment of knee OA. These treatments include, but are not limited to platelet-rich plasma (PRP), autologous conditioned plasma (ACP), bone marrow concentrate (BMC), and mesenchymal stem cells (MSC). (2) We describe a

---

Disclosure Statement: The authors have nothing to disclose.
[a] Bluetail Medical Group, St Louis, MO, USA; [b] Bluetail Medical Group, Naples, FL, USA; [c] 17300 North Outer 40 Drive, Suite 201, Chesterfield, MO 63005, USA; [d] Bluetail Medical Group, Columbia, MO, USA
* Corresponding author. 17300 North Outer 40 Drive, Suite 201, Chesterfield, MO 63005.
E-mail address: Dcranemd@gmail.com

Phys Med Rehabil Clin N Am 27 (2016) 985–1002
http://dx.doi.org/10.1016/j.pmr.2016.07.004
1047-9651/16/© 2016 Published by Elsevier Inc.

new model of knee OA that fills the gap in our understanding of it as a purely traumatic and/or inflammation-induced cartilage degenerative condition, to a current model of multinodal pathophysiology. The goal of this new model of OA is to provide physicians, stem cell scientists, and physical therapy and movement specialists with a new paradigm on which to perform tissue engineering, thus providing a scaffold to understand on what layer/level new therapies and studies will take place. (3) Graft choice and patient selection in the current state of understanding of the treatment of knee OA in a tissue engineering model with orthobiologics is discussed. (4) We present a sample treatment algorithm and decision "nest" (or multinodal decision tree) as it pertains to the decision on how to proceed with patient care in this complex problem.

PREVALENCE OF DISEASE

Knee OA represents a large and progressively worsening problem for the developed world. The rates of progression follow other diseases of lifestyle, and indeed affect a large portion of the population in the United States with current prevalence of 280 in 1000 patient population aged greater than 45 years of age. This is approximately 26.9 million US adults, which is believed to be a conservative estimate (prevalence data from 2005, up from 21 million in 1990).[2] With the annual total knee replacement percentage expected to increase by 601% by 2030,[3] we as a society will require a better understanding of pathophysiology, as well as an improved and earlier detection and treatment model of knee OA, to reduce the current progression of total joint arthroplasty. With the cost of total knee arthroplasty or joint replacement hovering around US$57,000, and with a reported mortality rate of approximately 0.25% (or 1 in 400 patients), and complications ranging from deep venous thrombosis to infection to persistent pain,[4] a more sustainable treatment model will be necessary to effectively deal with this growing public health problem.

CURRENT ORTHOBIOLOGIC TREATMENT OPTIONS

There are many treatments that now fit this overarching label (also known as regenerative injection therapies or biocellular grafts, depending on use). These options include (in order of appearance over the past decades) whole blood therapy, traditional prolotherapy, PRP, ACP or autologous conditioned serum, bone marrow aspirate concentrate, adipose biocellular autograft (as whole lipoaspirate without manipulation or stromal vascular fraction of adipose [SVF]), MSC allograft cellular concentrates, amniotic cellular concentrates, cord-derived cellular concentrates, interleukin receptor antagonist receptor peptides, and alpha 2 macroglobulins. This number of treatments can leave the clinician bewildered with regard to what treatment paradigm to offer the patient suffering with knee OA. This article focuses on the use of ACP, PRP, BMC, and briefly on whole lipoaspirate in the treatment of knee OA; as they have been, and remain, the most well-studied and prevalent grafts of current use. This article does not focus in on the growth factor cellular preparations constituted with amnion or cord-derived cells.

To help the reader, the author will put a shorthand delineation of graft composition after each reference that will include (A) the cellular concentration of autograft product (ie, ACP, PRP, BMC, or MSC), (B) the leukocyte concentration consisting of leukocyte-rich (LR) or leukocyte-poor (LP) platelet concentrated product (or unknown), (C) high red cell hemoglobin concentration (8%–15% heme or + heme) or low hemoglobin concentration (2%–7% heme or -heme) or unknown, and (D) the presence or absence of a matrix (+mtx or −mtx, or unknown). Examples may look like (BMC + PRP LR + heme −mtx) or (ACP LP −mtx). Leukocyte concentrations will be defined as

LP or LR and this will be understood to correlate with a granulocyte or neutrophil deficient product with a high mononuclear cellular concentration.[5–7] For this discussion, ACP is defined as a concentrated platelet product with platelets 2- to 3-fold greater than baseline that is LP in nature. PRP will be considered 4- to 6-fold fold greater than platelet baseline and either LR or LP (if known) and high or low hematocrit concentration (if known). BMC is BMC with concentrations of platelets and human MSCs[8–11] along with the addition of PRP from peripheral blood draw (if known). Adipose-derived cells will be designated Ad-MSC if they are obtained from a source that requires collagenase for processing or cell expansion. From the author's perspective, this shorthand makes it easier to correlate studies and determine the orthobiologic autograft used because there exists no standardized nomenclature to date to define the different preparations or the use of the term "PRP."

Platelet-rich Plasma and Knee Osteoarthritis Clinical Trials or Studies: Metaanalyses

In a level I systematic review and metaanalysis performed by Chang and colleagues in 2014, the effectiveness of PRP in treating cartilage degenerative pathology in knee joints was explored. For this metaanalysis, the investigators included single-arm prospective studies, quasiexperimental studies, and randomized controlled trials that used PRP to treat knee chondral degenerative lesions. Eight single-arm studies, 3 quasiexperimental studies, and 5 randomized controlled trials were identified, comprising 1543 participants. PRP injections in patients with knee degenerative pathology showed continual efficacy for 12 months compared with their pretreatment condition. The effectiveness of PRP was likely better and more prolonged than that of hyaluronic acid (HA). Patients with less severe OA achieved superior outcomes as opposed to those with advanced OA.[12]

In another level I metaanalysis of PRP use in knee OA using LR or LP products performed by Riboh and colleagues in 2015,[13] clinical outcomes and rates of adverse reactions between LP-PRP and LR-PRP preparations were compared. For this metaanalysis, the MEDLINE, EMBASE, and Cochrane databases were reviewed. The primary outcome was the incidence of local adverse reactions. Secondary outcomes were the changes in International Knee Documentation Committee (IKDC) subjective score and Western Ontario and McMaster Universities Osteoarthritis Index (WOMAC) score between baseline and final follow-up measurements. Included in the analysis were 6 randomized controlled trials (evidence level 1) and 3 prospective comparative studies (evidence level 2) with a total of 1055 patients. Injection of LP-PRP resulted in significantly better WOMAC scores than did injection of HA (mean difference, −21.14; 95% CI, −39.63 to −2.65) or placebo (mean difference, −17.84; 95% CI, −34.95 to −0.73). No such difference was observed with LR-PRP (mean difference, −14.28; 95% CI, −44.80 to 16.25). All treatment groups resulted in equivalent IKDC subjective scores. Subsequent analysis showed that LP-PRP was the highest ranked treatment for both measures of clinical efficacy (WOMAC and IKDC). Finally, PRP injections resulted in a higher incidence of adverse reactions than HA (odds ratio, 5.63; 95% CI, 1.38–22.90), but there was no difference between LR-PRP and LP-PRP (odds ratio, 0.78; 95% CI, 0.05–11.93). These reactions were nearly always local swelling and pain, with a single study reporting medical side effects including syncope, dizziness, headache, gastritis, and tachycardia (17 of 1055 total patients).[13]

Meheux and colleagues performed a level I systematic review of level I studies in 2015. Studies were evaluated to determine (1) whether PRP injection significantly improves validated patient-reported outcomes in patients with symptomatic knee OA at 6 and 12 months after injection, (2) differences in outcomes between PRP and corticosteroid injections or viscosupplementation or placebo injections at 6 and 12 months after injection, (3) and similarities and differences in outcomes based on the PRP formulations used in the analyzed studies. In this review, a quality assessment of all articles was performed using the Modified Coleman Methodology Score (average, 83.3/100), and outcomes were analyzed using 2-proportion z-tests. Six articles (739 patients, 817 knees, 39% males, mean age of 59.9 years, with 38 weeks average follow-up) were analyzed. All studies met minimal clinically important difference criteria and showed significant improvements in statistical and clinical outcomes, including pain, physical function, and stiffness, with PRP. All but 1 study showed significant differences in clinical outcomes between PRP and HA or PRP and placebo in pain and function. Average pretreatment WOMAC scores were 52.36 and 52.05 for the PRP and HA groups, respectively ($P = .420$). Mean posttreatment WOMAC scores for PRP were significantly better than for HA at 3 to 6 months (28.5 and 43.4, respectively; $P = .0008$) and at 6 to 12 months (22.8 and 38.1, respectively; $P = .0062$). None of the included studies used corticosteroids. This review suggests that, in patients with symptomatic knee OA, PRP injections result in significant clinical improvements up to 12 months after injection. There is limited evidence for comparing LR-PRP versus LP-PRP or PRP versus steroids per this review. The authors were therefore unable to evaluate the third stated objective as noted.[14]

Autologous Conditioned Plasma and Knee Osteoarthritis Clinical Trials or Studies

In a level I RCT study published by Smith in 2016, ACP proved to be an efficacious treatment for knee OA in a small group of patients studied. This was a US Food and Drug Administration–sanctioned, double-blind, randomized, controlled trial designed to determine the safety and efficacy of LP-ACP for knee OA treatment. The study was designed as a feasibility trial regulated by the US Food and Drug Administration. Thirty patients were included in the study. These patients were randomized to receive either ACP (n = 15) or saline placebo (n = 15) for a series of 3 weekly injections. WOMAC scores served as the primary efficacy outcome measure. Patients were followed for 1 year. Results showed no adverse events for ACP administration. Furthermore, the results demonstrated no difference in baseline WOMAC scores between the 2 groups. However, in the ACP group, WOMAC scores at 1 week were decreased significantly compared with baseline scores, and the scores for this group remained significantly lower throughout the study duration. At the study conclusion (12 months), subjects in the ACP group had improved their overall WOMAC scores by 78% from their baseline score, compared with 7% for the placebo group (Smith PA[7]; ACP LP –heme –mtx). In another small randomized, controlled trial study performed by Cerza and associates in 2013, a total of 120 patients affected by clinically and radiographically documented knee OA were evaluated. OA scores were graded using the Kellgren–Lawrence radiographic classification scale. The 120 patients were randomized into 2 study groups: 60 patients received 4 intraarticular injections of PRP (ACP LP –heme –mtx) and 60 patients received 4 intraarticular injections of HA. All patients were evaluated with the WOMAC score before the infiltration and at 4, 12, and 24 weeks after the first injection. Results showed that treatment with a local injection of ACP had a significant effect shortly after the final infiltration with a continuously improving sustained effect up to 24 weeks (WOMAC score, 65.1 and 36.5 in the HA and ACP groups, respectively; $P<.001$). In the HA group, the worst results were obtained for grade III knee OA, whereas the clinical results obtained in the ACP group did not show any difference in terms of the grade of knee arthrosis. The mean WOMAC scores for grade III knee OA were 74.85 in the HA group and 41.20 in the ACP group ($P<.001$; ACP LP –heme –mtx).[7]

In a level IV small case series reported by Filardo and colleagues in 2014, ACP use for the treatment of knee OA was studied. The aim of the study was to describe the clinical results obtained after intraarticular injection of an ACP preparation for the treatment of knee OA. In this study, 45 patients (mean age, 59 years; mean body mass index, 27 kg/m^2) were included and treated with a cycle of 3 weekly injections of ACP. Six patients were affected by bilateral symptomatic OA; therefore, 51 knees in total were treated. The patients were divided into 2 groups: those affected by early to moderate OA and those affected by severe OA. The patients were submitted to baseline evaluation, and evaluation after a mean follow-up of 14.5 months (range, 6–24). Outcome measures used included IKDC-subjective, the EuroQual Visual Analog Scale, Tegner, and Knee Injury and Osteoarthritis Outcome (KOOS) scores. The overall clinical outcome was positive and the treatment proved to be safe. In the early or moderate OA group, the IKDC-subjective score increased from 36.4 at the baseline evaluation to 57.3 at the follow-up ($P<.0005$) and a similar trend was shown by the EuroQual Visual Analog Scale, and Tegner and KOOS scores. Although an improvement was also recorded in the severe OA group, the clinical outcome of the patients in this group was significantly poorer, and they reported less benefit. In the early to moderate OA group, body mass index and longer symptom duration before treatment were found to be correlated with clinical outcome (ACP LP –heme –mtx).[15]

Platelet-rich Plasma and Knee Osteoarthritis Clinical Trials or Studies: Randomized Controlled Trials or Case Series

In a small level I randomized, controlled trial performed by Sanchez and colleagues in 2012, 176 patients were randomized to receive PRP or HA in 3 weekly injections with pain and function scores followed to 24 weeks. Of patients receiving PRP, 38% had a 50% decrease in WOMAC pain score at 24 weeks compared with 24% of patients receiving HA (P value 0.044; unknown platelet or leukocyte concentrations -mtx).[16,17] Another study performed by Vaquerizo and colleagues, 2013 compared the efficacy and safety of 3 injections of PRP versus 1 single intraarticular injection of HA as a treatment for reducing symptoms in patients with knee OA. Ninety-six patients with symptomatic knee OA were randomly assigned to receive PRP (3 injections on a weekly basis) or 1 infiltration with Durolane HA (Bioventus, Hoofddorp, The Netherlands). The primary outcome measures were a 30% decrease and a 50% decrease in the summed score for pain, physical function, and stiffness subscales of the WOMAC and Lequesne scores from baseline to weeks 24 and 48, respectively. Treatment with PRP was significantly more efficient than treatment with HA in reducing knee pain and stiffness and improving physical function in patients with knee OA. The rate of response to PRP was significantly higher than the rate of response to HA for all the scores including pain, stiffness, and physical function in patients at 24 and 48 weeks. Adverse events were mild and evenly distributed between the groups (unknown platelet or leukocyte concentration –mtx).[18]

Bone Marrow Concentrate and Human Mesenchymal Stem Cell Clinical Studies

In a prospective case series published in July 2015, Oliver and colleagues evaluated the clinical efficacy of autologous intraarticular BMC with autologous lipoaspirate as a treatment option for knee OA. Additionally, BMC samples from a patient population subset were sent for outside laboratory analysis. Seventy patients diagnosed with Kellgren-Lawrence stage 2 to 4 knee OA were analyzed. Data regarding adverse events and KOOS metrics were obtained at baseline, 90 days, and 180 days. Samples of BMC from 11 patients were sent to an outside source for laboratory analysis. Adverse events were limited to transient pain and swelling of the treated joint. The mean reported KOOS changes from before the procedure to 180 days after the procedure were as follows: pain, +18.1; activities of daily living, +15.6; symptoms, +17.3; quality of life, +20.3; and sports/recreation +18.1. Laboratory analysis of the samples demonstrated statistically significant increases in concentration of platelets, interleukin-1 receptor antagonist (IL-1Rra and IL-1β). This ratio of IL-1ra to IL-β has been shown to alleviate the degenerative effects of IL-1. The increase in the IL-1ra/IL-1β ratio was statistically significant at 193.54 when processed with a 2% hematocrit setting, and 720.62 when processed with a 15% hematocrit. The group concluded that intraarticular injection of autologous BMC and lipoaspirate in patients diagnosed with knee OA demonstrates encouraging results for positive outcomes in pain and function without complication, in addition to showing elevations of antiinflammatory levels of IL-1ra (BMC LP ± heme + mtx).[19,20]

Vangsness and colleagues in 2014 published a randomized, double-blind, controlled study using adult human MSCs delivered via intraarticular injection to the knee after partial medial meniscectomy. In this study, 55 patients from 7 institutions underwent partial medial meniscectomy. A single superolateral knee injection was given within 7 to 10 days after the meniscectomy. Patients were then randomized to 1 of 3 treatment groups: group A, in which patients received an injection of 50×10^6 allogeneic MSCs; group B, 150×10^6 allogeneic MSCs; and the control group, a sodium hyaluronate (HA/hyaluronan) vehicle control. Patients were followed to evaluate safety, meniscus regeneration, the overall condition of the knee joint, and clinical outcomes at intervals through 2 years. Evaluations included sequential MRI scans. The results showed no ectopic tissue or safety issues. Significantly increased meniscal volume (defined a priori as a 15% threshold) determined by quantitative MRI was noted in 24% of patients in group A and 6% in group B at 12 months after meniscectomy ($P = .022$). No patients in the control group met the 15% threshold for increased meniscal volume. Overall, patients with osteoarthritic changes who received MSCs experienced a significant reduction in pain compared with those who received the control, on the basis of assessments by visual analog scale (MSC unknown leuk, -heme –mtx).[21]

In a level II, randomized controlled trial published by Saw and colleagues in 2013, histologic and MRI evaluation of articular cartilage regeneration in patients with chondral lesions treated by arthroscopic subchondral drilling followed by postoperative intraarticular injections of HA with and without peripheral blood stem cells (PBSC) was evaluated. The PBSC were harvested through apheresis after filgrastim (recombinant human granulocyte colony-stimulating factor) stimulation. Fifty patients ages 18 to 50 years with International Cartilage Repair Society (ICRS) grade 3 and 4 lesions of the knee joint underwent arthroscopic subchondral drilling. Twenty-five patients each were randomized to the control (HA) and the intervention (PBSC plus HA) groups. Both groups received 5 weekly injections commencing 1 week after surgery. Three additional injections of either HA or PBSC plus HA were given at weekly intervals 6 months after surgery. Subjective IKDC scores and MRI scans were obtained preoperatively and postoperatively at serial visits. Second-look arthroscopy and biopsy was performed at 18 months on 16 patients in each group. Biopsy specimens using 14 components of the ICRS Visual Assessment Scale II (ICRS II) were graded and a total score was obtained. MRI scans at 18 months were assessed with a morphologic scoring system. The total ICRS II histologic scores for the control group averaged 957, whereas the intervention group averaged 1066 ($P = .022$). On evaluation of the MRI morphologic scores, the control group averaged 8.5 and the intervention group averaged 9.9 ($P = .013$). The mean 24-month IKDC scores for the control and intervention groups were 71.1 and 74.8, respectively ($P = .844$). There were no notable adverse events. The authors concluded that arthroscopic subchondral drilling into grades 3 and 4 chondral lesions with postoperative intraarticular injections of autologous PBSC in combination with HA resulted in an improvement of the quality of articular cartilage repair over the same treatment without PBSC as shown by histologic and MRI evaluation (MSC unknown leuk –heme + mtx).[1]

Autologous Conditioned Plasma Laboratory Studies

One study done by Sundman and colleagues was designed to look at the effects of PRP or high molecular weight HA on the expression of anabolic and catabolic genes as well as the secretion of nociceptive and inflammatory mediators in knee OA. This controlled laboratory study used synovium and cartilage harvested from patients undergoing total knee arthroplasty that were cocultured with media of PRP or HA. The results showed that inflammatory cytokines and interleukins and matrix metalloproteinases such as tumor necrosis factor-α, IL-6, and matrix metalloproteinase-13 concentrations decreased in ACP and HA preparations compared with control cultures. Neither platelet nor leukocyte concentration had a significant effect on outcome measurements (gene or protein expression data) in cartilage or synoviocytes in this model. These results indicated that PRP acts to stimulate endogenous HA production and decrease cartilage catabolism (ACP LP -mtx for the PRP-labeled cohort).[22]

In another study of ACP for use in cartilage growth, Sakata and colleagues in 2015 performed a controlled laboratory study, which evaluated superficial zone protein (SZP) production after use of ACP. SZP is known as a boundary lubricant in articular cartilage, plays a role in reducing friction and wear, and is involved with cartilage homeostasis. In using cells isolated from articular cartilage, synovium, and the anterior cruciate ligament (ACL) from 12 patients undergoing ACL reconstruction, they found that PRP stimulated proliferation of SZP cells derived from articular cartilage, synovium, and the ACL. It also significantly enhanced SZP secretion from synovium and cartilage-derived cells while reducing the friction coefficient compared with saline or HA. An unexpected finding was the presence of SZP in the PRP preparation (ACP LP allograft cells).[23]

Adipose Orthobiologic Clinical Studies

In 2016, Koh and colleagues published a level II prospective randomized comparative study evaluating Ad-MSC with microfracture (group 1) versus microfracture alone (group 2) with a 2-year follow-up. This study used Ad-MSCs with fibrin glue and microfracture in 40 patients versus microfracture alone in 40 patients with symptomatic knee ICRS grade III or IV cartilage defects. Preoperative MRI and quantitative and qualitative assessments of the repair tissue were carried out at 24 months by using the magnetic resonance observation of cartilage repair tissue scoring system with follow-up MRI. Clinical results were evaluated using the Lysholm score, the KOOS, and a 10-point visual analog score preoperatively and postoperatively at 3 months, 12 months, and the last follow-up visit. Group 1 included 26 patients (65%) who had complete cartilage coverage of the lesion at follow-up compared with 18 patients (45%) in group 2. Significantly better signal intensity was observed for the repair tissue in group 1, with 32 patients (80%) having normal or nearly normal signal intensity (ie, complete cartilage coverage of the lesion) compared with 28 patients (72.5%) in group 2. The mean clinical follow-up period was 27.4 months (range, 26–30). The improvements in the mean KOOS pain and symptom subscores were significantly greater at follow-up in group 1 than in group 2 (pain, 36.6 ± 11.9 in group 1 and 30.1 ± 14.7 in group 2 [P = .034]; symptoms, 32.3 ± 7.2 in group 1 and 27.8 ± 6.8 in group 2 [P = .005]). However, the improvements in the other subscores were not different between groups 1 and 2 (activities of daily living, 38.5 ± 12.8 and 37.6 ± 12.9, respectively [P = .767]; sports and recreation, 33.9 ± 10.3 and 31.6 ± 11.0, respectively [P = .338]; and quality of life, 38.4 ± 13.1 and 37.8 ± 12.0, respectively [P = .650]). Among the 80 patients, second-look arthroscopies were performed in 57 knees (30 in group 1 and 27 in group 2), and biopsy procedures were performed during these arthroscopies for 18 patients in group 1 and 16 patients in group 2. The second-look arthroscopies showed good repair tissue quality with slightly better safranin O and collagen II staining in group 1, although no intergroup difference was observed. Age, lesion size, duration of symptoms before surgery, mechanism of injury, and combined procedures were not correlated with clinical results (Ad-MSC + heme + mtx).[24]

In a multicenter case control study published in 2015 by Michalek and colleagues, the authors studied the use of SVF cells in a single injection in 1128 patients with OA of multiple joint structures. The design of the study was to evaluate the safety and clinical efficacy of freshly isolated autologous SVF cells in a case control study. Patients with grade 2 to 4 degenerative OA were selected. A total of 1128 patients underwent standard liposuction under local anesthesia and SVF cells were isolated and prepared for application into 1 to 4 large joints. A total of 1856 joints, mainly knee and hip joints, were treated with a single dose of SVF cells. These were processed using Cellthera Kit I or II from the Czech Republic containing good manufacturing practices-grade collagenase. Grafts were assessed for total nucleated cell counts, although a portion was culture expanded for colony-forming unit evaluation. Overall, 1114 patients were followed for 12.1 to 54.3 months (median 17.2 months) for safety and efficacy. Modified KOOS/HOOS Clinical Scores were used to evaluate clinical effect and was based on pain, nonsteroid analgesic usage, limping, extent of joint movement, and stiffness evaluation before and at 3, 6, and 12 months after treatment. No serious side effects, systemic infection, or cancer was associated with SVF cell therapy. Reportedly most patients gradually improved 3 to 12 months after the treatment. At least 75% score improvement was noticed in 63% of patients, and at least 50% score improvement was documented in 91% of patients 12 months after SVF cell therapy. Obesity and a higher grade of OA were associated with slower healing (Ad-MSC LP –heme –mtx).[25]

In 2014, Vilar and colleagues published a veterinary study entitled Assessment of the effect of Intraarticular Injection of Autologous Adipose-Derived Mesenchymal Stem Cells in Osteoarthritic Dogs Using a Double-blinded Force Platform Analysis. In this study, 10 lame dogs suffering from severe hip OA were enrolled as the active treatment group with 5 other animals for the control group. Outcomes were based on force platform analysis because this has been consistently used to verify and quantify the efficacy of different therapeutic strategies for the treatment of OA in dogs, including MSC associated with plasma rich in growth factors, but never with Ad-MSC alone. In the study, a biopsy of 20 g of subcutaneous fat tissue (4–5 cm³) was collected from the animal along with 120 mL of blood for preparation in a commercial kit. Immediately after sample collection, fat biopsy and blood (in an anticoagulant container) were sent at 4°C for cell isolation and to the Fat-Stem Laboratory used for processing. The fat was processed with collagenase and by centrifugation, and 30 million Ad-MSCs were subsequently administered in a single injection. Results were analyzed to detect a significant increase in peak vertical force and vertical impulse (from force plate measurements) in treated dogs. Mean values of peak vertical force and vertical impulse were improved significantly within the first 3 months after treatment in the OA group, increasing 9% and 2.5% body weight, respectively, at day 30. After this, the effect seemed to decrease, reaching initial values and tapering off over the ensuing 60 days (reportedly a 90 day effect; Vilar JM and colleagues[26]; Ad-MSC LP –heme –mtx).[26]

In another animal model using rabbit knees, Mehrabani and colleagues in 2015 used Ad-MSCs to evaluate treatment of full-thickness femoral articular cartilage defects. In this study, 2 Million cells suspended in culture medium (DMEM) were supplemented with 10% fetal bovine serum and transplanted using a single injection into the articular cartilage defect of the femoral articular cartilage. The cells were injected into the knee joint of 6 rabbits with 6 rabbits used as controls. Findings on subsequent dissection showed that, in the cell therapy group after transplantation, no abnormal gross findings were noticed. Neoformed tissues in cell-treated groups were translucent with a smooth and intact surface and less irregularity. In cell-treated group after 8 weeks after transplantation, the overall healing score of experimental knees were superior when compared with other groups (Ad-MSC unk leuk –heme + mtx).[27]

A NEW MODEL OF OSTEOARTHRITIS

The way we understand OA in today's medical space is different than what this author was taught in medical school 20 years ago, which was a "wear and tear" model with its notable cartilage loss and osteophyte/spur formation. As we proceed to better understand the causes and effects of chronic inflammation, and the model for this inflammation leading to collagen loss and microinstability to macroinstability; the progressive degradation of the synovial nutrition and loss of articular cartilage needs to be further developed and defined. This has led to a new multinodal model of OA, which this author prefers to call the "balloon, boing-boing, and bioreactor" model of joint homeostasis or pathology. These roughly correlate as: "balloon"—the joint capsule and surrounding myotendinous and fascial support structures of the knee; "boing-boing"—the mechanotransduction and bioinduction of the meniscus and knee articular cartilage; and "bioreactor"—the health, or lack thereof, of the synovial nutrition and lubrication functions as well as the cellular repletion structures of the knee. These are more than just fanciful terminology. We will be using the interplay of these dynamic structural and biologic biotensegrity elements, as well as the biologic homeostasis mechanisms, to help define and decide treatment algorithms further on in this article.

The "Balloon"

It has long been understood that providing muscular stabilizing support to a knee joint with OA provided benefits in pain and function in most patients.[28–36] Unfortunately, muscles and their tendinous attachments are both inhibited after injury and after surgery, and are fatigable structural stabilizers. This support wanes with progressive use, or with pain-induced muscle inhibition.[16,37] Numerous providers in the past have noted the stabilizing effect (or the lack thereof) of the joint capsule in their treatment protocol of knee OA.[38–41] Unfortunately, the orthopedic literature has a paucity of studies in this area. This may be owing to the prior inability to study dynamic models with modalities such as musculoskeletal ultrasound, while focusing instead on static imaging such as radiographic imaging or MRI studies. With the use of musculoskeletal ultrasound imaging, we can now see a more dynamic picture of microinstability and/or macroinstability in both mild and severe OA. The findings on musculoskeletal ultrasound imaging in a skilled provider's hands can predict the diagnosis of OA at a similar fashion to that of plain radiographs. Unfortunately, the findings on plain film images or MRI studies represent late OA in almost all cases, when the disease course is much more fixed and difficult to change. There has also been a recent improvement in the understanding of certain areas of the capsule in relation to joint stability. This improvement has been well-described recently in the medial capsule/medial meniscus relationship, with significant increases in joint cartilage shear load and in bone marrow lesions and bone cysts with medial meniscal extrusion.[42–45] There are also strong neuropathic pain signals that occur in knees with capsule and meniscal pathology. In 1 study, meniscal lesions, particularly extrusion, were found to be among the strongest risk factors for neuropathic pain in knee OA patients.[46] This was true for both medial and lateral meniscal lesions. As for structures in the lateral compartment, the anterior lateral ligament of the knee, which had been considered only a fascial thickening in prior anatomic dissections, has been found to provide significant internal rotatory support (possibly to the function of the ACL in translation and rotation).[47] We now have a better understanding of meniscus ligament/capsular stability and the resulting meniscus extrusion with capsular dysfunction. This concept is being addressed with new and novel surgical and orthobiologic techniques, either separately or in combination. The therapeutic evaluation and management of biomechanics is changing owing to the progressing body mass index/obesity epidemic in the developed world. A disease of lifestyle, in addition to the decline of proper biomechanics with the subsequent development of postural movement, stability, and strength dysfunctions seems to be a factor in disease progression. These upper level biomechanics will only be discussed briefly, because their role is an entire study in itself.

The "Boing-boing"

This model represents mechanotransduction and biotransduction of the soft cartilage and articular cartilage of the joint. In the meniscus, this is obtained with both the hoop stress model of force transduction to offload a vertical compressive or shear load, and the intricate connection of the meniscus with the medial and lateral joint capsules through direct or indirect collagen connections and meniscotibial ligament insertions. In the lateral meniscus, the relation of the meniscus with the lateral collateral ligament, anterolateral ligament, and lateral capsule knee structures all contribute to cartilage health and capsular stability, even though the lateral meniscus is thought not to be intimately tied to the lateral capsule itself. In our clinic and in other studies published, the dynamic and static evaluation of patients shows that a high prevalence of knee OA cases start with the breakdown of the joint capsule and cartilage interface (or the "balloon/boing-boing" interface). This factor causes subsequent progression of acute and chronic inflammation, cellular depletion, macroinstability with spur formation, and progressive cartilage loss (**Fig. 1**).[48,49] For example, in patients older than 65 years, the rate of degenerative meniscal tears is 60%. Root tears are observed in 28% of medial meniscal tears. One-half of the compressive load in the knee is transferred by the menisci in extension, whereas up to 85% of the load is transferred at 90° of flexion. The collagen orientation makes this load bearing possible by converting the compressive forces to tensile forces.[42,45] Resection of only 15% to 34% of a meniscus may increase contact pressure by more than 350%. It is also known that normal knees have 20% better shock-absorbing capacity than knees after meniscectomy.[45] It therefore behooves the practitioner to save as much functional tissue as our current treatment and science allows.

The "Bioreactor"

This represents the cellular state of the synovium (with its nutritional and lubrication functions) in addition to the current state of the joint to repair and turn over articular cartilage and cellular structures on a variable basis based on age.[23,50–54] This model of synovial nutrition and joint health is in a very rapid state of flux at the present. We have noted a more complex model of inflammation, with notable and measurable degenerative cytokines, metalloproteinases, and inflammatory mediators within the joint as OA progresses.[55–57] The current treatments for knee OA typically consist of

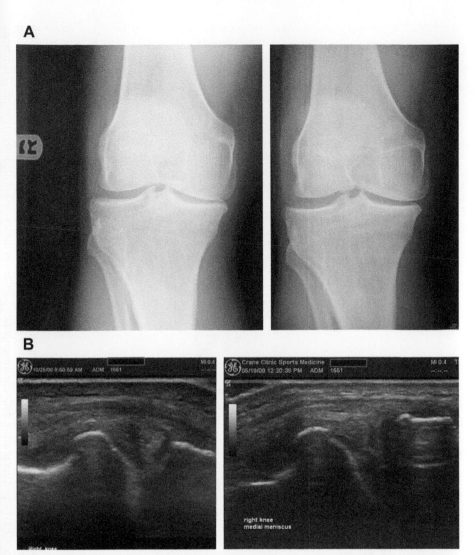

Fig. 1. (*A*) Weight-bearing radiograph and (*B*) corresponding musculoskeletal ultrasound pictures taken in comparison 6 months apart. This 40-year-old patient is status post orthobiologic treatment with bone marrow concentrate plus lipoaspirate matrix for the treatment of right knee medial compartment osteoarthritis with severe medial meniscus degeneration and medial meniscal extrusion (bone marrow concentrate plus lipoaspirate + heme + matrix). Posttreatment, the patient's medial compartment was supported by a medial unloader brace for this time frame. In the author's opinion, tibiofemoral compartment widening can only occur in the process of healing the capsule and meniscotibial and meniscofemoral ligaments. (*Courtesy of* Dr. David Crane, MD, Crane Clinic for Sports Medicine.)

downregulating inflammation with the use of nonsteroidal anti-inflammatory drugs, corticosteroids, or other nutraceuticals such as vitamin D, fish oil, or glucosamine; or in providing nutrition and lubrication to the joint in the form of HA supplementation. Changing the course of knee OA disease is very difficult with our current model of treatment. Indeed, without changing the mechanotransduction and/or joint stability,

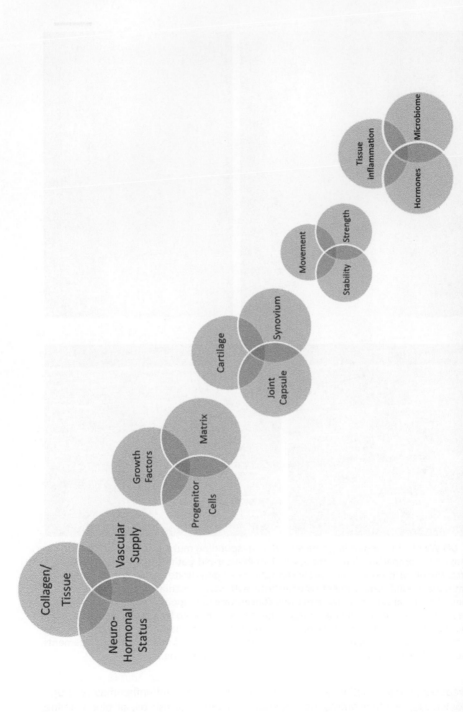

Fig. 2. Multinodal decision nest. Multiple factors require consideration when working on an orthobiologic model of tissue engineering. These factors can be nested together in groups to help the practitioner define on what level/node they are working. Ultimately they coalesce inside one another, and together provide tissue homeostasis. This model has helped our practice define and manipulate portions of the treatment algorithm to improve outcomes.

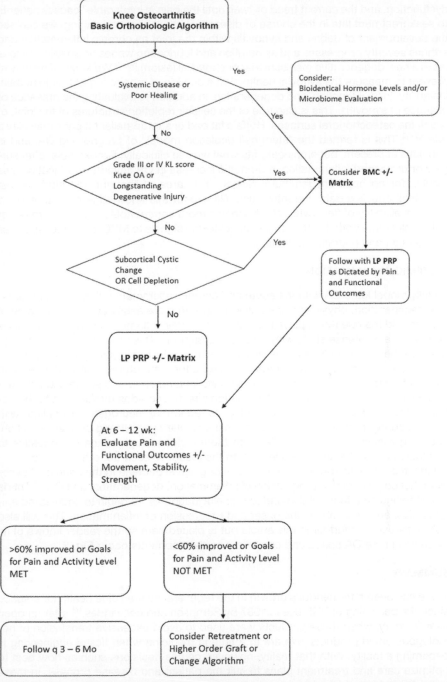

Fig. 3. Basic orthobiologic treatment algorithm for knee osteoarthritis (OA). BMC, bone marrow concentrate; LP, leukocyte poor; PRP, platelet-rich plasma.

the possibility of abating inflammation, in our opinion, is remote. This is why the typical treatment option after failing physical therapy and corticosteroids or HA is to move directly to total joint arthroplasty. In addition, early arthritis has very little pain and dysfunction, and the current trend of "wait until the pain is intolerable" causes patients to seek treatment late in the course of disease. With ultrasound imaging, we can see the development of debris and synovitis within the joint as chronic inflammation and arthritis severity progresses and as nutrition and lubrication wanes or acutely changes (as in a new degenerative meniscal tear or chondral lesion).[58,59] We know of no way at present to measure the synovial health status outside of monitoring further joint pain, instability, loss of function, and degeneration, in addition to evaluating the presence or absence of synovitis. This is also true of the cellular repletion structures of the joint, of which the osteochondral surfaces, Hoffa's fat pad or suprapatellar fat pads may play a role.[60–62] This is termed the "stem cell depletion model" of progressing OA, and is nebulous at present, but empirically fits what we see clinically. For example, after surgery or prolonged inflammation, a dramatic increase in OA severity and function loss results, for no apparent structural reason. This area of thought and study is just emerging, and few data currently exist. We expect this knowledge base to expand as the availability of flow cytometry becomes more commonplace, and we are better able to elucidate both the chemokine and cytokine signals to MSC, and other stem cell proliferation and migration pathways.

SYSTEMIC INFLAMMATION

To fully model knee OA with the acute and chronic inflammation that drives progressive degeneration, physicians are now looking with more acuity at the microbiome of the gut, and the role that it plays in local and systemic inflammation induction. This is now an area of intense study with widespread support. This process has been recognized by the functional/integrative medicine community but largely ignored by the allopathic medical community to date. See **Fig. 2** for a structured multinodal decision "nest" of factors that may drive tissue specific inflammation and subsequent degeneration. In this model, systemic inflammation affects and adds dysfunction to the homeostasis of the local tissues leading to abnormal neurogenic signaling with associated hormone dysfunction, abnormal vascular support and cellular depletion, and progressing degeneration. Because there is not enough space to do justice to this topic herein, the author will leave it to the reader to seek out other sources.

Last, there is also some question of oral or gingival bacteria in the knee joint synovium that could lead to a progression of inflammation, degeneration, and OA.[38] This is a burgeoning area that will demand further elucidation as we begin to understand epigenomics, and what drives the onset and progression of inflammation. This will also not be focused on further in this article but is placed here so the reader knows of its existence in the OA space and can follow as developments occur **Fig. 3**.

SUMMARY

There has been a tremendous growth in the regenerative medicine health care space since the beginning of PRP use in 1987 by Sampson and colleagues,[63] after an open heart surgery, when these products were used to avoid excessive transfusion of homologous blood products. We are at a time in medicine when tissue engineering is becoming a reality. With that reality, however, comes decisions such as how best to optimize care and treatment plans to suit the patient and disease process. In these early days of orthobiologics, we are starting to see a pattern of studies emerge that seem to support the safety of these products as defined in this article. We also see a pattern that seems to support orthobiologics in the treatment of knee OA for 1 year or possibly longer, depending on the age of the patient and disease severity. The current bewildering array of orthobiologic treatments and combinations will be a barrier of entry for many providers and patients. The physician community will thus be charged with ensuring proper algorithm development and optimization, further trials to document long-term effectiveness and safety, and whether medical care cost savings may be realized.

REFERENCES

1. Saw KY, Anz A, Siew-Yoke Jee C, et al. Articular cartilage regeneration with autologous peripheral blood stem cells versus hyaluronic acid: a randomized controlled trial. Arthroscopy 2013;29(4):684–94.
2. Arthritis-related statistics. Centers for Disease Control and Prevention. Available at: http://www.cdc.gov/arthritis/data_statistics/arthritis-related-stats.htm. Accessed July 1, 2016.
3. Singh J. Epidemiology of knee and hip arthroplasty: a systematic review. Open Orthop J 2011;5:80–5.
4. Sakellariou V, Poultsides LA, Ma Y, et al. Risk assessment for chronic pain and patient satisfaction after total knee arthroplasty. Orthopedics 2016;39(1):55–62.
5. Martin GM, Thornhill TS, Katz JN. Complications of total knee arthroplasty. UpToDate; September 2016.
6. Mascarenhas R, Saltzman B, Fortier L, et al. Role of platelet-rich plasma in articular cartilage injury and disease. J Knee Surg 2014;28(1):003–10.
7. Smith PA. Intra-articular autologous conditioned plasma injections provide safe and efficacious treatment for knee osteoarthritis: an FDA-sanctioned, randomized, double-blind, placebo-controlled clinical trial. Am J Sports Med 2016; 44(10):884–91.
8. Hernigou P, Beaujean F. Treatment of osteonecrosis with autologous bone marrow grafting. Clin Orthop Relat Res 2002;405:14–23.
9. Hernigou P, Lachaniette CHF, Delambre J, et al. Biologic augmentation of rotator cuff repair with mesenchymal stem cells during arthroscopy improves healing and prevents further tears: a case-controlled study. Int Orthop 2014;38(9): 1811–8.
10. Hernigou P, Merouse G, Duffiet P, et al. Reduced levels of mesenchymal stem cells at the tendon–bone interface tuberosity in patients with symptomatic rotator cuff tear. Int Orthop 2015;39(6):1219–25.
11. Hernández-Molina G, Reichenbach S, Zhang B, et al. Effect of therapeutic exercise for hip osteoarthritis pain: Results of a meta-analysis. Arthritis Rheum 2008; 59(9):1221–8.
12. Chang K-V, Hung C-Y, Aliwarga F, et al. Comparative effectiveness of platelet-rich plasma injections for treating knee joint cartilage degenerative pathology: a systematic review and meta-analysis. Arch Phys Med Rehabil 2014;95(3):562–75.
13. Riboh JC, Saltzman BM, Yanke AB, et al. Effect of leukocyte concentration on the efficacy of platelet-rich plasma in the treatment of knee osteoarthritis. Am J Sports Med 2016;44(3):792–800.
14. Meheux CJ, Mcculloch PC, Lintner DM, et al. Efficacy of intra-articular platelet-rich plasma injections in knee osteoarthritis: a systematic review. Arthroscopy 2016;32(3):495–505.
15. Filardo G, Kon E, Di Matteo B, et al. Leukocyte-poor PRP application for the treatment of knee osteoarthritis. Joints 2013;1(3):112–20.

16. Sánchez M, Fiz N, Azofra J, et al. A randomized clinical trial evaluating plasma rich in growth factors (PRGF-Endoret) versus hyaluronic acid in the short-term treatment of symptomatic knee osteoarthritis. Arthroscopy 2012;28(8):1070–8.

17. Uth K. Stem cell application for osteoarthritis in the knee joint: a minireview. World J Stem Cells 2014;6(5):629.

18. Vaquerizo V, Plasencia MÁ, Arribas I, et al. Comparison of intra-articular injections of plasma rich in growth factors (PRGF-Endoret) versus durolane hyaluronic acid in the treatment of patients with symptomatic osteoarthritis: a randomized controlled trial. Arthroscopy 2013;29(10):1635–43.

19. Oliver KS, Bayes M, Crane D, et al. Clinical outcome of bone marrow concentrate in knee osteoarthritis. J Prolotherapy 2015;7:937–46.

20. Pak J, Lee JH, Kartolo WA, et al. Cartilage regeneration in human with adipose tissue-derived stem cells: current status in clinical implications. Biomed Res Int 2016;2016:1–12.

21. Vangsness CT Jr, Farr J 2nd, Boyd J, et al. Adult human mesenchymal stem cells delivered via intra-articular injection to the knee following partial medial meniscectomy: a randomized, double-blind, controlled study. J Bone Joint Surg Am 2014;96(2):90–8.

22. Sundman EA, Cole BJ, Karas V, et al. The anti-inflammatory and matrix restorative mechanisms of platelet-rich plasma in osteoarthritis. Am J Sports Med 2013; 42(1):35–41.

23. Sakata R, McNary SM, Miyatake K, et al. Stimulation of the superficial zone protein and lubrication in the articular cartilage by human platelet-rich plasma. Am J Sports Med 2015;43(6):1467–73.

24. Koh Y-G, Kwon O-R, Kim Y-S, et al. Adipose-derived mesenchymal stem cells with microfracture versus microfracture alone: 2-year follow-up of a prospective randomized trial. Arthroscopy 2016;32(1):97–109.

25. Michalek J, Moster R, Lukac L, et al. Autologous adipose tissue-derived stromal vascular fraction cells application in patients with osteoarthritis. Cell Transplant 2015. http://dx.doi.org/10.3727/096368915x686760.

26. Vilar JM, Batista M, Morales M, et al. Assessment of the effect of intraarticular injection of autologous adipose-derived mesenchymal stem cells in osteoarthritic dogs using a double blinded force platform analysis. BMC Vet Res 2014;10(1):143.

27. Mehrabani D, Babazadeh M, Tanideh N, et al. The healing effect of adipose-derived mesenchymal stem cells in full-thickness femoral articular cartilage defects of rabbit. Int J Organ Transplant Med 2015;6:165–75.

28. Bartels E, Lund H, Hagen K, et al. Aquatic exercise for the treatment of knee and hip osteoarthritis. Cochrane Database Syst Rev 2005. http://dx.doi.org/10.1002/14651858.cd005523.

29. Berger CE, Kröner AH, Kristen K-H, et al. Transient bone marrow edema syndrome of the knee: clinical and magnetic resonance imaging results at 5 years after core decompression. Arthroscopy 2006;22(8):866–71.

30. Black LL, Gaynor J, Gahring D, et al. Effect of adipose-derived mesenchymal stem and regenerative cells on lameness in dogs with chronic osteoarthritis of the coxofemoral joints: a randomized, double-blinded, multicenter, controlled trial. Vet Ther 2007;8(4):272–84.

31. Cerza F, Carni S, Carcangiu A, et al. Comparison between hyaluronic acid and platelet-rich plasma, intra-articular infiltration in the treatment of gonarthrosis. Am J Sports Med 2012;40(12):2822–7.

32. Escalante Y, García-Hermoso A, Saavedra J. Effects of exercise on functional aerobic capacity in lower limb osteoarthritis: a systematic review. J Sci Med Sport 2011;14(3):190–8.
33. Felson DT, Chalsson CE, Hill CL, et al. The association of bone marrow lesions with pain in knee osteoarthritis. Ann Intern Med 2001;134(7):541.
34. Fransen M, Mcconnell S, Harmer AR, et al. Exercise for osteoarthritis of the knee. Cochrane Database Syst Rev 2015;(1):CD004376.
35. Frisbie DD, Kisiday JD, Kawcak CE, et al. Evaluation of adipose-derived stromal vascular fraction or bone marrow-derived mesenchymal stem cells for treatment of osteoarthritis. J Orthop Res 2009;27(12):1675–80.
36. Uthman OA, Windt DAVD, Jordan JL, et al. Exercise for lower limb osteoarthritis: systematic review incorporating trial sequential analysis and network meta-analysis. BMJ 2013;347:f5555.
37. Hart JM, Pietrosimone B, Hertel J, et al. Quadriceps activation following knee injuries: a systematic review. J Athletic Train 2010;45(1):87–97.
38. Ehrlich GD, Hu FZ, Sotereanos N, et al. What role do periodontal pathogens play in osteoarthritis and periprosthetic joint infections of the knee? J Appl Biomater Funct Mater 2014;12(1):13–20.
39. Rabago D, Patterson JJ, Mundt M, et al. Dextrose prolotherapy for knee osteoarthritis: a randomized controlled trial. Ann Fam Med 2013;11(3):229–37.
40. Reeves KD, Hassanein KM. Long term effects of dextrose prolotherapy for anterior cruciate ligament laxity. Altern Ther Health Med 2003;9(3):52–6.
41. Reeves KD, Hassanein K. Randomized prospective double-blind placebo-controlled study of dextrose prolotherapy for knee osteoarthritis with or without ACL laxity. Altern Ther Health Med 2000;6(2):68–74, 77–80.
42. Insall JH, Scott WN, editors. Surgery of the knee. 3rd edition. Philadelphia: WB Saunders Co; 2001.
43. Scott W. Intraosseous hyperpressure of the patella as a cause of anterior knee pain. Medscape Gen Med 1999;1(1):1272–4.
44. Jo CH, Lee YG, Shin WH, et al. Intra-articular injection of mesenchymal stem cells for the treatment of osteoarthritis of the knee: a proof-of-concept clinical trial. Stem Cells 2014;32(5):1254–66.
45. Vaziri A, Nayeb-Hashemi H, Singh A, et al. Influence of Meniscectomy and Meniscus Replacement on the Stress Distribution in Human Knee Joint. Ann Biomed Eng 2008;36(8):1335–44.
46. Roubille C, Raynauld J-P, Abram F, et al. The presence of meniscal lesions is a strong predictor of neuropathic pain in symptomatic knee osteoarthritis: a cross-sectional pilot study. Arthritis Res Ther 2014;16(6):507.
47. Claes S. The anterolateral ligament of the knee. Herentals (Belgium): kneeMOTION; 2014.
48. Kijowski R, Stanton P, Fine J, et al. Subchondral bone marrow edema in patients with degeneration of the articular cartilage of the knee joint 1. Radiology 2006;238(3):943–9.
49. Koh Y-G, Jo S-B, Kwon O-R, et al. Mesenchymal stem cell injections improve symptoms of knee osteoarthritis. Arthroscopy 2013;29(4):748–55.
50. Fox AJS, Bedi A, Rodeo SA. The basic science of articular cartilage: structure, composition, and function. Sports Health 2009;1(6):461–8.
51. Fransen M, Mcconnell S. Land-based exercise for osteoarthritis of the knee: a metaanalysis of randomized controlled trials. J Rheumatol 2009;36(6):1109–17.
52. Fuller E, Smith M, Little C, et al. Zonal differences in meniscus matrix turnover and cytokine response. Osteoarthritis Cartilage 2012;20(1):49–59.

53. Gobbi A, Karnatzikos G, Mahajan V, et al. Platelet-rich plasma treatment in symptomatic patients with knee osteoarthritis. Sports Health 2012;4(2):162–72.
54. Grote W, Delucia R, Waxman R, et al. Repair of a complete anterior cruciate tear using prolotherapy: a case report. Int Musculoskelet Med 2009;31(4):159–65.
55. Lohmander LS, Hoerrner LA, Lark MW. Metalloproteinases, tissue inhibitor, and proteoglycan fragments in knee synovial fluid in human osteoarthritis. Arthritis Rheum 1993;36(2):181–9.
56. Nalbant S, Martinez J, Kitumnuaypong T, et al. Synovial fluid features and their relations to osteoarthritis severity: new findings from sequential studies. Osteoarthritis Cartilage 2003;11(1):50–4.
57. Nixon AJ, Dahlgren LA, Haupt JL, et al. Effect of adipose-derived nucleated cell fractions on tendon repair in horses with collagenase-induced tendinitis. Am J Vet Res 2008;69(7):928–37.
58. Patil P, Dasgupta B. Role of diagnostic ultrasound in the assessment of musculoskeletal diseases. Ther Adv Musculoskelet Dis 2012;4(5):341–55.
59. Riecke B, Christensen R, Torp-Pedersen S, et al. An ultrasound score for knee osteoarthritis: a cross-sectional validation study. Osteoarthritis Cartilage 2014;22(10):1675–91.
60. Yun S, Ku S-K, Kwon Y-S. Adipose-derived mesenchymal stem cells and platelet-rich plasma synergistically ameliorate the surgical-induced osteoarthritis in Beagle dogs. J Orthop Surg Res 2016;11(1):9.
61. Liu Y, Buckley CT, Almeida HV, et al. Infrapatellar fat pad-derived stem cells maintain their chondrogenic capacity in disease and can be used to engineer cartilaginous grafts in clinically relevant dimensions. Tissue Eng Part A 2014;20(21–22):3050–62.
62. Zuk PA, Zhu M, Mizuno H, et al. Multilineage cells from human adipose tissue: implications for cell-based therapies. Tissue Eng 2001;7(2):211–28.
63. Sampson S, Gerhardt M, Mandelbaum B. Platelet rich plasma injection grafts for musculoskeletal injuries: a review. Curr Rev Musculoskelet Med 2008;1(3–4):165–74.

Regenerative Treatments for Spinal Conditions

Angelie Mascarinas, MD, Julian Harrison, BS, Kwadwo Boachie-Adjei, BS, CPH, Gregory Lutz, MD*

KEYWORDS

- Spine • Regenerative • Intradiscal • Platelet rich plasma • Mesenchymal stem cells
- Fibrin • Annular fissure • Low back pain

KEY POINTS

- Low back pain is a common and expensive cause of disability.
- Nonhealing annular fissures are the most common cause for low back pain.
- Early treatment of painful annular fissures may also help prevent progression to spinal deformity, stenosis, and disability.
- Intradiscal platelet rich plasma, mesenchymal stem cells, and fibrin are promising therapeutic options for intervertebral disc degeneration.
- Regenerative treatments may offer a more cost-effective solution for refractory discogenic pain and perhaps avoid expensive surgery altogether.

INTRODUCTION

Although there are many causes of low back pain, most experts agree that the beginning of the end of the spine starts with an injury to the intervertebral disc (IVD). When the disc begins to fail, the "degenerative cascade" begins and the subsequent sequelae of facet loading, spinal deformity, stenosis, and nerve root compression ensue.[1] Adult spinal deformity is increasingly common in the aging population, with prevalence as high as 68% in adults older than 60 years.[2] Adult spinal deformity is also a debilitating disease that greatly affects quality of life. Studies have shown that adults with scoliosis score significantly lower in self-reported outcome measures, such as the 36-item Short Form Health Survey (SF-36) questionnaire, compared with the general US population, including physical functioning, vitality, social functioning, emotional role, physical role, and mental health.[3] Adult spinal deformity has a similar

Conflicts of Interest: Dr G. Lutz is the Chief Medical Advisor for Biorestorative Therapies, LLC. The authors have no other financial interests to disclose.
Department of Physiatry, Hospital for Special Surgery, 429 East 75th Street, 3rd Floor, New York, NY 10021, USA
* Corresponding author.
E-mail address: LutzG@hss.edu

global burden as well. In fact, a prospective multicenter international database including 8 industrialized countries found that patients with adult spinal deformity actually have lower health-related quality of life scores when compared with patients with common chronic conditions. such as self-reported arthritis, chronic lung disease, congestive heart failure, and diabetes.[4]

The rising health care costs, the physical impact, and functional decline related to adult spinal deformity engender a need for more preventive measures and cost-effective treatments, such as preventive and regenerative interventions. Despite spending billions of dollars in various treatments, both surgical and nonsurgical current treatments have failed to meet patient expectations and curb the ever-escalating health care costs related to managing this condition. The concepts of cutting out discs, fusing the spine, burning disc nerve endings, and injecting steroids around inflamed structures all fail to address the underlying pathophysiology and do little to change the natural history of disc degeneration. It is our opinion that we need to be less aggressive with our surgical treatment of the spine, and more aggressive with intervening earlier in the disease process with regenerative treatments. Hopefully this approach will not only lead to better patient outcomes, but also to a more sustainable, cost-efficient way to manage this significant societal burden. In this article, we focus our review on the current literature that exists regarding the clinical and translational studies on regenerative treatments for healing the IVD.

DISCOGENIC PAIN

The IVD is composed of a central nucleus pulposus, consisting of hydrophilic proteoglycan and type II collagen, and the outer annulus fibrosus, made of a fibrous ring of mostly type I collagen.[5,6] Due its intrinsic hydrostatic pressure, the nucleus pulposus can bear heavy compressive loads, whereas the annulus fibrosus resists heavy tensile stresses.[7] Biomechanical studies have shown that torsion and flexion contribute to degenerative changes in the lumbar discs.[8] Disc herniations can be due to progressive degenerative changes from repetitive stress, or acute in nature due to trauma.[8] With repetitive stress, the annulus fibrosus fibers swell and disrupt as the annulus fibrosus undergoes myxomatous degeneration and cyst formation.[8] At the same time, the nucleus pulposus dehydrates, turns fibrotic, and eventually undergoes necrosis and herniation. The nucleus pulposus can herniate through annular fissures or endplate disruptions. The adult IVD is the largest avascular structure in the human body and relies on passive diffusion from adjacent endplate vessels for nutrition,[9] resulting in poor inherent healing potential. In fact, only 3% of disc bulges and 38% of focal protrusions resolve spontaneously.[10] Broad-based disc protrusions, extrusions, and sequestrations have a better prognosis, with approximately 75% to 100% resolving spontaneously.[10]

Nonhealing annular fissures of the IVD have been implicated as one of the major causes for chronic low back pain. A concomitant upregulation of proinflammatory cytokines, such as interleukin-1 (IL-1) and tumor necrosis (TNF) alpha, leads to chemical sensitization of the rich network of nerve fibers that supply the outer annulus fibrosus, resulting in pain with normal activities of daily living.[11–13] As the degenerated disc cells upregulate IL-1 expression, the native disc cells also increase matrix degrading enzyme production expression.[5] TNF-alpha expression from the degenerated tissue also upregulates matrix degrading enzymes and stimulates nerve ingrowth. Furthermore, annular fissures may also contribute to a chemical radiculitis due to the release of inflammatory mediators into the epidural space.[14] As the IVDs degenerate, there is loss of disc space height, and subsequent loading onto the posterior elements.[15] When the disc degenerates asymmetrically, spinal deformity and stenosis ensue.

   Considering the pathophysiology of disc degeneration, regenerative treatments need to focus on either stimulating production of extracellular matrix, or inhibiting the cytokines that upregulate matrix degrading enzymes. In turn, as the regenerative treatments slow down or reverse disc degeneration, the subsequent loss of disc space height, increased loading on posterior elements, and spinal stenosis also may be prevented.

PLATELET RICH PLASMA

The solution for IVD regeneration and inhibition of matrix degrading enzymes may be found in platelet rich plasma (PRP). PRP is acquired from an autologous sample of blood that is centrifuged to increase the platelet concentration up to 3 to 8 times the normal concentration in whole blood.[16] At the same time, PRP also contains amplified levels of growth factors and cytokines, which stimulate tissue healing. The alpha granules in platelets also secrete growth factors that are essential for tissue repair, such as basic fibroblast growth factor (b-FGF), epithelial growth factor, insulinlike growth factor (IGF-1), platelet-derived growth factor, and vascular endothelial growth factor.[17] The growth factors also increase collagen content, promote endothelial regeneration, and stimulate angiogenesis.[17,18]

INTRADISCAL PLATELET RICH PLASMA
Intradiscal Platelet Rich Plasma: In Vitro and In Vivo Studies

Clinicians have hypothesized that placing a high concentration of growth factors, such as in PRP, directly at the site of collagen injury can allow the growth factors to act as humoral mediators to induce the natural healing cascade[19] (**Box 1**). An in vitro study of PRP-infused human IVD cultures supports this hypothesis and exhibited nucleus pulposus proliferation and differentiation as well as upregulated proteoglycan synthesis.[20] Animal models of experimentally injured IVD treated with intradiscal PRP have also demonstrated restoration of normal cellular architecture and disc height.[21,22] Furthermore, PRP may also have an anti-inflammatory effect. An in vitro study found that cytokine (TNF-alpha and IL-1) induced proinflammatory degrading enzymes and mediators were suppressed with the addition of PRP into the collagen matrix of human nucleus pulposus cells.[23] A rabbit model with degenerated IVDs injected intradiscally

---

Box 1
Benefits of platelet rich plasma (PRP)

- Increased platelet concentrations 3 to 10 times over whole blood
- Platelets secrete growth factors (basic fibroblast growth factor, epithelial growth factor, insulinlike growth factor-1, platelet-derived growth factor, vascular endothelial growth factor)
   ○ Increase collagen content
   ○ Endothelial regeneration
   ○ Stimulate angiogenesis
- Suppress proinflammatory cytokines (tumor necrosis factor-alpha and interleukin-1)
- Reduce apoptosis
- Concentrated fibrinogen content

with PRP-impregnated gelatin hydrogel microspheres resulted in significantly higher water content determined by MRI, which corresponded with increased intradiscal proteoglycan content, upregulated mRNA precursors for type II collagen, and significantly reduced apoptotic nucleus pulposus cells.[24] Similarly, in a percutaneous annulus puncture-induced degenerated disc rat model, discs treated with PRP had fewer inflammatory cells, higher preservation of normal morphology, and higher fluid content in T2 MRI compared with sham at 4 weeks postinjection.[21]

Intradiscal Platelet Rich Plasma: Clinical Studies

A recent double-blind randomized control trial (RCT) involving intradiscal PRP injections of patients with chronic moderate to severe lumbar discogenic pain, has demonstrated improvement in functional and pain scores.[25] This study involved 47 participants randomized to receive a single injection of autologous PRP (29 in the treatment group) or contrast agent alone (18 in the control group) into symptomatic degenerative IVDs. The patients included were those with low back pain persisting for at least 6 months and refractory to conservative treatment, including oral medications, rehabilitation therapy, and/or injection therapy (**Box 2**). Before the intradiscal PRP procedure, a caudal epidural injection was trialed to determine if the patient with presumed discogenic low back pain would receive therapeutic benefit from the caudal injection. A prospective cohort study has shown that patients with at least 3 months of axial low back pain associated with central disc protrusions at L4–5 and/or L5–S1 do experience improvements in pain, function, and satisfaction after receiving caudal epidural steroid injections (Lee J, Nguyen E, Harrison J, et al. Fluoroscopically guided caudal epidural steroid injections for axial low back pain as a result of central disc protrusions: a prospective outcome study. Pain Med. Submitted for publication). The subjects who had relief of low back pain after the caudal injection then were considered for inclusion in the intradiscal PRP randomized control study.

Furthermore, there was strict selection criteria for included IVDs. Only the IVD heights of at least 50% of normal and with disc protrusion less than 5 mm on MRI or computerized tomography were included in the study. Disc extrusions, sequestered discs, and spinal stenosis at the levels investigated were excluded. The symptomatic discs were found via provocative discography performed on the day of the intradiscal PRP injection. Only grade 3 or 4 annular fissures as determined by discography were included. At 8 weeks, the intradiscal control (contrast only) group was allowed to cross over to receive intradiscal PRP if they failed to show improvement.

At 8 weeks, there were statistically significant improvements in pain (Numeric Rating Scale [NRS] for best pain), function (Functional Rating Index [FRI]), and patient satisfaction (North American Spine Society Outcome Questionnaire) in the intradiscal PRP group as compared with the control groups. In addition to the RCT, a longitudinal

---

Box 2
Selection for intradiscal PRP injection

- Low back pain greater than 6 months
- *Failed conservative treatment*: oral medications, physical therapy, injections
- *Transient relief following caudal epidural steroid injection*
- *MRI*: disc heights of at least 50% of normal, disc protrusion <5 mm
- *Provocative discography*: grade 3 or 4 annular fissures and <2 mL filling of contrast into annular fissure

analysis of the intradiscal PRP treatment group at 6 months, 1 year, and 2 years was conducted. This revealed continued improvement in the NRS best pain, FRI function, and SF-36, and clinically significant improvement sustained at 2 years postinjection for NRS worst pain, FRI function, SF-36 pain and function (reference both of our articles here). No adverse events of neurologic injury, progressive disc herniation, or disc space infection occurred throughout the course of the study.

The investigators concluded that PRP is a safe and sustainable treatment option for lumbar discogenic pain. This study demonstrated improved functional outcomes after intradiscal PRP, but the regenerative properties of PRP in the IVD is still inferred. The next step in our research will be a prospective cohort study of intradiscal PRP that will include sequential MRI of the spine to ascertain improvements in disc space height, healing of high-intensity zones (HIZs), resorption of focal protrusions, and possible improvement in Pfirrmann scores.[26] A case report with the same investigators demonstrated positive increased T2 nuclear signal intensity on MRI of IVD 1 year after intradiscal PRP injections, which correlated with improvement in the patient's low back pain and ability to return to running (**Fig. 1**) (JR Harrison, RJ Herzog, GE Lutz. Increased nuclear T2 signal intensity following intradiscal platelet rich plasma: a case report, Submitted to PM&R).

The investigators in this randomized control study described their technique for intradiscal PRP injection with 1 to 2 mL of autologous PRP and a double-needle extrapedicular technique, immediately after contrast administration for discography (**Box 3**). The patient is positioned prone on the fluoroscopy table after receiving 1 g cephazolin at 30 minutes before the procedure. After sterile preparation and local anesthesia, a 25-gauge needle is advanced through a 20-gauge needle introducer into the midportion of the suspected disc levels using anteroposterior and lateral

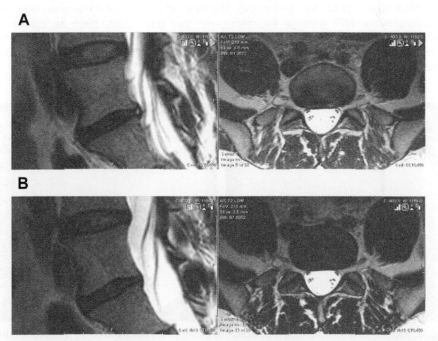

Fig. 1. Axial and sagittal MRIs depicting L4–5 and L5–S1 IVDs before (A) and 1 year after (B) intradiscal PRP injection at L5–S1.

Box 3
Intradiscal PRP injection technique

1. *1 g intravenous cephazolin* 30 minutes before injection
2. *Local anesthesia* with consideration of *intravenous sedation*
3. *Double-needle technique* (20-gauge needle introducer and 25-gauge needle) via extrapedicular technique (**Fig. 2**)
4. *1 to 2 mL contrast* injected intradiscally to confirm concordant low back pain; and contrast filling of annular fissure (<2 mL)
5. *PRP 1 to 2 mL* injected intradiscally slowly over 2 to 3 minutes

---

fluoroscopic imaging to confirm proper needle positioning. Thereafter, 1 to 2 mL of contrast agent is injected into the disc and the participant endorses concordant or discordant pain reproduction of low back pain. Only the discs that produce concordant pain and exhibit the contrast filling an annular fissure with incomplete annular disruption (<2 mL) are injected with PRP. No extension tubing is used during the injection. If more than one disc reproduces concordant pain, then the 3 to 4 mL of PRP obtained is divided into each of the affected discs.

Another recent prospective study[27] also found improvement in pain on the visual analog scale (VAS) and function based on the Oswestry Disability Index (ODI) after a single intradiscal PRP injection at one or multiple lumbar spinal discs. The investigators defined a successful outcome as 30% improvement in ODI and 50% improvement in VAS, which was achieved in 47% of patients in their preliminary 6-month results. This study involved 22 patients with discogenic back pain and a pain intensity of at least 40 mm of 100 mm on the VAS. The injected discs were determined either by discography or MRI findings for discogenic low back pain, such as disc HIZ, decreased disc signal on T2 sequence, disc protrusion, or type 1 or 2 endplate Modic changes. The investigators also ruled out other sources of low back pain with facet and sacroiliac joint blocks.

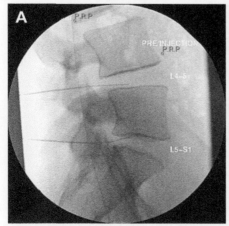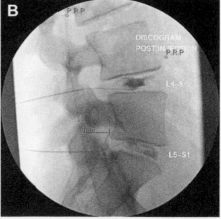

Fig. 2. Sagittal fluoroscopic images of a patient undergoing L4–5 and L5–S1 provocative discography before (*A*) and after injection of contrast at both levels and subsequent injection of PRP at L5–S1 (*B*).

The investigators of this study used a single-needle technique via a posterolateral extrapedicular approach into the disc nucleus. These investigators also used 1 mL of contrast to ensure intranuclear placement. The main differences in technique in this study compared with the RCT, is that 0.5 mL of 4% lidocaine for anesthesia and gentamicin for discitis prophylaxis were also injected intradiscally. Prior studies have indicated that anesthetics and antibiotics can decrease IVD cell synthesis in vitro.[28–30] Another limitation of this study is that the subjects paid out of pocket for the procedures, unlike in the RCT, which was completely funded. The study institution's research and education fund paid for the procedure and related fees, whereas the PRP kits were donated by the PRP centrifuge company.[25] Paying out of pocket for the treatment may be a source of bias, because the subjects may have a perceived investment in the treatment.

STEM CELL TREATMENTS IN THE SPINE

Stem cell treatments offer another promising solution for regenerative treatments in the spine. Autologous sources for stem cell treatments that have been studied in the spine thus far include native disc cells, adipose-derived and bone marrow–derived mesenchymal stem cells.[31] However, it has proven difficult to isolate pure nucleus pulposus cells without fibroblasts and macrophages.[32] Furthermore, the centrifugation process of autologous stem cells derived from bone marrow do not contain a high concentration of pure homogeneous mesenchymal stem cells, as there is also adherence to plastic during the process.[31] Mesenchymal stem cells may serve as the ideal cell source for IVD degeneration, as they can differentiate into nucleus pulposus–like cells and promote extracellular matrix synthesis. Mesenchymal stem cells may also influence nucleus pulposus cell function to secrete anabolic growth factors via paracrine signaling between the native and injected cells.[5]

There is currently ongoing research focusing on the optimum mixture of growth factors needed to stimulate differentiation into nucleus pulposus–like phenotype. Mesenchymal stem cells have been shown to differentiate into IVD-like phenotypes with induction by ascorbate, dexamethasone and transforming growth factor-beta.[33] Bone marrow–derived and adipose-derived mesenchymal stem calls stimulated with growth differentiation factor 6 (GDF6) have demonstrated increased nucleus pulposus marker genes and secrete an extracellular matrix that is more proteoglycan rich with a micromechanical composition most similar to the nucleus pulposus in 3-dimensional culture.[34] Animal models have established that autologous bone marrow mesenchymal cells survive and replicate within 8 to 48 weeks after transplantation.[35] Because mesenchymal cells have a relatively short survival time, a biomaterial scaffold may enhance the differentiation and viability of mesenchymal cells in the desired location (**Box 4**).

Box 4
Beneficial properties of mesenchymal stem cells

- Easy to harvest and culture
- Biocompatible
- Self-renewing
- Can differentiate into nucleus pulposus–like cells
- Enhanced extracellular matrix production
- Secrete anabolic factors

Intradiscal Stem Cell Treatments: In Vivo Studies

In vivo studies of implanted mesenchymal stem cells have shown enhanced matrix production, predominantly with glycosaminoglycan synthesis, as well as increased disc hydration and disc height. An in vivo model was used to study the differentiation status of mesenchymal stem cells transplanted to the nucleus pulposus of degenerative discs in rabbits.[36] At 48 weeks posttransplantation, significant augmentation of proteoglycan content and cell-associated matrix molecules, like type II collagen, chondroitin sulfate, and nucleus pulposus phenotypic markers, were seen in biochemical and gene expression analyses.

Similarly, an in vivo sheep model showed increased nucleus pulposus proteoglycan synthesis in IVDs injected with mesenchymal progenitor cells combined with pentosane polysulfate and embedded in a gelatin/fibrin scaffold.[37] The sheep in this study underwent standardized microdiscectomy and then the spines underwent MRI, biochemical, and histologic analysis at 6 months postoperatively. Interestingly, the discs with scaffolding and mesenchymal cells had better MRI imaging Pfirrmann scores compared with the discs injected with scaffolding alone.

An in vivo model of mice with severely degenerated discs implanted with adipose-derived stromal cells intradiscally also found positive radiographic findings.[38] At 7 weeks posttreatment, MRI spine imaging displayed increased disc signal intensity in the treated mice compared with the nontreated controls.

Intradiscal Stem Cell Treatments: Clinical Studies

A prospective, controlled, randomized, multicenter study titled Euro Disc Randomized Trial comparing autologous disc chondrocyte transplantation plus discectomy with discectomy alone has found promising results for autologous intradiscal stem cell treatment.[32,39] This study had a high sample size of 112 patients. Autologous disc chondrocytes were sequestered intraoperatively during the open discectomy. Thereafter, the sequestered disc material was expanded in culture and reinjected into the disc in a fluoroscopically guided procedure after 12 weeks. This study found a clinically significant reduction in low back pain scores, with regard to the Oswestry Low Back Pain Disability Questionnaire, Quebec Back Pain Disability Scale, and VAS at 2 years in the patients who received autologous disc cell transplantation after discectomy compared with those who had discectomy alone. Furthermore, the MRI for the treatment group revealed retained disc hydration when compared with the adjacent levels that had undergone discectomy without autologous disc chondrocyte transplantation. Specifically, the treatment group had 41% normal fluid content, whereas the discectomy alone group had only 25% normal fluid content. However, MRI found no significant differences in the mean IVD heights between the 2 groups.

Allogeneic mesenchymal stem cells, cultured from other patients, also have been studied. Intradiscal allogeneic mesenchymal stem cells are currently being explored in a phase 2, randomized controlled study.[40] Single-level mildly degenerated lumbar IVDs were selected. Preliminary data show that a greater number of patients treated with intradiscal mesenchymal stem cells reported greater than or equal to 50% reduction in low back pain compared with controls at 12 months after injection. Specifically, of the patients treated with intradiscal mesenchymal stem cells, 69% reported this successful outcome, compared with only 33% of control patients.

INTRADISCAL FIBRIN INJECTIONS

Intradiscal fibrin injections have the potential to ameliorate several concerns hindering successful treatment of degenerated and injured IVDs. Intradiscal fibrin injection targeted at injured annulus fibrosis benefits in treating IVD-related symptoms assuming 1 or all of the following 3 premises are true: (1) tears within the annulus fibrosis initiate the inflammatory and autoimmune cascade, (2) autologous nucleus pulposus instigates radiculopathy and radiculitis through its contact with adjacent descending spinal nerves, and (3) intradiscal injections of mesenchymal stem cells and PRP may possess the ability to improve disc pathology, yet their efficacy may be hindered by their leakage from targeted IVDs through annulus fibrosis tears. If these premises are true, sealing IVD tears may alleviate symptoms of internal disc disruption, and radiculopathy.

Injected fibrin sealant serves to occupy rents within tears of the lamella of the torn annulus fibrosis, thus functioning as a physical barrier between inflammatory constituents and the disc's nociceptors. Furthermore, fibrin sealant functions as a barrier, potentially limiting outflow of nucleus pulposus and associated inflammatory constituents onto dura, meninges, and descending spinal nerves. Logic dictates benefit would be derived from sealing fissures within the annulus fibrosis, thus stopping the outflow of IVD contents. More specifically, inflammatory components form when centrally located nucleus pulposus flows through tears of the annulus fibrosis. This instigates the expression of interleukins, cytokines, and other inflammatory and autoimmune cascade constituents.[41,42] Additionally, flow or extravasation of nucleus pulposus outside the torn annulus fibrosis causes injury to the adjacent descending spinal nerves,[6,43–47] and these inflammatory components on the spinal nerve affect structures as distant as the thalamus.[48] In addition to IVD disruption causing axial and extremity symptoms, through both inflammatory and autoimmune constituents stimulating annular nociceptors within the disc, and through leakage outside the disc ("leaky disc syndrome"), respectively, another potentially problematic issue results with treatment using intradiscal biologics such as mesenchymal stem cells and PRP. There exists potential for diminished efficacy and iatrogenic tissue growth caused by leakage of the injected biologics meant to repair the damaged disc. One investigation injected radiolabeled bone marrow mesenchymal stem cells into rabbit degenerated IVDs with the objectives of determining their effect and fate. Outcomes at 9 weeks following injection of radiolabeled mesenchymal stem cells into the disc's nucleus pulposus revealed no radiolabeled mesenchymal stem cells within the disc. More disconcerting, however, was visual and radiographic observation of new, large anterolateral osteophytes, and these osteophytes contained the radiolabeled mesenchymal stem cells.[49]

Fibrin may be the ideal biomaterial scaffold to enhance the differentiation and viability of mesenchymal cells in IVDs. Fibrin has been studied as a scaffold for repair of degenerated IVDs. Fibrin can act as a space filler of disc defects, retaining cells and facilitating cell growth and formation of new tissue.[50] Fibrin is a biocompatible composite hydrogel of fibrinogen and thrombin that acts as a hemostatic agent, sealant, and cell carrier.[51] Fibrin facilitates cell attachment because of its numerous binding sites for integrins.[51]

Intradiscal Fibrin: Translational Studies

In vitro and in vivo studies on intradiscal fibrin have displayed the many valuable characteristics of fibrin. Fibrin is easily modifiable to take on the ideal characteristics of disc cells and act as a potential adhesive for annulus repair. An in vitro study has found that fibrin gels composed of 250 mg/mL of fibrin and 0.25:1 or 0.5:1 genipin:fibrin showed a shear behavior similar to native annulus fibrosus.[52] Fibrin also may play an anti-inflammatory and anticatabolic role. An vitro study of fibrin embedded with human and porcine annulus fibrosus cells cultured in type I collagen beads and stimulated with IL-1 alpha demonstrated increased synthesis of anti-inflammatory cytokine IL-455. Meanwhile, fibrin embedded with human and porcine nucleus pulposus cells resulted in reduced secretion of proinflammatory cytokines.[53] Similarly, intradiscal fibrin prevented disc degeneration and stimulated proteoglycan content recovery in denucleated IVDs in a minipig model.[54] In a randomized, controlled investigation, approximately 120 porcine discs were treated with either normal saline or concentrated fibrin with aprotinin. In one investigation, statistical significance was demonstrated in all categories comparing fibrin treatment with normal saline. Intradiscal fibrin versus normal saline was demonstrated superior in all categories, including morphologic and histologic growth, proteoglycan composition, cytokine content, and mechanical properties with pressure and volume testing (**Box 5**).[54]

Intradiscal Fibrin Injections: Clinical Studies

Intradiscal fibrin has been effectively used as a sealant in a prospective study on patients with chronic lumbar pain.[55] Fibrin is a drug approved by the Food and Drug Administration (FDA), and at the time of this writing, its intradiscal injection is an off-label use of an FDA-approved drug.

Prior human cadaveric studies confirmed that the intradiscal flow patterns of fibrin sealant into annular fissures closely approximate the distribution of intradiscal contrast. Fifteen adults with chronic discogenic pain at a single or contiguous 2 lumbar disc levels were included and confirmed via provocation discography. The volume and pressure-controlled Biostat Delivery Device system (BIOSTAT BIOLOGIX, Spinal Restoration Inc., Austin, Texas) was used to percutaneously deliver 1.0 to 4.0 mL of Biostat Biologix fibrin sealant into the selected IVDs. The injector stopped injecting when the sustained delivery pressure reached or exceeded 100 psi, the minimum pressure found to cause annular rupture based on biomechanical studies.[56]

There was clinically significant pain relief and function in a high percentage of patients at 26 weeks. Clinically significant pain relief, defined as at least 30% reduction in low back pain VAS, was achieved in 87% of subjects at 26 weeks postinjection. Clinically significant improvements in function, defined as at least 30% reduction in Roland-Morris Disability Questionnaire score, was achieved in 73% of subjects at 26 weeks postinjection. This improvement was sustained at 52 weeks in 73% of subjects and slightly decreased to 60% of subjects at 104 weeks. With regard to global improvement in low back pain, 85% of subjects responded that their pain was better or much better compared with baseline at 52 weeks, and 54.5% of subjects at 104 weeks. However, long-term conclusions were confounded by the loss of subjects at extended follow-up (2 at 52 weeks and 4 subjects at 104 weeks). Furthermore, there

---

Box 5
Beneficial properties of fibrin

- Biocompatible
- Hemostatic
- Space filler and sealant
- Cell carrier
- Numerous binding sites for integrins
- Anticatabolic: reduced secretion of proinflammatory cytokines
- Anti-inflammatory: increased synthesis of interleukin-4

were 3 adverse events during the study, including a case of discitis and 2 cases of lumbar muscle spasms within 1 week after treatment.

Fibrin has been safely used as a scaffold for allogeneic cells in an intradiscal clinical trial. A prospective study on allogeneic juvenile chondrocyte cells injected intradiscally with commercial fibrin under fluoroscopic guidance has demonstrated improved functional outcome scores as well as improvements on MRI.[57] Fifteen patients received a single percutaneous intradiscal injection of 1 to 2 mL of juvenile chondrocytes with approximately 10^7 chondrocyte cells/mL with fibrin carrier. Single-level L3–S1 degenerated discs with Pfirrmann Grades III–IV were selected for injection. At 12 months postinjection, patients had significant improvement in ODI, NRS, and SF-36. At the 6-month follow-up, 10 of 13 patients who had an MRI showed improvements, with 3 showing improved disc contour or height, and 89% had improved or resolved HIZs. No adverse events like discitis or neurologic deterioration occurred during the study.

FUTURE CONSIDERATIONS

Further research is needed to better determine which patients are the ideal candidates for regenerative treatments, the ideal number of treatments, single-level versus multiple-level intradiscal injections, and to elucidate the ideal injectate (PRP or mesenchymal stem cells) with or without scaffolding like fibrin to provide the best environment for cell growth. Perhaps there are certain biomarkers or MRI variations that could serve as prognostic indicators for ideal candidates for these treatments. The exact number and frequency of intradiscal injections have yet to be confirmed in literature. Furthermore, single-level versus multilevel intradiscal injections have not yet been compared in clinical studies. Upcoming clinical trials should focus on verifying the optimal PRP concentration and composition that promotes IVD regeneration. Both intradiscal PRP studies presented in this article used a centrifuge that concentrates platelets to 5 times the concentration in whole blood. Yet there are many other centrifuge systems that can concentrate the platelets to 8 to 10 times that of whole blood, and thus result in higher levels of growth factors, and perhaps also improved regenerative ability. Based on the studies presented previously, perhaps a combination of PRP and mesenchymal stem cells and the use of fibrin:genipin gels as a scaffold will result in the most favorable injectate.

Current intradiscal therapies have focused on targeting the nucleus pulposus. Perhaps injecting the annulus fibrosus in addition to the nucleus pulposus may also reveal additional benefits. There may also be a role for injectable regenerative therapies to augment surgical treatments at the time of intervention and serve as a protective tool against post-procedural IVD degeneration. In fact, the Euro Disc Randomized Trial described previously supports that autologous disc cell transplantation resulted in greater pain reduction and improved disc fluid content on MRI after discectomy.[39]

SUMMARY

Low back pain is a universal and disabling chronic condition that has significantly contributed to rising health care costs. IVD degeneration is the leading cause of back pain and is also often the precursor to the degenerative cascade of facet arthropathy, spinal deformity, and stenosis. Treatments targeting the painful annular fissures early on may also help prevent progression of spinal deformity and disability. Interventions that hinder ongoing cell degradation or that supplement anabolic cell production are necessary cost-effective treatments for low back pain, as the current epidural injection options offer only transient relief and current surgical options cost exorbitantly more. Surgeries themselves may contribute to adjacent-level degeneration, as seen in spinal fusions.[58] Regenerative treatments may also offer a great solution for those refractory to pain management and injections and those who prefer to avoid surgery. The existing translational and clinical studies presented in this article provide supportive evidence for regenerative treatments for discogenic pain, including intradiscal PRP, mesenchymal stem cell, and fibrin treatments. These studies are paving the way to the future of spine medicine, which is shifting toward regenerative biologic treatments and away from spinal fusion surgeries for discogenic low back pain.

REFERENCES

1. Yong-Hing K, Kirkaldy-Willis WH. The pathophysiology of degenerative disease of the lumbar spine. Orthop Clin North Am 1983;14(3):491–504.

2. Schwab F, Dubey A, Gamez L, et al. Adult scoliosis: prevalence, SF-36, and nutritional parameters in an elderly volunteer population. Spine (Phila Pa 1976) 2005; 30(9):1082–5.

3. Schwab F, Dubey A, Pagala M, et al. Adult scoliosis: a health assessment analysis by SF-36. Spine (Phila Pa 1976) 2003;28(6):602–6.

4. Pellise F, Vila-Casademunt A, Ferrer M, et al, European Spine Study Group. Impact on health related quality of life of adult spinal deformity (ASD) compared with other chronic conditions. Eur Spine J 2015;24:3–11.

5. Richardson SM, Kalamegam G, Pushparaj P, et al. Mesenchymal stem cells in regenerative medicine: focus on articular cartilage and intervertebral disc regeneration. Methods 2016;99:69–80.

6. Cornefjord M, Olmarker K, Rydevik R, et al. Mechanical and biochemical injury of spinal nerve roots: a morphological and neurophysiological study. Eur Spine J 1996;5(3):187–92.

7. Roberts S, Evans H, Trivedi J, et al. Histology and pathology of the human intervertebral disc. J Bone Joint Surg Am 2006;88(Suppl 2):10–4.

8. Kadow T, Sowa G, Vo N, et al. Molecular basis of intervertebral disc degeneration and herniations: what are the important translational questions? Clin Orthop Relat Res 2015;473:1903–12.

9. Bogduk N. Clinical anatomy of the lumbar spine and sacrum. 4th edition. New York: Elsevier; 2005. p. 147–8.

10. Jensen TS, Albert HB, Soerensen JS, et al. Natural course of disc morphology in patients with sciatica: an MRI study using a standardized qualitative classification system. Spine (Phila Pa 1976) 2006;31(14):1605–12 [discussion: 1613].

11. Weiler C, Nerlich AG, Bachmeier BE, et al. Expression and distribution of tumor necrosis factor alpha in human lumbar intervertebral discs: a study in surgical specimen and autopsy controls. Spine 2005;30:44–53.

12. Le Maitre CL, Freemont AJ, Hoyland JA. The role of interleukin-1 in the pathogenesis of human intervertebral disc degeneration. Arthritis Res Ther 2005;7: R732–45.

13. Hoyland JA, Le Maitre CL, Freemont AJ. Investigation of the role of IL-1 and TNF in matrix degradation in the intervertebral disc. Rheumatology 2008;47:809–14.

14. Peng B, Wu W, Li Z, et al. Chemical radiculitis. Pain 2007;127:11–6.

15. Inoue N, Espinoza Orías AA. Biomechanics of Intervertebral Disc Degeneration. The Orthopedic Clinics of North America 2011;42(4):487–99. http://dx.doi.org/10.1016/j.ocl.2011.07.001.

16. Nguyen RT, Borg-Stein J, Mcinnis K. Application of platelet-rich plasma in muscu-loskeletal and sports medicine: an evidence based approach. PM R 2011;3: 226–50.

17. Sampson S, Gerhardt M, Mandelbaum B. Platelet rich plasma injection grafts for musculoskeletal injuries: a review. Curr Rev Musculoskelet Med 2008;1:165–74.

18. Podd D. Platelet-rich plasma therapy: origins and applications investigated. JAAPA 2012;25(6):44–9.

19. Foster TE, Puskas BL, Mandelbaum BR, et al. Platelet-rich plasma: from basic science to clinical applications. Am J Sports Med 2009;37(11):2259–72.

20. Chen WH, Lo WC, Lee JJ, et al. Tissue-engineered intervertebral disc and chon-drogenesis using human nucleus pulposus regulated through TGF-beta1 in platelet-rich plasma. J Cell Physiol 2006;209(3):744–54.

21. Gullung GB, Woodall JW, Tucci MA, et al. Platelet-rich plasma effects on degen-erative disc disease: analysis of histology and imaging in an animal model. Evid Based Spine Care J 2011;2(4):13–8.

22. Obata S, Akeda K, Imanishi T, et al. Effect of autologous platelet-rich plasma-re-leasate on intervertebral disc degeneration in the rabbit anular puncture model: a preclinical study. Arthritis Res Ther 2012;14(6):R241.

23. Kim HJ, Yeom JS, Koh YG, et al. Anti-inflammatory effect of platelet-rich plasma on nucleus pulposus cells with response of TNF-α and IL-1. J Orthop Res 2014; 32:551–6.

24. Sawamura K, Ikeda T, Nagae M, et al. Characterization of in vivo effects of platelet-rich plasma and biodegradable gelatin hydrogel microspheres on de-generated intervertebral discs. Tissue Eng Part A 2009;15:3719–27.

25. Tuakli-Wosornu YA, Terry A, Boachie-Adjei K, et al. Lumbar intradiskal platelet-rich plasma (PRP) injections: a prospective, double-blind, randomized controlled study. PM R 2016;8(1):1–10.

26. Pfirrmann CW, Metzdorf A, Zanetti M, et al. Magnetic resonance grade of lumbar intervertebral disc degeneration. Spine 2001;26:1873–8. http://dx.doi.org/10.1097/00007632-200109010-00011.

27. Levi D, Horn S, Tyszko S, et al. Intradiscal platelet-rich plasma injection for chronic discogenic low back pain: preliminary results from a prospective trial. Pain Med 2016;17:1010–22.

28. Chee AV, Ren J, Lenart BA, et al. Cytotoxicity of local anesthetics and nonionic contrast agents on bovine intervertebral disc cells cultured in a three-dimensional culture system. Spine J 2014;14(3):491–8.

29. Hoelscher GL, Gruber HE, Coldham G, et al. Effects of high antibiotic concentra-tion on human intervertebral disc cell proliferation, viability, and metabolism in vitro. Spine 2000;25(15):1871–7.

30. Iwasaki K, Sudo H, Yamada K, et al. Cytotoxic effects of radiocontrast agent io-trolan and anesthetic agents bupivacaine and lidocaine in three-dimensional cul-tures of human intervertebral disc nucleus pulposus cells: identification of apoptotic pathways. PLoS One 2014;9(3):e92442.

31. DePalma MJ, Gasper JJ. Cellular supplementation technologies for painful spine disorders. PM R 2015;7(4 Suppl):S19–25.

32. Meisel HJ, Siodla V, Ganey T, et al. Clinical experience in cell-based therapeutics: disc chondrocyte transplantation. A treatment for degenerated or damaged inter-vertebral discs. Biomol Eng 2007;24(1):5–21.

33. Steck E, Bertram H, Abel R, et al. Induction of intervertebral disc-like cells from adult mesenchymal stem cells. Stem Cells 2005;23:403–11.

34. Clarke LE, McConnell JC, Sherratt MJ, et al. Growth differentiation factor 6 and transforming growth factor-beta differentially mediate mesenchymal stem cell differentiation, composition, and micromechanical properties of nucleus pulposus constructs. Arthritis Res Ther 2014;16(2):R67.
35. Yim RL, Lee TJ, Bow CH, et al. A systematic review of the safety and efficacy of mesenchymal stem cells for disc degeneration: insights and future directions for regenerative therapeutics. Stem Cells Dev 2014;23(21):2553–67.
36. Sakai D, Mochida J, Iwashina T, et al. Differentiation of mesenchymal stem cells transplanted to a rabbit degenerative disc model: potential and limitations for stem cell therapy in disc regeneration. Spine (Phila Pa 1976) 2005;30(21): 2379–87.
37. Oehme D, Ghosh P, Shimmon S, et al. Mesenchymal progenitor cells combined with pentosane polysulfate mediating disc regeneration at the time of microdiscectomy: a preliminary study in an ovine model. J Neurosurg Spine 2014;20(6): 657–69.
38. Marfia G, Campanella R, Navone SE, et al. Potential use of human adipose mesenchymal stromal cells for intervertebral disc regeneration: a preliminary study on biglycan-deficient murine model of chronic disc degeneration. Arthritis Res Ther 2014;16(5):457.
39. Hohaus C, Ganey TM, Minkus Y, et al. Cell transplantation in lumbar spine disc degeneration disease. Eur Spine J 2008;17(Suppl 4):S492–503.
40. DePalma MJ. International Spine Intervention Society, Annual Scientific Meeting, Orlando (FL), July 30, 2014.
41. Kang JD, Georgescu HI, McIntyre-Larkin L, et al. Herniated lumbar intervertebral discs spontaneously produce matrix metalloproteinases, nitric oxide, interleukin-6, and prostaglandin E2. Spine (Phila Pa 1976) 1996;21(3):271–7.
42. Tian P, Li ZJ, Fu X, et al. Role of interleukin-17 in chondrocytes of herniated intervertebral lumbar discs. Exp Ther Med 2015;10(1):81–7.
43. Olmarker K, Rydevik B. New information concerning pain caused by herniated disk and sciatica. Exposure to disk tissue sensitizes the nerve roots. Lakartidningen 1998;95(49):5618–22.
44. Olmarker K, Nordborg C, Larsson K, et al. Ultrastructural changes in spinal nerve roots induced by autologous nucleus pulposus. Spine (Phila Pa 1976) 1996; 21(4):411–4.
45. Cuellar JM, Montesano PX, Carstens E. Role of TNF-alpha in sensitization of nociceptive dorsal horn neurons induced by application of nucleus pulposus to L5 dorsal root ganglion in rats. Pain 2004;110(3):578–87.
46. Kang JD, Stefanovic-Racic M, McIntyre LA, et al. Toward a biochemical understanding of human intervertebral disc degeneration and herniation. Contributions of nitric oxide, interleukins, prostaglandin E2, and matrix metalloproteinases. Spine (Phila Pa 1976) 1997;22(10):1065–73.
47. Kato K, Kikuchi S, Konno S, et al. Participation of 5-hydroxytryptamine in pain-related behavior induced by nucleus pulposus applied on the nerve root in rats. Spine (Phila Pa 1976) 2008;33(12):1330–6.
48. Brisby H, Hammer I. Thalamic activation in a disc herniation model. Spine (Phila Pa 1976) 2007;32(25):2846–52.
49. Vadalà G, Sowa G, Hubert M, et al. Mesenchymal stem cells injection in degenerated intervertebral disc: cell leakage may induce osteophyte formation. J Tissue Eng Regen Med 2012;6:348–55.
50. Ahmed TA, Dare EV, Hincke M. Fibrin: a versatile scaffold for tissue engineering applications. Tissue Eng Part B Rev 2008;14(2):199–215.

51. Colombini A, Ceriani C, Banfi G, et al. Fibrin in intervertebral disc tissue engineering. Tissue Eng Part B Rev 2014;20(6):713–21.
52. Schek RM, Michalek AJ, Iatridis JC. Genipin-crosslinked fibrin hydrogels as a potential adhesive to augment intervertebral disc annulus repair. Eur Cell Mater 2011;21:373–83.
53. Buser Z, Liu J, Thorne KJ, et al. Inflammatory response of intervertebral disc cells is reduced by fibrin sealant scaffold in vitro. J Tissue Eng Regen Med 2014;8(1): 77–84.
54. Buser Z, Kuelling F, Liu J, et al. Biological and biomechanical effects of fibrin injection into porcine intervertebral discs. Spine (Phila Pa 1976) 2011;36(18): E1201–9.
55. Yin W, Pauza K, Olan WJ, et al. Intradiscal injection of fibrin sealant for the treatment of symptomatic lumbar internal disc disruption: results of a prospective multicenter pilot study with 24-month follow-up. Pain Med 2014;15(1):16–31.
56. Lencana SM. Lumbar intervertebral disc herniation following experimental intradiscal pressure increase. Acta Neurochir (Wien) 2000;142:669–76.
57. Coric D, Pettine K, Sumich A, et al. Prospective study of disc repair with allogeneic chondrocytes presented at the 2012 Joint Spine Section Meeting. J Neurosurg Spine 2013;18:85–95.
58. Zhang C, Berven SH, Fortin M, et al. Adjacent segment degeneration versus disease after lumbar spine fusion for degenerative pathology: a systematic review with meta-analysis of the literature. Clin Spine Surg 2016;29(1):21–9.

Orthopedic Surgical Options for Joint Cartilage Repair and Restoration

David J. Ruta, MD[a],*, Arturo D. Villarreal, MD[b],
David R. Richardson, MD[b]

KEYWORDS

- Articular cartilage • Microfracture • Osteochondral • Autograft • OAT • Allograft
- Autologous chondrocyte implantation (ACI) • Juvenile particulated

KEY POINTS

- Articular cartilage has limited intrinsic healing ability. The goal of surgical intervention is joint preservation through cartilage repair or restoration.
- Bone marrow stimulation, whole-tissue transplantation, and cell-based strategies are broad treatment concepts for these injuries. Technique variations exist within each division.
- Substantial differences often exist among interventions regarding the size of injury that can be addressed, anatomic location, technical considerations, cost, and expectations. These differences warrant transparent discussion with patients about specific goals of treatment and require at least a basic understanding of available surgical options.

INTRODUCTION

Articular surface injuries present a common and challenging problem for the musculoskeletal physician. This difficulty is secondary to the complex structure of articular cartilage and its limited natural capacity for regeneration.[1–3] Furthermore, these injuries frequently occur in a younger patient population with potential for significant effects on quality of life.[4] Many nonoperative treatment modalities are widely used and typically considered first-line management, though this depends on the size, location, and other injury characteristics. For persistently symptomatic or larger articular injuries, surgical intervention often can provide substantial improvement in symptoms and functional capacity.[1]

There are no commercial/financial conflicts of interest among the authors or external sources of funding to report.
a St. Luke's Department of Orthopedics & Sports Medicine, Duluth, MN, USA; b Department of Orthopaedic Surgery & Biomedical Engineering, University of Tennessee-Campbell Clinic, Memphis, TN, USA
* Corresponding author. 1012 E. Second Street, Level 5, Duluth, MN 55805.
E-mail address: david.j.ruta@gmail.com

Phys Med Rehabil Clin N Am 27 (2016) 1019–1042
http://dx.doi.org/10.1016/j.pmr.2016.06.007
1047-9651/16/© 2016 Elsevier Inc. All rights reserved.

pmr.theclinics.com

Surgical options for chondral and osteochondral injury range from procedures traditionally considered primary or reparative to traditionally secondary or restorative. These procedures include open reduction and internal fixation, bone marrow stimulation, whole-tissue transplantation, and cell-based strategies.[5] The purpose of these techniques is surface reconstitution, with the ideal goal of mature, organized, hyaline cartilage. Some interventions achieve this better than others.

Many of these techniques are performed arthroscopically or with arthroscopic assistance. Vast research has been reported on this broad and evolving field, much of which is from the knee literature. Earlier interventions have naturally received more attention and rigorous study than more recent ones. Many newer developments remain in the early stages of determining indications and long-term outcomes, some with little support for efficacy. Accordingly, reviews of more recently developed interventions are more superficial, though with anticipation of what their potential may hold.

Evaluation of outcomes has been largely through comparative studies of various surgical methods, as the natural history of articular lesions remains poorly defined.[2] In addition, a paucity of randomized controlled trials has made robust comparisons between techniques statistically challenging, and results must be interpreted in this context.[5-8]

With an increasingly large area of injury, arthritic severity, or advancing age, definitive management often is arthroplasty or arthrodesis. There are exceptions to this with the capabilities of bulk osteochondral allografting. As arthroplasty and arthrodesis are considered neither reparative nor restorative, their role is not included in this review.

Of note, considerations of periarticular biomechanical factors, such as malalignment adjacent to the injured joint and soft-tissue deficiencies (meniscus, labrum, and so forth) are extremely important. Although outside the scope of this article, these can strongly influence whether joint salvage will be successful or predicted to fail and must always receive careful consideration in surgical decision-making. These procedures may be performed in a staged or concomitant fashion. Independent of whether these complicating factors are present, transparent discussion between the physician and patient regarding goals is required. This discussion allows review of evidence-based outcomes and provides insight into specific expectations of this typically younger, physically active population.

INDICATIONS

Considering the several joints most commonly affected by chondral injuries and their differing anatomic structure, function, and weight-bearing demands, this injury group represents a heterogeneous population. However, broad, generalized indications for chondral and osteochondral interventions may be inferred from this vast body of investigation. These indications are largely extrapolated from knee literature, though frequently applied to other joints, serving as their framework. Most investigators agree that indications include patient age ranging from skeletal maturity (depending on the procedure) to 40 to 50 years, well-preserved adjacent cartilage surfaces with minimal or no surrounding signs of osteoarthritis, noninflammatory arthritis, focal full-thickness cartilage defects (Modified Outerbridge or International Cartilage Repair Society [ICRS] grade 3 or 4), and patient ability and willingness to participate in a rigorous postoperative physical therapy regimen[2,3,9,10] (Table 1). Defect depth and area guide the decision on surgical technique. A joint-specific example of such considerations for the knee is shown in Table 2. More than one defect may be surgically treated, though outcomes have not been as successful if the lesions are "bipolar" or "kissing (present in the same area, on opposing surfaces of the joint)."[3,11,12]

Table 1
Classification of articular cartilage lesions by severity

Grade	Outerbridge	Modified Outerbridge	ICRS
0	Normal cartilage	Intact cartilage	Intact cartilage
I	Softening and swelling	Chondral softening or blistering with intact surface	Superficial (soft indentation or superficial fissures and cracks)
II	Fragmentation and fissures in area <0.5-in diameter	Superficial ulceration, fibrillation, or fissuring <50% of depth of cartilage	Lesion less than half the thickness of articular cartilage
III	Fragmentation and fissures in area >0.5-in diameter	Deep ulceration, fibrillation, fissuring, or chondral flap >50% of cartilage without exposed bone	Lesion more than half the thickness of articular cartilage
IV	Exposed subchondral bone	Full-thickness wear with exposed subchondral bone	Lesion extending to subchondral bone

Abbreviation: ICRS, International Cartilage Repair Society.
From Canale ST, Beaty JH. Campbell's operative orthopaedics. 12th edition. Philadelphia: Mosby; 2013. p. 2183.

An important consideration must always be the potential for direct repair of a displaced fragment with open reduction and internal fixation (ORIF). Preoperative imaging will determine if this may be possible. If so, this should always be attempted so as to preserve patients' native articular surface (**Fig. 1**). The described lateral inverted osteochondral fracture of the talus (LIFT) lesion is an example of an injury that may be suitable for this technique[13] (**Fig. 2**). The surgeon must ensure that required implants are available at the time of surgery, both for ORIF and an alternative technique if needed. The need for an operative backup plan often accompanies these injuries. The following surgical interventions are indicated when direct reduction and fixation are not possible or have been attempted and failed.

Table 2
Operative treatment of articular cartilage lesions

Lesion Size	Operative Treatment
≤1.0 cm	Observation Abrasion chondroplasty Microfracture Osteochondral autograft transfer
1.0–2.0 cm	Abrasion chondroplasty Microfracture Osteochondral autograft transfer
2.0–3.5 cm	Fresh osteochondral allograft Autologous chondrocyte implantation
3.5–10.0 cm	Autologous chondrocyte implantation
Multiple (2 or 3)	Autologous chondrocyte implantation

From Canale ST, Beaty JH. Campbell's operative orthopaedics. 12th edition. Chapter 45. Philadelphia: Mosby; 2013. p. 2052–211.

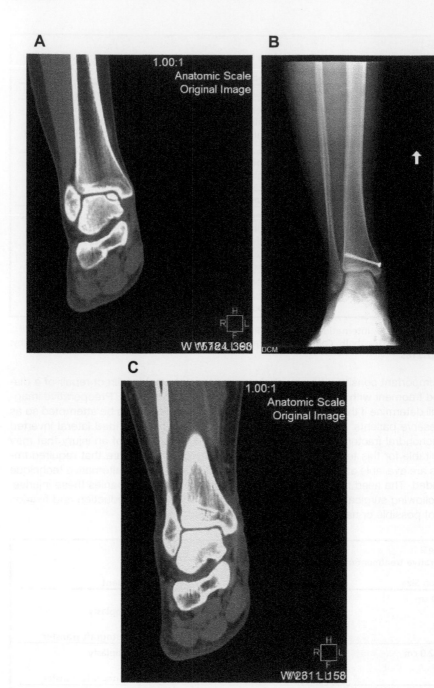

Fig. 1. (*A*) Preoperative computed tomography (CT) of nondisplaced medial talar dome fragment. (*B*) Postoperative radiograph after ORIF with bioabsorbable radiolucent compression screws using a medial malleolar osteotomy, thereby preserving native articular cartilage. The osteotomy was fixed with 2 partially threaded screws as shown. (*C*) Follow-up CT confirming healed talar fragment. Malleolar screws have been removed.

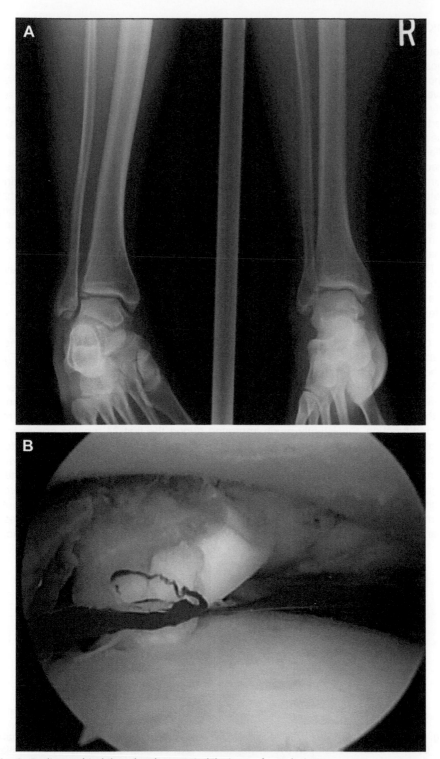

Fig. 2. Radiographic (*A*) and arthroscopic (*B*) views of LIFT lesion.

MICROFRACTURE

Bone marrow stimulation, most commonly with a microfracture (MF) technique, is the most frequently performed first-line surgical management of a small full-thickness chondral defect.[5,14] Rationale for this includes its straightforward and minimally invasive technique, low cost, and low morbidity compared with other interventions.[15] Usually performed arthroscopically, MF involves debridement of the defect to stable and vertical margins, removal of the calcified cartilage layer, and systematic penetration of the subchondral plate with an awl, drill, or pick (**Fig. 3**). This technique achieves medullary bleeding, which releases undifferentiated mesenchymal stem cells and associated growth factors into the defect.[16–18] As a stable, maximally filling clot has been correlated with success of this procedure,[19] it is important that medullary bleeding be confirmed intraoperatively on tourniquet release.[16,20] The technique requires that a sufficient number and depth of channels be produced without altering the subchondral osseous architecture.[21] The clot matures to produce a repaired layer containing some type II cartilage but largely one of fibrocartilage characteristics, especially on analysis 1 year postoperatively.[5,22,23]

The resultant fibrocartilage is a limitation of the technique, as long-term studies have reported inferior wear properties compared with hyaline cartilage and degeneration of this repaired layer with time.[14,24,25] Although the fibrocartilage resulting from MF is inferior to native cartilage, a recent meta-analysis failed to show clear inferiority of MF to more advanced interventions, such as whole-tissue or cell-based techniques, as discussed later.[6] Although there is a large body of data available within the knee literature, there still remains a paucity of long-term outcome studies following MF in other joints, such as the ankle and hip.[9,14]

Most investigators agree with MF as the first-line surgical treatment of full-thickness defects less than 2.5 cm^2 in the knee,[1,14,26,27] 1.5 cm^2 in the talus,[28,29,30] and 4.0 cm^2 in the hip.[9,31] A systematic review of 28 studies with more than 3100 knee patients reported function consistently much improved during the first 24 months postoperatively.[32] More recently, 2 studies reported retained improvement and 7 reported deterioration in 47% to 80% of patients; however, postoperative functional scores still remained higher than preoperative scores. The 9 studies that included MRI reported highly variable degrees of cartilage filling the defect, with functional outcomes scores highly correlated with percentage of fill. Other identified factors predicting good outcomes included age less than 40 years, symptoms less than 12 months, defect less than 4 cm^2, body mass index (BMI) less than 30 kg/m^2, and no previous surgical

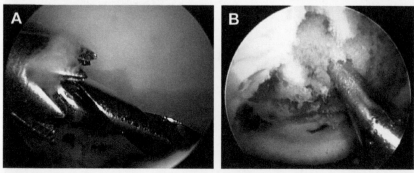

Fig. 3. Arthroscopic views of drill (*A*) and awl (*B*) used for marrow stimulation. (*From* Canale ST, Beaty JH. Campbell's operative orthopaedics. 12th edition. Chapter 45. Philadelphia: Mosby; 2013. p. 2052–211.)

intervention. Histology reports were varied, with a statistical trend toward fibrocartilage as compared with autologous chondrocyte implantation (ACI) ($P = .08$). There was no statistical correlation between histology and clinical outcomes scores, but an association was found between improved histologic appearance and lower failure rate. Revision rates were significantly higher in more methodically strict studies, reported at a mean 8 to 38 months after MF.[33]

Several studies have documented significantly better clinical outcomes following MF in younger patients,[5,34,35] especially those younger than 40 years.[36] Steadman and colleagues[15] identified this in one of the first reports on long-term MF outcomes. In 71 knees followed for 11 years, all in patients aged less than 45 years, they found age to be an independent predictor of functional improvement.

MF in athletes has yielded similar results.[37] Mithoefer and colleagues[34] described deterioration of 47% of elite athletes' knee function at an average of 41 months with only 44% returning to high-impact sports and 57% of these at their preoperative level. Schuman and colleagues[38] reported that 45% of 38 patients with talar osteochondral defects were limited or unable to return to sport at a mean 4.8 years following marrow stimulation. Fourteen of 17 professional hockey players returned to play by 2 years following hip MF, though with decreased number of games played and points scored.[39] With an increasing focus on utilization of health care dollars, Miller and colleagues[40] recently analyzed 3 level 1 or 2 studies with 10-year follow-up, reporting lower initial cost with femoral condyle MF, followed by diminishing savings and overall near-equivalent cost with other techniques for return to play. Contributing to this were cumulative reoperation rates of 28.6% and 12.5% after MF and osteochondral autograft, respectively.

A recent systematic review of 12 arthroscopic hip MF reports including 267 patients with femoroacetabular impingement[31] and 2.5-year follow-up indicated significant improvement for Outerbridge 4 defects. Variability in outcome measures prevented more specific analyses. Similarly, pooled analyses of talar MF is lacking, given individual study variability,[7] though reported long-term outcomes at a mean of 10 years postoperatively have shown 65% of 82 patients with no or mild symptoms. Thirty-three percent have since increased one stage of radiographic arthritis.[24]

Despite limitations of questionable durability and reports of a higher failure rate for cell-based techniques following a failed MF compared with primary cell-based intervention, MF remains the most commonly used first-line surgery.[12,41] This point is especially true considering a lack of clear superiority of any one treatment thus far.[6,33,42,43]

Based on a report of a significantly higher ACI failure rate when done after MF,[44] caution is warranted in using marrow stimulation (with or without augmentation) for larger defects likely to require future ACI surgery, commonly with an area greater than 2.5 cm^2.[33,44]

OSTEOCHONDRAL AUTOGRAFT/MOSAICPLASTY

Bone-to-bone healing has been shown to more reliably integrate than cartilage alone,[1] making osteochondral transplantation an attractive option for chondral or osteochondral defects.[5,14,32] Osteochondral autograft transplantation (OAT) is commonly referenced using various terminology, including the proprietary Osteochondral Autograft Transfer System (OATS) (Arthrex, Naples, FL) and mosaicplasty, the latter denoting transplantation of multiple grafts side by side in a mosaic-type fashion. OAT is a single-stage procedure of harvesting cylindrical osteoarticular plugs of healthy articular cartilage and underlying subchondral bone from an expendable area (typically lesser-weight-bearing portions of an ipsilateral femoral condyle) and transplanting to the symptomatic defect[45] (**Fig. 4**). It is performed both open and arthroscopically. As with microfracture, any unstable area is first debrided back to healthy margins

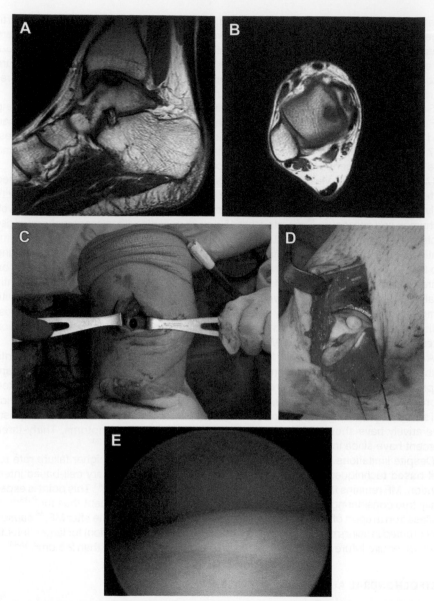

Fig. 4. (*A, B*) Preoperative MRI demonstrating large, uncovered osteochondral lesion of talar dome. (*C*) Osteochondral autograft harvest from ipsilateral knee. (*D*) Graft in place after medial malleolar osteotomy. (*E*) Second-look arthroscopy 15 months postoperatively, showing good incorporation of graft with articular surface restoration.

and then measured to determine the size and number of plugs necessary. The transplanted grafts quickly incorporate to render a restored surface of viable, mature, hyaline cartilage. As one would expect, the single-stage nature and immediate restoration have produced more rapid improvement compared with ACI.[5] Donor sites naturally heal with cancellous bone and overlying fibrocartilage.[5]

OAT indications include failure of bone marrow stimulation or primary use for relatively small to moderately sized areas (<3 cm^2 in knee)[1,44,46] of focal cartilage loss with compromised underlying subchondral bone, including unstable osteochondritis dissecans lesions.[14,47–49] Areas greater than 10 mm typically warrant multiple plugs.[2]

Limitations include limited graft availability; donor-site morbidity; technical factors, including surgical exposure; and differences between donor and recipient joint cartilage, including thickness, contour, and mechanical properties.[4] Reports of harvest-site knee pain have ranged from 0% to 37%.[47] Plugs with depth matched to the defect will be more stable before integration and more likely to heal than a relatively short plug that relies on press-fit frictional forces alone.[50,51] However, grafts left proud by 0.5 to 1.0 mm have shown a 50% increase in mean contact pressures, whereas those flush or slightly depressed restore near-normal contact pressures.[52,53] Care must be taken to achieve the most congruent orientation possible. Integrity of the repair may also be hindered by potential dead space between plugs in mosaicplasty or from graft subsidence on weight bearing.[54]

The exposure required for graft implantation in some locations is a limitation compared with the minimally invasive technique of MF and some cell-based techniques. Exposure for implantation can range from a mini-arthrotomy in the knee[5] to plafondplasty or malleolar osteotomy in the ankle[55] to surgical dislocation of the hip.[9] Likewise, risks of these approaches range from relatively minor to potential for significant morbidity. These risks include arthrofibrosis,[33] osteotomy nonunion,[56] and osteonecrosis of the femoral head.[9] These same approaches are commonly used for some cell-based techniques and allografting.

Long-term analysis of more than 1000 knee and talar mosaicplasty patients with small and medium-sized defects showed good to excellent clinical scores in 92% of femoral condyles, 87% of tibial lesions, 74% of patellar and/or trochlear defects, and 93% of talar implants. At least moderate donor-site complaints were reported in 3% of patients. Eighty-one of 98 follow-up arthroscopies showed congruent gliding surfaces with hyaline cartilage on histology at the transplant site and fibrocartilage at donor sites.[57] Follow-up MRI reports vary, some with excellent fill and congruency within 1 mm in 84% of knees at mean 32.4 months.[58] Other reports of quantitative T2 MRI talar analysis at a mean of 24.8 months have shown persistent differences from native controls.[59]

Gudas and colleagues[32] reported long-term results of a level 1 prospective randomized controlled trial comparing all-arthroscopic OAT to MF in knees of 60 elite athletes (mean age 24.3 years) with 95% follow-up at mean 10.4 years. The average lesion size was 2.8 cm^2 and included both osteochondral and articular-only lesions. Although both groups had decreased clinical scores compared with controls, both still showed significant improvement compared with presurgery scores. The OAT group had significantly better results at the final follow-up ($P<.005$). Fourteen percent of OAT patients had required another operation compared with 38% of MF patients ($P<.05$). The same physical activity level was maintained in 75% of OAT patients but only 37% of MF patients. MRI at 10 years showed complete defect filling in 75% of the OAT group and 35% of the MF group ($P<.05$). Patients aged less than 25 years at the time of surgery showed persistently higher clinical scores at the final follow-up compared with older patients ($P<.05$). Regardless of procedure, defects smaller than 2 cm^2 were associated with a significantly higher rate of return to sports ($P = .04$). Although both techniques allowed a high rate of return to sports, these long-term results support a higher rate of return to preinjury athletic level, maintenance of activity, and lower failure rate with OAT in athletes.

A recent systematic review of OAT outcomes,[60] including 607 patients in 9 level 1 and 2 studies, showed better clinical results from OAT/mosaicplasty when compared with MF, with better maintenance of preoperative activity level, higher rate of return to sports, and fewer reoperations. In comparing OAT with ACI, neither was clearly superior, though a greater failure rate at 10 years was found in the OAT group. The data suggested that OAT may show the most reliable benefit for lesions smaller than 2 cm^2.

OSTEOCHONDRAL ALLOGRAFT

Osteochondral allografting (OCA) uses the same concept of osseous healing and immediate single-stage mature hyaline surface restoration as osteochondral autografting, with the added benefits of a cadaveric source and, therefore, no harvest-site morbidity, much-increased available donor area, and ability to precisely match architecture.[61,62] OCA may be performed in a mosaicplasty fashion (**Fig. 5**) as with OAT or as a bulk allograft (**Fig. 6**). If performed in bulk, the resultant surface is uniform, avoiding potential dead space as with mosaicplasty, which allows use for defects of greater area as well as restoration of large areas of deficient underlying bone stock.

This open surgical technique can be used for a failed previous reparative procedure or as a bulk primary reconstruction for large defects (ie, >2.0–2.5 cm^2),[3,42] including osteonecrosis with segmental collapse,[63] large cystic areas or unreliable underlying structure,[1,14,64] and localized posttraumatic arthritis.[65] A substantial area may be replaced, including an entire femoral condyle in the knee,[3,66] subtotal talar dome,[29,65] and nearly half of the humeral head.[64] When used in carefully selected patients, this technique has the potential to improve functionality and delay or possibly avoid arthrodesis or arthroplasty. OCA remains the only restorative option to address

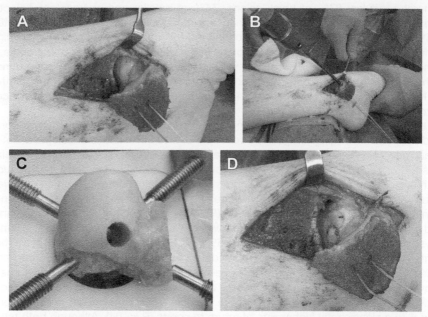

Fig. 5. (A) Intraoperative view of large talar dome lesion following malleolar osteotomy. (B) Reaming of damaged recipient site. (C) Allograft talus after harvest of size- and location-matched osteochondral plug. (D) Allografts in place with mosaicplasty technique for optimal fill.

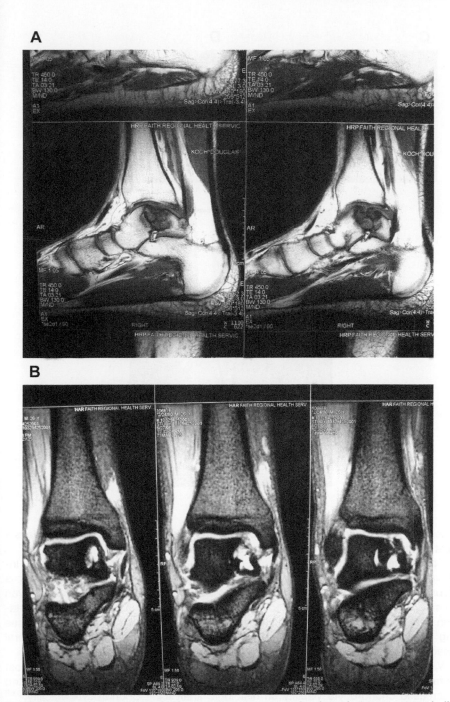

Fig. 6. (*A*, *B*) Preoperative MRI showing very large, cystic, talar dome lesion, requiring bulk allograft. (*C*) Intraoperative view after partial talectomy to remove entire lesion. (*D*) Matching location between excised fragment and donor allograft. (*E*) Postoperative non–weight-bearing radiograph with allograft in place. Graft settling often occurs once weight bearing is initiated.

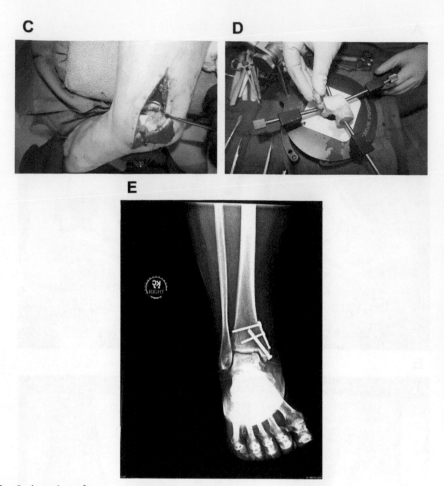

Fig. 6. (*continued*).

failed cell-based therapy or large osteochondritis dissecans lesions[3] and also plays a vital role in reconstruction following tumor resection.[66,67]

Specific techniques of OCA are joint dependent, but the general methodology involves first ensuring availability of a size-matched donor allograft. The lesion is debrided to clearly define its margins and is then resected. Great attention is given to matching the allograft implant to the resected specimen, in both size and orientation. The allograft is inserted with either a press-fit technique or internal fixation (see **Fig. 6**). The latter is more commonly used for larger grafts, including partial humeral head, talar dome, or knee hemicondyle.[64,66]

Various storage methods have been investigated, with fresh allograft the most commonly used.[14] Fresh-frozen and cryopreserved grafts have both demonstrated decreased chondrocyte viability on histologic analysis.[14] Chondrocyte viability[66,68] and incorporation of host bone[3] directly correlate with the success of OCA. Other characteristics associated with favorable long-term outcomes include preservation of the extracellular matrix, robust mechanical stability at the time of implantation, and complete replacement of the graft with host bone, which occurs by creeping substitution.[5] Fresh allografts are maintained in a temperature-controlled environment while undergoing a screening process, which must be both thorough and efficient, given that chondrocyte viability in fresh grafts has been shown to diminish with time.[41] The surgeon and patients are both bound by this time-dependent relationship, requiring flexibility in surgical scheduling.

Limitations of OCA include the cost and availability of allograft tissue, chondrocyte viability following storage, size and contour matching, increased technical difficulty, and the potential for host rejection of the cadaveric graft.[66]

Similar to the previously discussed techniques, available evidence suggests that patients most suitable for OCA are younger (<50 years), without evidence of adjacent osteoarthritis,[9] with larger defects (ie, >2.0–2.5 cm^2 up to 10 cm^2 in large joints), or with substantial subchondral bone compromise.[9,61,62] A defect of this nature can significantly influence quality of life in a younger population, in whom arthroplasty is a poor alternative.[69–71] Likewise, MF and OAT have had suboptimal results in lesions greater than 2 cm^2.[32,43] ACI remains an option for larger lesions in the younger population, although it is multistage and less predictable with certain defect characteristics, such as an unshouldered talar lesion.[3]

Levy and colleagues[72] reported OCA efficacy for both primary and salvage intervention. One hundred twenty-nine knees (121 patients) undergoing femoral condyle OCA showed 82% survivorship at 10 years, 74% at 15 years, and 66% at 20 years. Similar results ranging from 84.5% to 100% at 5 years and 71% to 90% at 10 years have also been reported.[3] In the series by Levy and colleagues,[72] lesions stemming from corticosteroid-induced osteonecrosis produced worse results, a finding supported in other joints as well.[73] Poor results also have been reported with bipolar, large (>10 cm^2), and increasingly chronic lesions and those in the context of primary osteoarthritis or inflammatory arthropathy.[3,4,11]

Younger patients improve more predictably. Murphy and colleagues[74] reported 39 OCA patients (43 femoral condyles) aged 18 years or younger. At 10 years, there was 90% survival with 88% good to excellent clinical outcomes scores and 4 of the 5 failures were salvaged with a revision allograft.

Fresh OCA is used frequently for large talar lesions (>1.5 cm^2) not suitable for other interventions, with moderate success in some subtotal dome defects.[75] Raikin[65] prospectively evaluated 15 patients after fresh allografting of cystic lesions with a volume of 3 cm^3 or greater at a mean follow-up of 44 months. Although clinical function and pain scores were improved, there were radiographic findings of graft resorption in 10 (67%) and joint space narrowing in 9 ankles (60%). Two (13%) required conversion to ankle arthrodesis.

More recently, Haene and colleagues[76] reported allografting 17 ankles with a mean lesion volume of 3.4 cm^3 (range 1.0–10.9 cm^3). The mean follow-up was 4.1 years, with 10 (59%) reporting good to excellent outcome scores, 2 (12%) showing failure of graft incorporation on computed tomography, and overall 5 (29%) ankles considered failures, with 2 requiring reoperation.

Although these studies illustrate the guarded outcomes with use in large-volume talar lesions, this procedure provides a viable option to delay more permanent procedures, such as total ankle arthroplasty or arthrodesis.

AUTOLOGOUS CHONDROCYTE IMPLANTATION/MATRIX AUTOLOGOUS CHONDROCYTE IMPLANTATION

Introduced in the mid-1990s,[77] the goal of ACI is to achieve chondral restoration with hyaline-like cartilage rather than fibrocartilage. Different from previously discussed techniques, the chondral surface is produced in vivo, following transplantation of the patient's own chondrocytes. The process requires a 2-staged procedure, the first involving harvest of chondrocytes (200–300 mg), typically from lesser weight-bearing areas of the distal femur (**Fig. 7**). The harvest site is similar to that used for OAT, though without the need for cylindrical plug harvest, given the cell-based nature of the intervention.[2] The chondrocytes undergo in vitro culture expansion with techniques developed to maintain the chondrocyte phenotype while yielding an increased volume. The second implantation surgery was initially described as an open procedure involving harvest and suturing of a transferred periosteal patch to the defect, under which the cultivated cells were injected. Reports of periosteal patch hypertrophy, cell leakage, uneven transplant distribution, and other unwanted outcomes led to the addition of a structured augment.[5,14]

The second-generation technique involves suspended cultured chondrocytes with a covering of bioabsorbable porcine type-I/III collagen membrane on implantation. The third-generation technique involves implantation on cell-seeded scaffolds, termed *matrix-associated ACI* (MACI).[9,78,79] Various matrices have been described, including type-I collagen gel and hyaluronic acid-based membrane.[80] These matrices are applied through a mini-arthrotomy or with arthroscopic techniques, thereby decreasing the technical difficulty of the procedure while assisting with maintenance of chondrocyte phenotype in vitro and avoiding the morbidity and restrictions that accompany periosteal patch harvest.[5,9]

Although ACI/MACI is largely used following failure of a previous intervention, most commonly bone marrow stimulation,[1] there have been reports of improved outcomes following primary use in larger defects. Minas and colleagues[58] reported ACI to fail at 3 times the rate in defects previously treated with MF compared with nontreated

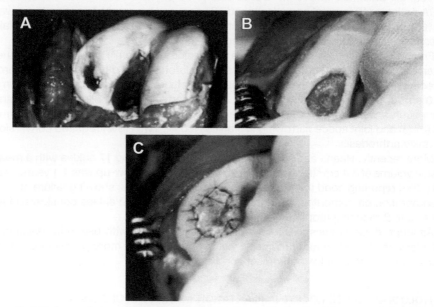

Fig. 7. ACI (second-stage surgery, first-generation technique). (*A*) Large, full-thickness femoral condyle defect with otherwise well-maintained articular surfaces. (*B*) After debridement. (*C*) Previously harvested and expanded chondrocytes are injected deep to sutured periosteal patch. (*From* Canale ST, Beaty JH. Campbell's operative orthopaedics. 12th edition. Philadelphia: Mosby; 2013. p. 2186.)

defects. Most investigators agree that chondrocyte transplantation is best reserved as a second-line option behind MF for lesions of less than 2.5 cm^2 and as a primary option for larger defects. In either situation, advanced degenerative changes are a contraindication.[1,81,82]

Limitations include the need for a 2-stage procedure, increased cost and technical demands, and the long recovery required to allow for transplanted chondrocyte maturation.[5]

Although systematic reviews have shown equivalent outcomes produced between first- and second-generation and between open and arthroscopic ACI techniques, complication rates have been higher with open, periosteal-associated, first-generation methods.[4,6,82]

Bentley and colleagues[63] reported a minimum 10-year follow-up of a controlled randomized study of 100 patients comparing ACI with OAT for treatment of large knee chondral lesions (>3.99 cm^2) with a mean of 1.5 previous surgeries. Those in the ACI group had significantly better functional outcome scores ($P = .02$) and a lower failure rate (17% vs 55%; $P<.001$). Biant and colleagues[83] reported a minimum 10-year follow-up of a prospective series of 104 patients with mean 477 mm^2 knee chondral defects and a mean 1.3 previous surgeries; 26% developed failure of the graft by 5.7 years. Of the surviving grafts, only 63% had excellent results and 25% had good results, though 98 of the 100 patients available at final follow-up would undergo the procedure again.

Some have reported follow-up MRI and histologic analysis both revealing cartilage similar to native controls and covering most of the former defect area.[77,84,85] The resulting layer has been termed *hyaline-like*, as the most superficial layer has still displayed some fibrocartilage properties.[2] However, using quantitative T2 MRI techniques to evaluate the 10-year follow-up of 71 ACI transplant sites, Salzmann and colleagues[86] found significantly decreased imaging scores ($P = .005$) compared with healthy femoral cartilage, despite significant improvement in clinical outcome scores from preoperative values. The investigators, therefore, reported only weak correlation between quantitative imaging and clinical function in this cohort.

Harris and colleagues[82] performed a systematic review of 13 level 1 and 2 studies comparing ACI with other techniques in 917 patients. Three of 7 studies favored ACI over MF up to 3 years, with MF outcomes deteriorating at 18 to 24 months. ACI and OAT showed equivalent short-term outcomes, though OAT patients recovered quicker. A more recent and comprehensive systematic review and meta-analysis[6] of 12 level 1 studies of 765 patients with a mean knee lesion size of 3.9 cm^2 found pooled analysis of ACI and marrow stimulation comparisons to show no difference in clinical outcomes ($P = .16$) or pain ($P = .33$) at 24 months. ACI and OAT comparisons were not suitable for pooled analysis, though 5 of 6 trials found no significant difference in functional outcomes between ACI and OAT. These investigators concluded that there were no significant differences among marrow stimulation, ACI, and OAT in clinical function or pain at the intermediate follow-up. Other systematic analyses have drawn similar conclusions.[2,87] This lack of clear superiority has prompted the recommendation that MF be considered the first-line management in most patients, given its low cost and ease of application.[2]

Long-term data from well-designed level 1 studies are warranted to better characterize outcomes and clarify indications for these various procedures. An example is a current level 1 clinical trial comparing ACI with simple chondral debridement in the knee, with initial data reports still pending.[88]

PARTICULATED JUVENILE ARTICULAR CARTILAGE ALLOGRAFT

Particulated juvenile articular cartilage allograft (PJAC) is a more recent development in cartilage repair. Currently, it is only available commercially as De Novo NT Natural Tissue Graft (Zimmer, Warsaw, IN). Since its introduction in 2007, it has been implanted in more than 10,000 patients.[89]

The allograft tissue consists of articular chondral fragments sized 1 mm^3, harvested from donors aged less than 13 years, though typically less than 2 years without fetal inclusion.[90,91] Juvenile articular cartilage has been shown to have higher proteoglycan content, express collagen type II and IX at significantly higher rates, and yield greater numbers of viable cells compared with adult articular cartilage.[90,92] Both open and arthroscopic techniques have been described. The technique involves preparing the defect with stable vertical margins down through the calcified cartilage layer. The chondral fragments are then applied, using one vial of PJAC per 2.5 cm^2 of defect. Application can be by mixture with fibrin glue in a foil mold of the defect and then inlaid if applied open or direct application of fragments into the defect, followed by fibrin glue if applied arthroscopically.[93] This glue is then allowed to dry for stabilization. Weight bearing is limited for approximately 6 weeks postoperatively, with gradual resumption of weight, strengthening, and then ultimately return to sport, as with other techniques.[90,94,95]

Benefits of PJAC include those of allograft use: relatively simple technique and an ability to treat larger lesions in a single-stage surgery without donor-site morbidity or need for involved surgical approaches for access (ie, malleolar osteotomy for talar access). It does not require violation of the subchondral plate, as with marrow stimulation techniques, which may compromise subsequent ACI outcomes.[58] Limitations include cost and limited outcomes literature.

Well-defined indications remain in evolution. Results are reported in case series and case reports.[96,97] Tompkins and colleagues[98] reported a retrospective series of 15 patellar defects in 13 patients with an average size of 2.4 cm^2. MRI at a mean 28.8 months showed 73% of patients with normal or near-normal repair and 80% with at least 90% coverage. Five patients showed graft hypertrophy. Despite improvement in several outcome scores, patients were not returning to their previous level of sport.[98] Farr and Yao[93] prospectively evaluated 25 knee lesions, including medial and lateral femoral condyles and trochlea. The average size was 2.7 cm^2. Knee outcome measures showed improvement at 2 years. Histologic analysis of 8 arthroscopy samples at 24 months showed a mixture of hyaline and fibrocartilage.[93]

Coetzee and colleagues[99] presented a multicenter series of 24 talar lesions with an average size of 125 ±75 mm^2 and a mean follow-up 16.2 months. Multiple outcome measures were used including American Orthopedic Foot and Ankle Society (AOFAS) Ankle-Hindfoot Scale. AOFAS scores greater than 80 were considered good/excellent. Based on the largest dimension, 10 to 15 mm was considered moderate and greater than 15 mm was considred large. In the moderate group, 12 of 13 had AOFAS scores greater than 80, whereas only 5 of 9 in the large-sized group reported these scores. Similar trends were seen in the other outcome measures.

FUTURE DIRECTIONS

Clinical trials comparing various articular restoration techniques remain ongoing.[100,101] These techniques include MF augmentation with bone marrow aspirate, increased stem cell availability, individual growth factors, altered cytokine profiles, and scaffold addition with the goal of improving the reparative tissue quality.[102–107] Implantation of cultured autologous nasal chondrocytes is another method under current investigation.[108] Although not all effects have been fully characterized or borne out clinically,[109] there have been encouraging results with autologous matrix-induced chondrogenesis. This procedure is a single-stage technique, adding an exogenous scaffold to MF to stabilize the clot. A recent systematic review[33] reported improved prolonged outcomes with the augment, though with a need for a more standardized technique and comparative studies. Stem cell techniques under active investigation include harvest from synovial brushings, bone marrow and peripheral blood mesenchymal stem cells, and adipose stem cells from infrapatellar fat.[110–113]

Distraction arthroplasty has been used for several years with moderate success, largely in younger patients (<45 years of age) with moderate to severe posttraumatic ankle arthritis.[114] The technique involves slight (approximately 5 mm) distraction of the tibiotalar joint using thin-wire external fixation, so as to minimize joint contact pressures. This technique may be performed as an augment, in conjunction with joint debridement, MF, or another previously discussed joint-preservation technique.[115] It is hypothesized that the increased joint space may facilitate improved cell proliferation and differentiation.[116] Both static and hinged applications have been described. The latter allows ankle motion while in place, which has demonstrated improved outcome scores compared with the static application[117], though these benefits may not be long-term.[118] Both typically allow full weight bearing while the frame is in place. Several series have reported improvement in clinical outcomes scores and pain while maintaining motion and reducing radiographic subchondral sclerosis.[114,117,119] Many of these reports indicate improvement in only a moderate number of patients, often with incomplete pain relief. Several reports indicate at least moderate rates of failure and conversion to ankle arthroplasty or arthrodesis.[118,120] Smith and colleagues[120] performed a comprehensive review of 30 articles evaluating treatment results of ankle distraction arthroplasty, reporting insufficient evidence for use of the technique across all of its several commonly accepted indications and concluding that additional high-quality studies are needed.

The KineSpring Knee Implant System (Moximed, Hayward, CA) is an extracapsular, subfascial, load-absorbing device that has had good preliminary results reported from its use in 53 patients with isolated medial knee osteoarthritis.[121] Although only 10 patients have reached the 12-month follow-up thus far, knee outcome subscales have shown significant improvement. Five of the 53 have required reoperation. This device remains under study.

SUMMARY

The limited natural capacity for articular cartilage to regenerate has led to a continuously broadening array of surgical interventions with the shared goals of joint preservation and restoration. Management is guided by the defect's location and characteristics in combination with patient's goals. Although the relationship of specific technique to defect size is joint dependent, most investigators agree with bone marrow stimulation as the first-line surgical treatment of small full-thickness defects. Cell-based techniques or whole-tissue transplantation as autograft or allograft are commonly used for failure of marrow stimulation or as primary treatment of larger defects. Articular surface restoration remains a broad and active area of clinical and basic science research.

REFERENCES

1. Moran CJ, Pascual-Garriido C, Chubinskaya S, et al. Restoration of articular cartilage. J Bone Joint Surg Am 2014;96:336–44.

2. Safran MR, Seiber K. The evidence for surgical repair of articular cartilage in the knee. J Am Acad Orthop Surg 2010;18:259–66.

3. Sherman SL, Garrity J, Bauer K, et al. Fresh osteochondral allograft transplantation for the knee: current concepts. J Am Acad Orthop Surg 2014;22:121–33.

4. Heir S, Nerhus TK, Røtterud JH, et al. Focal cartilage defects in the knee impair quality of life as much as severe osteoarthritis: a comparison of knee injury and osteoarthritis outcome score in 4 patient categories scheduled for knee surgery. Am J Sports Med 2010;38:231–7.

5. Bedi A, Freeley BT, Williams RJ 3rd. Management of articular cartilage defects of the knee. J Bone Joint Surg Am 2010;92:994–1009.

6. Mundi R, Bedi A, Chow L, et al. Cartilage restoration of the knee: a systematic review and meta-analysis of level 1 studies. Am J Sports Med 2016;44(7): 1888–95.

7. Hannon CP, Murawski CD, Fansa AM, et al. Microfracture for osteochondral lesions of the talus: a systematic review of reporting of outcome data. Am J Sports Med 2013;41:689–95.

8. Pinski JM, Boakye LA, Murawski CD, et al. Low level of evidence and methodologic quality of clinical outcome studies on cartilage repair of the ankle. Arthroscopy 2016;32:214–22.

9. El Bitar YF, Lindner D, Jackson TJ, et al. Joint-preserving surgical options for management of chondral injuries of the hip. J Am Acad Orthop Surg 2014;22: 46–56.

10. Mandelbaum BR, Browne JE, Fu F, et al. Articular cartilage lesions of the knee. Am J Sports Med 1998;26:853–61.

11. Meric G, Gracitelli GC, Görtz S, et al. Fresh osteochondral allograft transplantation for bipolar reciprocal osteochondral lesions of the knee. Am J Sports Med 2015;43:709–14.

12. Chahal J, Gross AE, Gross C, et al. Outcomes of osteochondral allograft transplantation in the knee. Arthroscopy 2013;29:575–88.

13. Dunlap BJ, Ferkel RD, Applegate GR. The "LIFT" lesion: lateral inverted osteochondral fracture of the talus. Arthroscopy 2013;29:1826–33.

14. Murawski CD, Kennedy JG. Operative treatment of osteochondral lesions of the talus. J Bone Joint Surg Am 2013;95:1045–54.

15. Steadman JR, Briggs KK, Rodrigo JJ, et al. Outcomes of microfracture for traumatic chondral defects of the knee: average 11-year follow-up. Arthroscopy 2003;19:477–84.

16. Murawski CD, Foo LF, Kennedy JG. A review of arthroscopic bone marrow stimulation techniques of the talus: the good, the bad, and the causes for concern. Cartilage 2010;1:137–44.

17. Takao M, Uchio Y, Kakimaru H, et al. Arthroscopic drilling with debridement of remaining cartilage for osteochondral lesions of the talar dome in unstable ankles. Am J Sports Med 2004;32:332–6.

18. Frisbie DD, Morisset S, Ho CP, et al. Effects of calcified cartilage on healing of chondral defects treated with microfracture in horses. Am J Sports Med 2006; 34:1824–31.

19. Frisbie DD, Oxford JT, Southwood L, et al. Early events in cartilage repair after subchondral bone microfracture. Clin Orthop Relat Res 2003;407:215–27.

20. Steadman JR, Rodkey WG, Rodrigo JJ. Microfracture: surgical technique and rehabilitation to treat chondral defects. Clin Orthop Rela Res 2001;(391 Suppl):S362–9.

21. Bae DK, Yoon KH, Song SJ. Cartilage healing after microfracture in osteoarthritic knees. Arthroscopy 2006;22:367–74.

22. Chuckpaiwong B, Berkson EM, Theodore GH. Microfracture for osteochondral lesions of the ankle: outcome analysis and outcome predictors of 105 cases. Arthroscopy 2008;24:106–12.

23. Furukawa T, Eyre DR, Koide S, et al. Biochemical studies on repair cartilage resurfacing experimental defects in the rabbit knee. J Bone Joint Surg Am 1980; 62:79–89.

24. Gobbi A, Nunag P, Malinowski K. Treatment of full thickness chondral lesions of the knee with microfracture in a group of athletes. Knee Surg Sports Traumatol Arthrosc 2005;13:213–21.

25. Mithoefer K, Williams RJ 3rd, Warren RF, et al. The microfracture technique for the treatment of articular cartilage lesions in the knee. A prospective cohort study. J Bone Joint Surg Am 2005;87:1911–20.

26. Nehrer S, Spector M, Minas T. Histologic analysis of tissue after failed cartilage repair procedures. Clin Orthop Relat Res 1999;365:149–62.

27. Shapiro F, Koide S, Glimcher MJ. Cell origin and differentiation in the repair of full-thickness defects of articular cartilage. J Bone Joint Surg Am 1993;75: 532–53.

28. Choi WJ, Park KK, Kim BS, et al. Osteochondral lesion of the talus: is there a critical defect size for poor outcome? Am J Sports Med 2009;37:1974–80.

29. Hannon CP, Smyth NA, Murawski CD, et al. Osteochondral lesions of the talus: aspects of current management. Bone Joint J 2014;96-B:164–71.

30. Polat G, Ersen A, Erdil ME, et al. Long-term results of microfracture in the treatment of talus osteochondral lesions. Knee Surg Sports Traumatol Arthrosc 2016; 24:1299–303.

31. McDonald AE, Bedi A, Horner NS, et al. Indications and outcomes for microfracture as an adjunct to hip arthroscopy for treatment of chondral defects in patients with femoroacetabular impingement: a systematic review. Arthroscopy 2016;32:190–200.

32. Gudas R, Gudaite A, Pocius A, et al. Ten-year follow-up a prospective, randomized clinical study of mosaic osteochondral autologous transplantation versus microfracture for the treatment of osteochondral defects in the knee joint of athletes. Am J Sports Med 2012;40:2499–508.

33. Mithoefer K, McAdams T, Williams RJ, et al. Clinical efficacy of the microfracture technique for articular cartilage repair in the knee: an evidence-based systematic analysis. Am J Sports Med 2009;37:2053–63.

34. Mithoefer K, Williams RJ 3rd, Warren RF, et al. High-impact athletics after knee articular cartilage repair: a prospective evaluation of the microfracture technique. Am J Sports Med 2006;34:1413–8.

35. Campbell AB, Pineda M, Harris JD, et al. Return to sport after articular cartilage repair in athletes' knee: a systematic review. Arthroscopy 2016;32:651–68.

36. Kreuz PC, Erggelet C, Steinwachs MR, et al. Is microfracture of chondral defects in the knee associated with different results in patients aged 40 years or younger? Arthroscopy 2006;22:1180–6.

37. Minhas SV, Kester BS, Larkin KE, et al. The effect of an orthopaedic surgical procedure in the National Basketball Association. Am J Sports Med 2016;44: 1056–61.

38. Schuman L, Struijs PA, van Dijk CN. Arthroscopic treatment for osteochondral defects of the talus. Results at follow-up at 2 to 11 years. J Bone Joint Surg Br 2002;84:364–8.

39. McDonald JE, Herzog MM, Philippon MJ. Performance outcomes in professional hockey players following arthroscopic treatment of FAI and microfracture of the hip. Knee Surg Sports Traumatol Arthrosc 2014;22:915–9.

40. Miller DJ, Smith MV, Matava MJ, et al. Microfracture and osteochondral autograft transplantation are cost-effective treatments for articular cartilage lesions of the distal femur. Am J Sports Med 2015;43:2175–81.

41. Williams SK, Amiel D, Ball ST, et al. Prolonged storage effects on the articular cartilage of fresh human osteochondral allografts. J Bone Joint Surg Am 2003;85:2111–20.

42. Harris JD, Brophy RH, Siston RA, et al. Treatment of chondral defects in the athlete's knee. Arthroscopy 2010;26:841–52.

43. Knutsen G, Drogset JO, Engebretsen L, et al. A randomized trial comparing autologous chondrocyte implantation with microfracture: findings at five years. J Bone Joint Surg Am 2007;89:2105–12.

44. Lee YH, Suzer F, Thermann H. Autologous matrix-induced chondrogenesis in the knee: a review. Cartilage 2014;5:145–53.

45. Hangody L, Ráthonyi GK, Duska Z, et al. Autologous osteochondral mosaicplasty. Surgical technique. J Bone Joint Surg Am 2004;86(Suppl 1):65–72.

46. Marcacci M, Kon E, Delcogliano M, et al. Arthroscopic autologous osteochondral grafting for cartilage defects of the knee: prospective study results at a minimum 7-year follow-up. Am J Sports Med 2007;35:2014–21.

47. Zengerink M, Struijs PA, Tol JL, et al. Treatment of osteochondral lesions of the talus: a systematic review. Knee Surg Sports Traumatol Arthrosc 2010;18: 238–46.

48. Berlet GC, Mascia A, Miniaci A. Treatment of unstable osteochondritis dissecans lesions of the knee using autogenous osteochondral grafts (mosaicplasty). Arthroscopy 1999;15:312–6.

49. Miniaci A, Tytherleigh-Strong G. Fixation of unstable osteochondritis dissecans lesions of the knee using arthroscopic autogenous osteochondral grafting (mosaicplasty). Arthroscopy 2007;23:845–51.

50. Kock NB, Van Susante JL, Buma P, et al. Press-fit stability of an osteochondral autograft: influence of different plug length and perfect depth alignment. Acta Orthop 2006;77:422–8.

51. Kock NB, Hannink G, van Kampen A, et al. Evaluation of subsidence, chondrocyte survival and graft incorporation following autologous osteochondral transplantation. Knee Surg Sports Traumatol Arthrosc 2011;19:1962–70.

52. Koh JL, Kowalski A, Lautenschlager E. The effect of angled osteochondral grafting on contact pressure: a biomechanical study. Am J Sports Med 2006;34: 116–9.

53. Fansa AM, Murawski CD, Imhauser CW, et al. Autologous osteochondral transplantation of the talus partially restores contact mechanics of the ankle joint. Am J Sports Med 2011;39:2457–65.

54. Kordás G, Szabó JS, Hangody L. Primary stability of osteochondral grafts used in mosaicplasty. Arthroscopy 2006;22:414–21.

55. Garras DN, Santangelo JA, Wang DW, et al. A quantitative comparison of surgical approaches for posterolateral osteochondral lesions of the talus. Foot Ankle Int 2008;29:415–20.

56. Lamb J, Murawski CD, Deyer TW, et al. Chevron-type medial malleolar osteotomy: a functional, radiographic and quantitative T2-mapping MRI analysis. Knee Surg Sports Traumatol Arthrosc 2013;21:1283–8.

57. Hangody L, Vásárhelyi G, Hangody LR, et al. Autologous osteochondral grafting—technique and long-term results. Injury 2008;39(Suppl 1):S32–9.
58. Minas T, Gomoll AH, Rosenberger R, et al. Increased failure rate of autologous chondrocyte implantation after previous treatment with marrow stimulation techniques. Am J Sports Med 2009;37:902–8.
59. Flynn S, Ross KA, Hannon CP, et al. Autologous osteochondral transplantation for osteochondral lesions of the talus. Foot Ankle Int 2016;37:363–72.
60. Lynch TS, Patel RM, Benedick A, et al. Systematic review of autogenous osteochondral transplant outcomes. Arthroscopy 2015;31:746–54.
61. Krych AJ, Lorich DG, Kelly BT. Treatment of focal osteochondral defects of the acetabulum with osteochondral allograft transplantation. Orthopedics 2011;34: e307–11.
62. Williams RJ 3rd, Ranawat AS, Potter HG, et al. Fresh stored allografts for the treatment of osteochondral defects of the knee. J Bone Joint Surg Am 2007; 89:718–26.
63. Bentley G, Blant LC, Vijayan S, et al. Minimum ten-year results of a prospective randomised study of autologous chondrocyte implantation versus mosaicplasty for symptomatic articular cartilage lesions of the knee. J Bone Joint Surg Br 2012;94(4):504–9.
64. Saltzman BM, Riboh JC, Cole BJ, et al. Humeral head reconstruction with osteochondral allograft transplantation. Arthroscopy 2015;31:1827–34.
65. Raikin SM. Fresh osteochondral allografts for large-volume cystic osteochondral defects of the talus. J Bone Joint Surg Am 2009;91:2818–26.
66. De Caro F, Bisicchia S, Amendola A, et al. Large fresh osteochondral allografts of the knee: a systematic clinical and basic science review of the literature. Arthroscopy 2015;31:757–65.
67. Maury AC, Safir O, Heras FL. Twenty-five-year chondrocyte viability in fresh osteochondral allograft. A case report. J Bone Joint Surg Am 2007;89:159–65.
68. Cook JL, Stannard JP, Stoker AM, et al. Importance of donor chondrocyte viability for osteochondral allografts. Am J Sports Med 2016;44(5):1260–8.
69. Keeney JA, Nunley RM, Baca GR, et al. Are younger patients undergoing THA appropriately characterized as active? Clin Orthop Relat Res 2015;473: 1083–92.
70. Keeney JA, Nunley RM, Wright RW, et al. Are younger patients undergoing THA appropriately characterized as active? Clin Orthop Relat Res 2014;472:1210–6.
71. Lonner JH, Hershman S, Mont M, et al. Total knee arthroplasty in patients 40 years of age and younger with osteoarthritis. Clin Orthop Relat Res 2000;380: 85–90.
72. Levy YD, Görtz S, Pulido PA, et al. Do fresh osteochondral allografts successfully treat femoral condyle lesions? Clin Orthop Relat Res 2013;471:231–7.
73. Meyers MH. Resurfacing of the femoral head with fresh osteochondral allografts: long-term results. Clin Orthop Relat Res 1985;197:111–4.
74. Murphy RT, Pennock AT, Bugbee WD. Osteochondral allograft transplantation of the knee in the pediatric and adolescent population. Am J Sports Med 2014;42: 635–40.
75. Gross CE, Adams SB, Easley ME, et al. Role of fresh osteochondral allografts for large talar osteochondral lesions. J Am Acad Orthop Surg 2016;24:e9–17.
76. Haene R, Qamirani E, Story RA, et al. Immediate outcomes of fresh talar osteochondral allografts for treatment of large osteochondral lesions of the talus. J Bone Joint Surg Am 2012;94:1105–10.

77. Battaglia M, Vannini F, Buda R, et al. Arthroscopic autologous chondrocyte implantation in osteochondral lesions of the talus: mid-term T2-mapping MRI evaluation. Knee Surg Sports Traumatol Arthrosc 2011;19:1376–84.
78. Jones CW, Willers C, Keogh A, et al. Matrix-induced autologous chondrocyte implantation in sheep: objective assessments including confocal arthroscopy. J Orthop Res 2008;26:292–303.
79. Goyal D, Goyal A, Keyhani S, et al. Evidence-based status of second- and third-generation autologous chondrocyte implantation over first generation: a systematic review of level I and II studies. Arthroscopy 2013;29:1872–8.
80. Haleem AM, Chu CR. Advances in tissue engineering techniques for articular cartilage repair. Oper Tech Orthop 2010;20:76–89.
81. Niemeyer P, Albrecht D, Andereya S, et al. Autologous chondrocyte implantation (ACI) for cartilage defects of the knee: a guideline by the working group "Clinical Tissue Regeneration" of the German Society of Orthopaedics and Trauma (DGOU). Knee 2016;23(3):426–35.
82. Harris JD, Siston RA, Pan X, et al. Autologous chondrocyte implantation: a systematic review. J Bone Joint Surg Am 2010;92:2220–33.
83. Biant LC, Bentley G, Vijayan S, et al. Long-term results of autologous chondrocyte implantation in the knee for chronic chondral and osteochondral defects. Am J Sports Med 2014;42:2178–83.
84. Giannini S, Buda R, Vannini F, et al. Arthroscopic autologous chondrocyte implantation in osteochondral lesions of the talus: surgical technique and results. Am J Sports Med 2008;36:873–80.
85. Quirbach S, Trattnig S, Marlovits S, et al. Initial results of in vivo high-resolution morphological and biochemical cartilage imaging of patients after matrix-associated autologous chondrocyte transplantation (MACT) of the ankle. Skeletal Radiol 2009;38:751–60.
86. Salzmann GM, Erdel B, Porichis S, et al. Long-term T2 and qualitative MRI morphology after first-generation knee autologous chondrocyte implantation: cartilage ultrastructure is not correlated to clinical or qualitative MRI outcome. Am J Sports Med 2014;42:1832–40.
87. Wasiak J, Clar C, Villanueva E. Autologous cartilage implantation for full thickness articular cartilage defects of the knee. Cochrane Database Syst Rev 2006;(3):CD003323.
88. Randsborg PH, Brinchmann J, Løken S, et al. Focal cartilage defects in the knee -a randomized controlled trial comparing autologous chondrocyte implantation with arthroscopic debridement. BMC Musculoskelet Disord 2016;17:117.
89. De Novo NT Longitudinal Data Collection (LDC) Knee Study (Zimmer Orthobiologics, Inc.) ClinicalTrials.gov NCT01329445. Available at: https://clinicaltrials.gov/ct2/show/NCT01329445?term=NCT01329445&rank=1. Accessed April 1, 2016.
90. Farr J, Tabet SK, Margerrison E, et al. Clinical, radiographic, and histological outcomes after cartilage repair with particulated juvenile articular cartilage: a 2-year prospective study. Am J Sports Med 2014;42:1417–25.
91. Cerrato R. Particulated juvenile articular cartilage allograft transplantation for osteochondral lesions of the talus. Foot Ankle Clin 2013;18:79–87.
92. Tompkins M, Adkisson HD, Bonner KF. DeNovo NT allograft. Oper Tech Sports Med 2013;21:82–9.
93. Farr J, Yao LQ. Chondral defect repair with particulated juvenile cartilage allograft. Cartilage 2011;2:3436–53.

94. Adams SB Jr, Demetracopoulos CA, Parekh SG, et al. Arthroscopic particulated juvenile cartilage allograft transplantation for the treatment of osteochondral lesions of the talus. Arthrosc Tech 2014;3:e533–7.

95. Griffin JW, Gilmore CJ, Miller MD. Treatment of a patellar chondral defect using juvenile articular allograft implantation. Arthrosc Tech 2013;2:e351–4.

96. Stevens HY, Shockley BE, Willett NJ, et al. Particulated juvenile articular cartilage implantation in the knee: a 3-year EPIC-μCT and histological examination. Cartilage 2014;5:74–7.

97. Kruse DL, Ng A, Paden M, et al. Arthroscopic De Novo NT(®) juvenile allograft cartilage implantation in the talus: a case presentation. J Foot Ankle Surg 2012; 51:218–21.

98. Tompkins M, Hamman JC, Diduch DR, et al. Preliminary results of a novel single-stage cartilage restoration technique: particulated juvenile articular cartilage allograft for chondral defects of the patella. Arthroscopy 2013;29:1661–70.

99. Coetzee JC, Giza E, Schon LC, et al. Treatment of osteochondral lesions of the talus with particulated juvenile cartilage. Foot Ankle Int 2013;34:1205–11.

100. Knee articular cartilage repair: cartilage autograft implantation system versus conventional microfracture (CAIS). Clinicaltrial.gov (NCT01498029). Available at: https://clinicaltrials.gov/ct2/show/NCT01498029?term=NCT01498029&rank=1. Accessed April 1, 2016.

101. A study to compare two techniques for articular cartilage repair: ACIC vs MCIC. Clinicaltrials.gov (NCT01984450). Available at: https://clinicaltrials.gov/ct2/show/NCT01984450?term=NCT01984450&rank=1. Accessed April 1, 2016.

102. HyaloFAST trial for repair of articular cartilage in the knee (Fast TRACK). Clinical trials.gov (NCT02659215). Available at: https://clinicaltrials.gov/ct2/show/NCT02659215?term=NCT02659215&rank=1. Accessed April 1, 2016.

103. Confirmatory study of NeoCart in knee cartilage repair. Clinicaltrials.gov (NCT01066702). Available at: https://clinicaltrials.gov/ct2/show/NCT01066702?term=NCT01066702&rank=1. Accessed April 1, 2016.

104. Biphasic cartilage repair implant (BcCRI) IDE clinical trial-Taiwan. Clinicaltrials.-gov (NCT01477008). Available at: https://clinicaltrials.gov/ct2/show/NCT01477008?term=NCT01477008&rank=1. Accessed April 1, 2016.

105. Safety and effectiveness study to evaluate NOVOCART 3D Plus compared to the microfracture to treat articular cartilage defects of the knee (N3D). Clinicaltrials.gov (NCT01656902). Available at: https://clinicaltrials.gov/ct2/show/NCT02203071?term=NCT02203071&rank=1. Accessed April 1, 2016.

106. Comparison of BioCartilage versus marrow stimulating procedure for cartilage defects of the knee. Clinicaltrials.gov (NCT02203071). Available at: https://clinicaltrials.gov/ct2/show/NCT02203071?term=NCT02203071&rank=1. Accessed April 1, 2016.

107. NOVOCART 3D for treatment of articular cartilage of the knee (N3D). Clinicaltrials.gov (NCT01957722). Available at: https://clinicaltrials.gov/ct2/show/NCT01957722?term=NCT01957722&rank=1. Accessed April 1, 2016.

108. Tissue engineered nasal cartilage for regeneration of articular cartilage (Nose2-Knee). Clinicaltrials.gov (NCT01605201). Available at: https://clinicaltrials.gov/ct2/show/NCT01605201?term=NCT01605201&rank=1. Accessed April 1, 2016.

109. Strauss EJ, Barker JU, Kercher JS, et al. Augmentation strategies following the microfracture technique for repair of focal chondral defects. Cartilage 2010;1: 145–52.

110. Synovium brushing to augmented microfracture for improved cartilage repair (AURA). Clinicaltrials.gov (NCT02696876). Available at: https://clinicaltrials.gov/ct2/show/NCT02696876?term=NCT02696876&rank=1. Accessed April 1, 2016.

111. Microfracture versus adipose derived stem cells for the treatment of articular cartilage defects. Clinicaltrials.gov (NCT02090140). Available at: https://clinicaltrials.gov/ct2/show/NCT02090140?term=NCT02090140&rank=1. Accessed April 1, 2016.

112. The use of autologous bone marrow mesenchymal stem cells in the treatment of articular cartilage defects. Clinicaltrials.gov (NCT00891501). Available at: https://clinicaltrials.gov/ct2/show/NCT00891501?term=NCT00891501&rank=1. Accessed April 1, 2016.

113. A study to compare two techniques for articular cartilage repair: cultured chondrocytes vs cultured BMAC (cultured). Clinicaltrials.gov (NCT01961973). Available at: https://clinicaltrials.gov/ct2/show/NCT01961973?term=NCT01961973&rank=1. Accessed April 1, 2016.

114. Barg A, Amendola A, Beaman DN, et al. Ankle joint distraction arthroplasty: why and how? Foot Ankle Clin 2013;18(3):459–70.

115. Tellisi N, Fragomen AT, Kleinman D, et al. Joint preservation of the osteoarthritic ankle using distraction arthroplasty. Foot Ankle Int 2009;30(4):318–25.

116. Yanai T, Ishii T, Chang F, et al. Repair of large full-thickness articular cartilage defects in the rabbit: the effects of joint distraction and autologous bone-marrow-derived mesenchymal cell transplantation. J Bone Joint Surg Br 2005;87(5):721–9.

117. Saltzman CL, Hillis SL, Stolley MP, et al. Motion versus fixed distraction of the joint in the treatment of ankle osteoarthritis: a prospective randomized controlled trial. J Bone Joint Surg Am 2012;94(11):961–70.

118. Nguyen MP, Pedersen DR, Gao Y, et al. Intermediate-term follow-up after ankle distraction for treatment of end-stage osteoarthritis. J Bone Joint Surg Am 2015;87(5):590–6.

119. Intema F, Thomas TP, Anderson DD, et al. Subchondral bone remodeling is related to clinical improvement after joint distraction in the treatment of ankle osteoarthritis. Osteoarthritis Cartilage 2011;19(6):668–75.

120. Smith NC, Beaman D, Rozbruch SR, et al. Evidence-based indications for distraction ankle arthroplasty. Foot Ankle Int 2012;33(8):632–6.

121. Madonna V, Condello V, Piovan G, et al. Use of the KineSpring system in the treatment of medial knee osteoarthritis: preliminary results. Joints 2016;3(3):129–35.

Rehabilitation Considerations in Regenerative Medicine

Penny L. Head, PT, MS, SCS, ATC, CSCS

KEYWORDS

- Regenerative rehabilitation • Mechanotransduction • Mechanotherapy
- Physical therapy • Platelet-rich plasma • Stem cell therapy

KEY POINTS

- Regenerative rehabilitation pairs exercise principles with regenerative therapies to facilitate the regeneration and repair of bone, muscle, cartilage, ligaments, tendons, nerves, and other musculoskeletal tissues.
- Mechanotherapies form one of the largest groups of interventions prescribed by physical therapists with nearly every intervention used introducing mechanical forces.
- A basic understanding of mechanotransduction and the impact of mechanical loading on cellular biology can guide the development of appropriate rehabilitation programs after regenerative therapies.
- Regenerative rehabilitation guides protocols for when to start therapy, types of stimuli administered, and graded exercise programs, taking into account biological factors and technologies designed to optimize healing potential.

INTRODUCTION

Regenerative medicine is an emerging, interdisciplinary field that combines advances in molecular biology, gene therapy, cellular therapy, and tissue engineering to replace or regenerate human cells, tissues, or organs.[1,2] The goal of regenerative medicine is to restore or establish normal function after loss from any cause, including congenital defects, injury, disease, or aging.[2,3] Given that physical rehabilitation shares the same goal, the combination of the 2 approaches may serve to enhance the desired treatment outcomes and could be transformative for individuals with previously untreatable injuries or disorders.[3,4]

Regenerative rehabilitation is defined by the American Physical Therapy Association as "the integration of principles and approaches from rehabilitation and regenerative

Disclosures: None.
Department of Physical Therapy, University of Tennessee Health Science Center, 930 Madison Avenue, Room 604, Memphis, TN 38163, USA
E-mail address: phead2@uthsc.edu

Phys Med Rehabil Clin N Am 27 (2016) 1043–1054
http://dx.doi.org/10.1016/j.pmr.2016.07.002
1047-9651/16/© 2016 Elsevier Inc. All rights reserved.
pmr.theclinics.com

medicine, with the ultimate goal of developing innovative and effective methods that promote the restoration of function through tissue regeneration and repair."[5] Regenerative rehabilitation pairs exercise principles (eg, loading, intensity, frequency, duration), with regenerative therapies to facilitate regeneration and repair of bone, muscle, cartilage, ligaments, tendons, nerves, and other musculoskeletal tissues. This concept requires an interdisciplinary approach between scientists, clinicians, and physical therapists (PTs). In addition, it requires PTs to develop an understanding of the impact of exercise on cellular and molecular biology.

After tissue injury, PTs use targeted exercise therapy to enhance the efficiency of the body's innate healing potential.[6] Properly designed rehabilitation programs can play a critical role in optimizing the incorporation of regenerative therapies into the native tissues. The role of PTs should not be confined to restoring function after tissue regeneration or repair has occurred, because we should also play an active role in facilitating regeneration and repair during the healing process.[1]

MECHANOTHERAPY

The term "mechanotherapy" was initially coined in the 19th century, and defined in the Oxford English Dictionary as "the employment of mechanical means for the cure of disease."[7,8] In 2009, Khan and Scott[7] proposed to update the definition to "the employment of mechanotransduction for the stimulation of tissue repair and remodeling" to highlight the cellular basis of therapeutic exercise prescription for tissue healing. This definition also recognized that injured and healthy tissues may respond differently to mechanical loads.[7]

In 2016, Thompson and colleagues[1] proposed to once again update the definition to "any intervention that introduces mechanical forces with the goal of altering molecular pathways and inducing a cellular response that enhances tissue growth, modeling, remodeling, or repair." This definition highlights the responsiveness to mechanical signals at a multisystem level (ie, molecular level, cellular level, and tissue level) and recognizes the influence of mechanical forces on the processes responsible for tissue development, maintenance, healing, and regeneration.[1]

Mechanotherapies form one of the largest groups of interventions prescribed by PTs. Nearly every intervention used in the practice of physical therapy introduces mechanical forces.[1] Such interventions, including but not limited to, exercise prescription, joint mobilization, soft tissue mobilization, muscle stretching, and even neuromuscular electrical stimulation, provide mechanical stimulation at both the cellular and tissue levels.[7,9] Developing insight into the molecular and cellular responses to the forces used in daily practice will allow PTs to increase understanding of therapeutic dosing and potentially improve clinical outcomes in patients undergoing regenerative therapies.

MECHANOTRANSDUCTION

Mechanotransduction refers to the physiologic process by which cells convert mechanical stimuli into cellular responses.[1,7,10] These cellular responses will, in turn, promote structural adaptation. Mechanotransduction consists of 3 distinct phases: (1) mechanocoupling, (2) cell–cell communication, and (3) the effector response. Mechanocoupling refers to a mechanical stimulus or load that causes physical perturbation to cells.[7] The perturbation may be direct or indirect and can trigger a variety of cellular responses depending on the type, magnitude, frequency, and duration of the load.[11–13] Cells may be exposed to an array of mechanical forces, including tension, compression, shear, hydrostatic pressure, vibration, and fluid shear. The tissue in which a cell resides, as well as the location of the cell within that tissue, will influence the types of mechanical stimuli to which the cell is exposed.[1] The mechanical stimuli are sensed by various mechanosensitive molecular mechanisms that transduce the signal intracellularly. These mechanisms may include cell surface receptors, integrins, focal adhesion complexes, stretch-activated ion channels, growth factor receptors, and the extracellular matrix, to name a few.[10,14-16]

The cell–cell communication phase, sometimes referred to as the signal propagation phase, involves the recruitment of cell signaling pathways and other means of signal spread (eg, cytoskeleton tension) for the biochemical conversion and propagation of the transmitted mechanical signal.[7,17] Just as there are multiple mechanosensitive mechanisms available to sense the mechanical stimulus, there are also multiple signaling pathways that a cell may use to create a biochemical response.[1] The cell signaling pathways are composed of a cascade of multiple potential cytosolic mediators that will transmit the biochemical signal from the cell surface to the effector endpoint.[9]

The final phase of mechanotransduction is the effector response. Once the biochemical signal is transmitted to the effector endpoint, changes in cellular biology occur. If the endpoint is the nucleus, the signal may induce expression of mechanosensitive genes.[1] If the endpoint is effector cells, changes may include an increase or decrease in intracellular tension, changes in adhesive properties, cytoskeletal reorganization, and/or modulation of cellular proliferation, differentiation, migration, and apoptosis.[18]

Eccentric exercise provides an excellent example of the potential impact of mechanotransduction on muscle repair or regeneration. Muscle regeneration depends on a functioning population of satellite cells.[19] Eccentric exercise has been shown to stimulate an array of cellular responses that have the potential to optimize the regenerative process in muscle by stimulating the activation and proliferation of satellite cells. Although the underlying mechanisms are still under investigation, recent studies demonstrate that interstitial nonmyogenic, nonsatellite stem cells, including pericytes, may play an important role in the regenerative process.[20,21]

Although nonmyogenic, pericytes have been shown to secrete a variety of beneficial growth factors and antiinflammatory cytokines (eg, insulinlike growth factor-1, interleukin-6, vascular endothelial growth factor, and hepatocyte growth factor) that activate satellite cells upon extraction from exercised muscle.[22] Valero and colleagues[23] demonstrated an increase in the accumulation of pericytes and an increase in satellite cell number in muscle after acute eccentric exercise in mice. Results of the study suggest that the pericytes upregulate the expression of stem cell markers when subjected to mechanical strain, potentially accounting for the significant increase in the accumulation of satellite cells in muscle after exercise. In addition, the authors demonstrated that pericytes indirectly stimulate new fiber synthesis after injection of muscle-resident mesenchymal stem cells, particularly when recipient mice are exercised immediately before injection. The results of this study provide evidence that coordinated communication between pericytes and satellite cells positively influence muscle regeneration after eccentric exercise.[23]

CLINICAL INTEGRATION OF MECHANOTRANSDUCTION

Recent advances in the field of regenerative medicine, including the use of plateletrich plasma (PRP), stem cell therapy, and tissue engineering provide promising strategies to enhance tissue repair after musculoskeletal injury. The success of these regenerative medicine technologies ultimately depends on the therapies being incorporated into the native tissue and creating a musculoskeletal tissue with enhanced mechanical characteristics.[1] Physical therapy has foundations in the use of targeted mechanical stimuli designed to enhance the intrinsic healing potential of tissue.[3] A basic understanding of mechanotransduction and the impact of mechanical loading on cellular biology can help to guide the development of appropriate rehabilitation programs after the application of regenerative therapies.

Eccentric exercise, as discussed, is 1 form of mechanotherapy that may serve to facilitate tissue healing in conjunction with regenerative therapies. A more recent strategy involving low-load resistance training with blood flow restriction (BFR), may potentially play a role in regenerative rehabilitation. This form of exercise, also referred to as strength training with vascular occlusion, has been shown to increase muscle hypertrophy and strength similar to heavy-load resistance training.[24] BFR training involves decreasing blood flow to a muscle using a wrapping device, such as a blood pressure cuff or specially designed restrictive straps. Muscle hypertrophy has been demonstrated during resistance exercises with intensities as low as 20% of 1 repetition maximum with moderate vascular restriction ($\sim$100 mm Hg).[25] In some studies, BFR training has been applied with high frequency (1–2 sessions per day) and short duration (1–3 weeks), resulting in significant increases in muscle size and strength.[26,27] This form of training could potentially be quite beneficial to patients after regenerative therapies that are unable to tolerate high-intensity resistance training ($\geq$70% 1 repetition maximum).

Although the underlying cellular mechanisms responsible for the adaptive changes in muscle size and strength are largely unknown, recent studies show increased protein synthesis after acute bouts of BFR training, accompanied by posttranslation regulation in the AKT/mammalian target of rapamycin pathway.[27,28] Nielsen and colleagues[26] demonstrated marked proliferation of satellite stem cells and increased number of myonuclei per myofiber with a short-term, high-frequency BFR training program using low-load resistance.

Platelet-Rich Plasma

The use of PRP injections is one of the most common applications of regenerative therapies for musculoskeletal injury. Although originally introduced in the 1970s, the use of PRP injections has increased significantly in recent years, especially for the treatment of sports-related ligament and tendon injuries.[29,30] Rehabilitation protocols after PRP therapy have not been well-outlined in the literature. Although physical therapy is often used after PRP injections, there is little clinical evidence regarding the optimal program design. Virchenko and Aspenberg[31] examined the relationship between mechanical stimulation and tendon healing after PRP injection in the transected Achilles tendons of rats. Results of this study indicated that although PRP improved the material properties of the tendon callus, the effects were lost when the tendon was unloaded mechanically. The authors concluded that mechanical stimulation may be necessary for PRP therapy to be successful. In addition, the study demonstrated that only the early phases of tendon regeneration were influenced by the platelets, stressing the importance of mechanical stimulation early in the process of healing.[31]

The results of the Virchenko and Aspenberg study have led to most rehabilitation protocols endorsing early controlled loading of the tissue after PRP therapy for tendinopathy.[32] Although several studies investigating the efficacy of PRP injection to promote tissue healing have demonstrated improvements in various outcome measures,[33–36] few have described the rehabilitation program or activity level of the involved subjects after PRP therapy. Those that provide a detailed description of post-PRP rehabilitation are often case reports or case series versus randomized controlled trials.[37,38] Although a common recommendation after PRP injection for the treatment of tendon pathology is the use of eccentric exercise, the timing of exercise implementation varies widely.[38–41]

Kaux and colleagues[38] described a standardized rehabilitation program based on submaximal eccentric exercise after PRP injection for patients with patellar tendinopathy. The protocol used 1 week of relative rest before initiating a progressive regimen of closed kinetic chain eccentric quadriceps strengthening performed 3 times per week.[38] Progression of eccentric exercise was based on pain threshold as recommended by Stanish.[42] Results of this case series indicated significant improvements for pain and function, as measured by the visual analog scale, the International Knee Document Committee scale, and the Victorian Institute of Sport Assessment scale.[38]

van Ark and colleagues[41] described a 5-phase rehabilitation program after PRP injection for patients with patellar tendinopathy. The goal of the initial 3 phases was to create conditions to optimize recovery. The final 2 phases focused on loading to optimize return to sport/activity. Gradual progression of the intensity of the exercise program was based on correct execution of exercises and a visual analog scale score of 50 or less on a scale of 0 to 100. Eccentric exercises were implemented in the third phase of the program and were initially performed only twice a week to allow the tendon to adapt to the load.[41] The protocol described by van Ark and colleagues incorporates both concentric and eccentric training, because the combination of both types of training may promote collagen synthesis.[43] In addition, the protocol integrated core stability exercises, because core muscle strength has been found to be important in the load distribution on the patellar tendon.[44] Results of this case-series demonstrated improvements in both pain and function as measured by the visual analog scale and Victorian Institute of Sport Assessment. The results also indicated a potential relationship between patient compliance and improvement in pain and function; the 3 patients with the highest self-reported program compliance demonstrated the greatest improvement in Victorian Institute of Sport Assessment scores, and the 1 patient who did not improve had the lowest self-reported compliance.[41]

Based on the study by Virchenko and Aspenberg,[31] it seems that tendon healing requires a combination of biological and mechanical factors. Rehabilitation after PRP therapy is necessary to provide the mechanical loading component. There are a number of important factors to consider when designing a rehabilitation program after PRP injection. In addition to addressing specific impairments the patient may have, interventions should facilitate the potential synergistic effects of mechanical loading and PRP therapy. Factors to be considered include timing of the initiation of physical therapy after PRP injection, type of exercise (eg, concentric vs eccentric loading), intensity, duration, and frequency. Although treatment should be individualized for each patient after PRP therapy, general guidelines are provided in **Table 1** for rehabilitation after PRP or stem cell therapy for tendon, ligament, and/or articular cartilage. In addition, the rehabilitation protocol after PRP injection for patellar tendinopathy as described by van Ark and colleagues[41] is detailed in **Box 1**.

Stem Cell Therapy

The use of stem cell injections for the purpose of tissue regeneration has received considerably more attention in the last decade.[45,46] Use of stem cells for this purpose is appealing because of their ability to differentiate into a variety of specialized musculoskeletal tissues including bone, cartilage, tendon, ligament, and muscle.[47,48] Key features determining the success of stem cell therapy once injected into the host tissue include the ability of the stem cells to survive and divide, migrate to the site of

Table 1
General guidelines for platelet-rich plasma/stem cell therapy

Phase I—(0–3 d)

Goals	• Protection of affected tissue/joint • Pain control
Precautions	• Limited immobilization and/or unloading of affected joint • Consider sling for shoulder/elbow pathologies • Consider unloading brace for knee osteoarthritis cellular therapies • Consider partial weight-bearing with crutches for lower extremity pathologies • Consider walking boot for ankle/foot pathologies
Suggested interventions	• Begin gentle PROM and AROM exercises out of the immobilizing device • Perform short duration (2–3 min), multiple times per day (3 times/d) • Taping techniques for tendon unloading
Criteria for progression	Minimal pain/discomfort (<50 on VAS) with AROM

Phase II—(3–14 d)

Goals	• Increase tissue tolerance to loading • Discontinue immobilization/unloading
Precautions	• Prevent overstressing affected tissue • Avoid shear stress if articular cartilage pathology • Gradually wean from immobilization • Gradually progress weight-bearing
Suggested Interventions	• Continue PROM and AROM activities for 3–5 min/session, 3–5 times a day • Begin submaximal isometric exercises for affected tendons/joints; maximal isometrics if ligament • Begin progressive loading for lower extremity pathologies (eg, weight shifting, aquatic exercise, zero-gravity treadmill) • Unloaded cycling/upper body ergometer • Well leg/arm conditioning exercises • Core stability exercises • Continuation of taping techniques to unload if tendon pathology
Criteria for progression	• Minimal pain (<50 on VAS) during exercise and ADLs • Pain should decrease after completion of exercise • Normal gait if lower extremity pathology

Phase III—(2–8 wk)

Goals	• Full ROM of affected joint • Increase tissue tolerance to loading • Improve strength/endurance
Precautions	• Avoid impact, high-intensity, or high-velocity activities (eg, jumping, running, throwing, heavy weight lifting) • Avoid postexercise/activity pain
Suggested interventions	• Joint mobilization as needed to restore normal joint arthrokinematics • Stretching of affected muscle–tendon unit (holding 30 s for 3–5 reps) • Progress to isotonic strengthening • Initiate eccentric strengthening with tendon pathology if symptoms allow (<50 on VAS); pain should subside within 24 h; 3–4 d/wk • Dynamic neuromuscular control drills • Cardiovascular exercise with progressive loading (eg, stationary bike, upper body ergometer, elliptical trainer, deep water running, zero gravity treadmill)

(continued on next page)

Table 1 (continued)	
Criteria for progression	• Full ROM • No pain with ADLs • Minimal pain with exercise activity
Phase IV—(≥8 wk)	
Goals	• Increase tolerance of tissue to loading • Good neuromuscular control with activity • Return to sport/work
Precautions	• Minimal pain with activity • Postactivity soreness resolves within 24 h
Suggested interventions	• Progressive strengthening with increased load • Daily eccentric exercises if tendon pathology • Progress neuromuscular control drills • Initiate and progress walk/run program if lower extremity pathology • Initiate and progress plyometric program is applicable to patient • Sport-specific training
Criteria for return to sport/work	• Full ROM • Strength within 85% of contralateral extremity • Good neuromuscular control with activity • No pain with activity

Abbreviations: ADL, activity of daily living; AROM, active range of motion; PROM, passive range of motion; ROM, range of motion; VAS, visual analog scale.

tissue injury, and ultimately differentiate into the targeted tissue of interest.[3] Although rehabilitation protocols after stem cell therapy have not been well-outlined in the literature, a number of studies provide evidence that exercise and physical activity are linked to the activation, mobilization, and differentiation of various types of stem cells.[49–51]

Tissues and cells in the human body are constantly exposed to a mechanical environment. This environment is significantly influenced and changed by exercise training.[52] The integration of exercise after stem cell therapy helps to recruit transplanted stem cells to the site of interest,[53] as well as stimulate activity of endogenous stem cells.[54] Ambrosio and colleagues[55] investigated the effect of exercise on stem cell transplantation to heal injured skeletal muscle in mice. Results of the study demonstrated that 5 weeks of daily treadmill running significantly increased the number of transplanted stem cells. In addition, the majority of the donor cells terminally differentiated toward a myogenic lineage. In the absence of mechanical loading via treadmill running, the transplanted stem cells failed to rapidly divide.[55]

Yamaguchi and colleagues[56] investigated the histologic effect of treadmill exercise on osteochondral defects in rats after intraarticular injection of stem cells. Using the Wakitani cartilage repair scoring system, results of the study demonstrated that exercise after stem cell injection significantly improved cartilage repair, especially at the 4-week timeframe. This study highlights the importance of exercise after stem cell therapy for the treatment of articular cartilage defects.[56]

Aoyama and colleagues[57] demonstrated the feasibility and safety of a 12-week rehabilitation program after mesenchymal stem cell transplantation augmented by vascularized bone grafting for the treatment of idiopathic osteonecrosis of the femoral head. Program design focused on improving hip joint function, avoiding collapse of the femoral head, and promoting bone formation from the transplanted stem cells. The

---

Box 1
Physical therapy program after platelet-rich plasma therapy for patellar tendinopathy

Phase 1—Inflammation/proliferation phase (0–2 weeks)

Inform and advise patient, rest, low load (1× week physical therapy)

Days 1 to 3: Inform and advise patient
- Rest
- Low load (walk with 2 crutches)
- Reduce pain (cryotherapy)

Days 4 to 7: Inform and advise patient
- Optimize ROM if necessary, combined with isometric exercises for m. quadriceps
- Increase activities of daily living with VAS pain score of less than 50

Days 7 to 14: Exercise
- Optimize knee flexion and extension combined with unloaded cycling (hometrainer)
- Walking: 100% load without crutches
- Home exercise program: m. quadriceps isometric contraction, active straight-leg raise, abduction side-lying (2× day, 3 × 20 reps, rest interval 30–60 s)

Pain score must not exceed 50 on the VAS scale during all exercises and activities of daily living

Phase 2—Proliferation phase (weeks 2–4)

More dynamic and active exercises (1 × 2 weeks physical therapy)
- Higher cycling intensity (build up load), goal: 20 to 30 minutes
- Home exercise program
  ○ Squats, calf extensions, single-leg squat with arm swing, abduction side-lying, cycling on home trainer (3 × 20 reps, rest interval 30–60 s)
  ○ Exercises have to be possible (need to be executed) in complete ROM
  ○ Closed chain exercises, mainly coordination and strength endurance; stability plays no major role yet
  ○ Light pain (VAS <50) allowed during exercises; however, the pain must decrease after the exercise

Phase 3—Remodeling phase (weeks 5–6)

Active exercises are expanded (2× week physical therapy)
- Eccentric exercises are integrated into the program
  Home exercise program (on days without supervised physical therapy): 2 days per week
  Single-leg squat on decline board (25°)
- Various exercises (strength endurance) to increase load capacity of lower extremity
  Including hometrainer warm-up, core stability exercises, lunges, abduction side-lying, squats and step-downs (3 × 15 reps, rest interval 30 s)
- Integrate core stability exercises (eg, prone bridge, side bridge)

A pain increase within 48 hours is allowed (VAS <50) but the pain must have disappeared after 48 hours. No leg extension in open chain.

Phase 4—Integration phase (weeks 7–8)

Exercises progressing to higher percent of 1 repetition maximum, 3 × 8 to 15 reps, rest interval 30 s, more muscular hypertrophy (2× week physical therapy)
- Daily eccentric training (2× day, 3 × 20 reps)
- Run-and-walk exercises of increasing intensity and difficulty (starting with interval walking/jogging, advancing to multidirectional, acceleration and deceleration running)
- Jump exercises with increasing difficulty (correct execution with controlled landing important; start with height jumps, progress to long jumps)
- Core stability with greater difficulty
- Sport-specific exercises at maximal and speed strength

Phase 5—Sport-specific phase (After 8th week)

- Daily eccentric training continues (2× day, 3 × 20 reps) until end of supervised physical therapy program (±12 weeks)

- Advance to more sport-specific exercises, for example, plyometric, a-lactic, multidirectional running, acceleration and deceleration

Abbreviations: ROM, range of motion; VAS, visual analog scale.
Data from van Ark M, van den Akker-Scheek I, Meijer LT, et al. An exercise-based physical therapy program for patients with patellar tendinopathy after platelet-rich plasma injection. Phys Ther Sport 2013;14(2):124–30.

rehabilitation program used a combination of passive and active range of motion, progressive weight-bearing, resistance training, and aerobic training, and used evidence from the literature for the progression of these interventions.[57]

Research indicates that implementation of targeted rehabilitation programs after stem cell therapy is necessary to maximize outcomes. Similar to the development of a rehabilitation program after PRP injection, there are a number of important factors to consider when designing a program after stem cell therapy. As stated, in addition to addressing specific impairments the patient may have, interventions should facilitate the potential synergistic effects of mechanical loading and stem cell therapy. Factors to be considered include timing of the initiation of physical therapy after stem cell injection, type of exercise (eg, concentric vs eccentric loading), intensity, duration, and frequency. Refer to **Table 1** for general rehabilitation guidelines after stem cell therapy.

SUMMARY

Rehabilitation coupled with regenerative medicine therapies has shown improved outcomes for tissue regeneration.[6] Regenerative rehabilitation seeks to guide protocols in terms of when to start therapy, types of stimuli administered, and graded exercise programs, while taking into account biological factors and technologies designed to optimize healing potential.[6] Although there are currently no evidence-based guidelines for rehabilitation after regenerative therapies, some fundamental physical therapy principles most likely apply. Immobilization after injury tends to have deleterious effects on musculoskeletal tissues, whereas mechanical loading promotes tissue healing and regeneration.[58–61] Integration of common physical therapy interventions such as passive and active range of motion, joint mobilization, soft tissue mobilization, and exercise prescription may provide beneficial effects after the application of regenerative therapies. Further research is needed to determine optimal rehabilitation protocols to enhance tissue healing and regeneration.

REFERENCES

1. Thompson WR, Scott A, Loghmani MT, et al. Understanding mechanobiology: physical therapists as a force in mechanotherapy and musculoskeletal regenerative rehabilitation. Phys Ther 2015;96(4):560–9.
2. Daar AS, Greenwood HL. A proposed definition of regenerative medicine. J Tissue Eng Regen Med 2007;1(3):179–84.
3. Ambrosio F, Wolf SL, Delitto A, et al. The emerging relationship between regenerative medicine and physical therapeutics. Phys Ther 2010;90(12):1807–14.
4. Perez-Terzic C, Childers MK. Regenerative rehabilitation: a new future? Am J Phys Med Rehabil 2014;93(11 Suppl 3):S73–8.

5. American Physical Therapy Association. Regenerative rehabilitation. Practice and patient care. Available at www.apta.org/RegenerativeRehab/. Accessed October 14, 2015.

6. Norland R, Muchnick M, Harmon Z, et al. Opportunities for regenerative rehabilitation and advanced technologies in physical therapy: perspective from academia. Phys Ther 2015;96(4):550–7.

7. Khan KM, Scott A. Mechanotherapy: how physical therapists' prescription of exercise promotes tissue repair. Br J Sports Med 2009;43(4):247–52.

8. Huang C, Holfeld J, Schaden W, et al. Mechanotherapy: revisiting physical therapy and recruiting mechanobiology for a new era in medicine. Trends Mol Med 2013;19(9):555–64.

9. Dunn SL, Olmedo ML. Mechanotransduction: relevance to physical therapist practice-understanding our ability to affect genetic expression through mechanical forces. Phys Ther 2015;96(5):712–21.

10. Ingber DE. Cellular mechanotransduction: putting all the pieces together again. FASEB J 2006;20(7):811–27.

11. Wall ME, Banes AJ. Early responses to mechanical load in tendon: role for calcium signaling, gap junctions and intercellular communication. J Musculoskelet Neuronal Interact 2005;5(1):70–84.

12. Chiquet M, Renedo AS, Huber F, et al. How do fibroblasts translate mechanical signals into changes in extracellular matrix production? Matrix Biol 2003;22(1):73–80.

13. Zhang H, Labouesse M. Signalling through mechanical inputs: a coordinated process. J Cell Sci 2012;125:3039–49.

14. Matthews BD, Overby DR, Mannix R, et al. Cellular adaptation to mechanical stress: role of integrins, Rho, cytoskeletal tension and mechanosensitive ion channels. J Cell Sci 2006;119:508–18.

15. Schwartz MA. Integrins and extracellular matrix in mechanotransduction. Cold Spring Harb Perspect Biol 2010;2(12):a005066.

16. Zollner AM, Holland MA, Honda KS, et al. Growth on demand: reviewing the mechanobiology of stretched skin. J Mech Behav Biomed Mater 2013;28:495–509.

17. Philp A, Hamilton DL, Baar K. Signals mediating skeletal muscle remodeling by resistance exercise: PI3-kinase independent activation of mTORC1. J Appl Physiol (1985) 2011;110(2):561–8.

18. Jaalouk DE, Lammerding J. Mechanotransduction gone awry. Nat Rev Mol Cell Biol 2009;10(1):63–73.

19. Zou K, De Lisio M, Huntsman HD, et al. Laminin-111 improves skeletal muscle stem cell quantity and function following eccentric exercise. Stem Cells Transl Med 2014;3(9):1013–22.

20. Dellavalle A, Maroli G, Covarello D, et al. Pericytes resident in postnatal skeletal muscle differentiate into muscle fibres and generate satellite cells. Nat Commun 2011;2:499.

21. Birbrair A, Zhang T, Wang ZM, et al. Role of pericytes in skeletal muscle regeneration and fat accumulation. Stem Cells Dev 2013;22(16):2298–314.

22. Boppart MD, De Lisio M, Zou K, et al. Defining a role for non-satellite stem cells in the regulation of muscle repair following exercise. Front Physiol 2013;4:310.

23. Valero MC, Huntsman HD, Liu J, et al. Eccentric exercise facilitates mesenchymal stem cell appearance in skeletal muscle. PLoS One 2012;7(1):e29760.

24. Loenneke JP, Wilson JM, Marin PJ, et al. Low intensity blood flow restriction training: a meta-analysis. Eur J Appl Physiol 2012;112(5):1849–59.

25. Loenneke JP, Young KC, Fahs CA, et al. Blood flow restriction: rationale for improving bone. Med Hypotheses 2012;78(4):523–7.

26. Nielsen JL, Aagaard P, Bech RD, et al. Proliferation of myogenic stem cells in human skeletal muscle in response to low-load resistance training with blood flow restriction. J Physiol 2012;590(17):4351–61.
27. Fujita S, Abe T, Drummond MJ, et al. Blood flow restriction during low-intensity resistance exercise increases S6K1 phosphorylation and muscle protein synthesis. J Appl Physiol (1985) 2007;103(3):903–10.
28. Fry CS, Glynn EL, Drummond MJ, et al. Blood flow restriction exercise stimulates mTORC1 signaling and muscle protein synthesis in older men. J Appl Physiol (1985) 2010;108(5):1199–209.
29. Foster TE, Puskas BL, Mandelbaum BR, et al. Platelet-rich plasma: from basic science to clinical applications. Am J Sports Med 2009;37(11):2259–72.
30. Ahmad Z, Howard D, Brooks RA, et al. The role of platelet rich plasma in musculoskeletal science. JRSM Short Rep 2012;3(6):40.
31. Virchenko O, Aspenberg P. How can one platelet injection after tendon injury lead to a stronger tendon after 4 weeks? Interplay between early regeneration and mechanical stimulation. Acta Orthop 2006;77(5):806–12.
32. Mishra A, Harmon K, Woodall J, et al. Sports medicine applications of platelet rich plasma. Curr Pharm Biotechnol 2012;13(7):1185–95.
33. de Vos RJ, Weir A, van Schie HT, et al. Platelet-rich plasma injection for chronic Achilles tendinopathy: a randomized controlled trial. JAMA 2010;303(2):144–9.
34. Sanchez M, Anitua E, Azofra J, et al. Comparison of surgically repaired Achilles tendon tears using platelet-rich fibrin matrices. Am J Sports Med 2007;35(2):245–51.
35. Peerbooms JC, Sluimer J, Bruijn DJ, et al. Positive effect of an autologous platelet concentrate in lateral epicondylitis in a double-blind randomized controlled trial: platelet-rich plasma versus corticosteroid injection with a 1-year follow-up. Am J Sports Med 2010;38(2):255–62.
36. Mishra A, Pavelko T. Treatment of chronic elbow tendinosis with buffered platelet-rich plasma. Am J Sports Med 2006;34(11):1774–8.
37. Cheatham SW, Kolber MJ, Salamh PA, et al. Rehabilitation of a partially torn distal triceps tendon after platelet rich plasma injection: a case report. Int J Sports Phys Ther 2013;8(3):290–9.
38. Kaux JF, Forthomme B, Namurois MH, et al. Description of a standardized rehabilitation program based on sub-maximal eccentric following a platelet-rich plasma infiltration for jumper's knee. Muscles Ligaments Tendons J 2014;4(1):85–9.
39. Filardo G, Kon E, Della Villa S, et al. Use of platelet-rich plasma for the treatment of refractory jumper's knee. Int Orthop 2010;34(6):909–15.
40. Dragoo JL, Wasterlain AS, Braun HJ, et al. Platelet-rich plasma as a treatment for patellar tendinopathy: a double-blind, randomized controlled trial. Am J Sports Med 2014;42(3):610–8.
41. van Ark M, van den Akker-Scheek I, Meijer LT, et al. An exercise-based physical therapy program for patients with patellar tendinopathy after platelet-rich plasma injection. Phys Ther Sport 2013;14(2):124–30.
42. Stanish WD, Rubinovich RM, Curwin S. Eccentric exercise in chronic tendinitis. Clin Orthop Relat Res 1986;(208):65–8.
43. Kongsgaard M, Kovanen V, Aagaard P, et al. Corticosteroid injections, eccentric decline squat training and heavy slow resistance training in patellar tendinopathy. Scand J Med Sci Sports 2009;19(6):790–802.
44. Kountouris A, Cook J. Rehabilitation of Achilles and patellar tendinopathies. Best Pract Res Clin Rheumatol 2007;21(2):295–316.

45. Giordano A, Galderisi U, Marino IR. From the laboratory bench to the patient's bedside: an update on clinical trials with mesenchymal stem cells. J Cell Physiol 2007;211(1):27–35.
46. Wong RS. Mesenchymal stem cells: angels or demons? J Biomed Biotechnol 2011;2011:459510.
47. Satija NK, Singh VK, Verma YK, et al. Mesenchymal stem cell-based therapy: a new paradigm in regenerative medicine. J Cell Mol Med 2009;13(11–12):4385–402.
48. Caplan AI. Adult mesenchymal stem cells for tissue engineering versus regenerative medicine. J Cell Physiol 2007;213(2):341–7.
49. Dreyer HC, Blanco CE, Sattler FR, et al. Satellite cell numbers in young and older men 24 hours after eccentric exercise. Muscle Nerve 2006;33(2):242–53.
50. Pietrangelo T, Di Filippo ES, Mancinelli R, et al. Low intensity exercise training improves skeletal muscle regeneration potential. Front Physiol 2015;6:399.
51. Svensson RB, Heinemeier KM, Couppe C, et al. The effect of aging and exercise on the tendon. J Appl Physiol (1985) 2016. [Epub ahead of print].
52. Wahl P, Brixius K, Bloch W. Exercise-induced stem cell activation and its implication for cardiovascular and skeletal muscle regeneration. Minim Invasive Ther Allied Technol 2008;17(2):91–9.
53. Palermo AT, Labarge MA, Doyonnas R, et al. Bone marrow contribution to skeletal muscle: a physiological response to stress. Dev Biol 2005;279(2):336–44.
54. Zhang J, Pan T, Liu Y, et al. Mouse treadmill running enhances tendons by expanding the pool of tendon stem cells (TSCs) and TSC-related cellular production of collagen. J Orthop Res 2010;28(9):1178–83.
55. Ambrosio F, Ferrari RJ, Distefano G, et al. The synergistic effect of treadmill running on stem-cell transplantation to heal injured skeletal muscle. Tissue Eng Part A 2010;16(3):839–49.
56. Yamaguchi S, Aoyama T, Ito A, et al. The effect of exercise on the early stages of mesenchymal stromal cell-induced cartilage repair in a rat osteochondral defect model. PLoS One 2016;11(3):e0151580.
57. Aoyama T, Fujita Y, Madoba K, et al. Rehabilitation program after mesenchymal stromal cell transplantation augmented by vascularized bone grafts for idiopathic osteonecrosis of the femoral head: a preliminary study. Arch Phys Med Rehabil 2015;96(3):532–9.
58. Hudelmaier M, Glaser C, Hausschild A, et al. Effects of joint unloading and reloading on human cartilage morphology and function, muscle cross-sectional areas, and bone density - a quantitative case report. J Musculoskelet Neuronal Interact 2006;6(3):284–90.
59. Lloyd SA, Lang CH, Zhang Y, et al. Interdependence of muscle atrophy and bone loss induced by mechanical unloading. J Bone Miner Res 2014;29(5):1118–30.
60. Schepull T, Aspenberg P. Early controlled tension improves the material properties of healing human Achilles tendons after ruptures: a randomized trial. Am J Sports Med 2013;41(11):2550–7.
61. Amiel D, Woo SL, Harwood FL, et al. The effect of immobilization on collagen turnover in connective tissue: a biochemical-biomechanical correlation. Acta Orthop Scand 1982;53(3):325–32.

Index

Note: Page numbers of article titles are in **boldface** type.

Phys Med Rehabil Clin N Am 27 (2016) 1055–1069
http://dx.doi.org/10.1016/S1047-9651(16)30091-2
1047-9651/16/$ – see front matter

1. Publication Title	2. Publication Number	3. Filing Date
PHYSICAL MEDICINE AND REHABILITATION CLINICS OF NORTH AMERICA	009 – 243	9/18/2016

4. Issue Frequency	5. Number of Issues Published Annually	6. Annual Subscription Price
FEB, MAY, AUG, NOV	4	$275.00

7. Complete Mailing Address of Known Office of Publication (Not printer) (Street, city, county, state, and ZIP+4®)

ELSEVIER INC.
360 PARK AVENUE SOUTH
NEW YORK, NY 10010-1710

Contact Person
STEPHEN R. BUSHING

Telephone (Include area code)
215-239-3688

8. Complete Mailing Address of Headquarters or General Business Office of Publisher (Not printer)

ELSEVIER INC.
360 PARK AVENUE SOUTH
NEW YORK, NY 10010-1710

9. Full Names and Complete Mailing Addresses of Publisher, Editor, and Managing Editor (Do not leave blank)

Publisher (Name and complete mailing address)

ADRIANNE BRIGIDO, ELSEVIER INC.
1600 JOHN F KENNEDY BLVD. SUITE 1800
PHILADELPHIA, PA 19103-2899

Editor (Name and complete mailing address)

LAUREN BOYLE, ELSEVIER INC.
1600 JOHN F KENNEDY BLVD. SUITE 1800
PHILADELPHIA, PA 19103-2899

Managing Editor (Name and complete mailing address)

PATRICK MANLEY, ELSEVIER INC.
1600 JOHN F KENNEDY BLVD. SUITE 1800
PHILADELPHIA, PA 19103-2899

10. Owner (Do not leave blank. If the publication is owned by a corporation, give the name and address of the corporation immediately followed by the names and addresses of all stockholders owning or holding 1 percent or more of the total amount of stock. If not owned by a corporation, give the names and addresses of the individual owners. If owned by a partnership or other unincorporated firm, give its name and address as well as those of each individual owner. If the publication is published by a nonprofit organization, give its name and address.)

Full Name	Complete Mailing Address
WHOLLY OWNED SUBSIDIARY OF REED/ELSEVIER, US HOLDINGS	1600 JOHN F KENNEDY BLVD. SUITE 1800 PHILADELPHIA, PA 19103-2899

11. Known Bondholders, Mortgagees, and Other Security Holders Owning or Holding 1 Percent or More of Total Amount of Bonds, Mortgages, or Other Securities. If none, check box ► ☐ None

Full Name	Complete Mailing Address
N/A	

12. Tax Status (For completion by nonprofit organizations authorized to mail at nonprofit rates) (Check one)
The purpose, function, and nonprofit status of this organization and the exempt status for federal income tax purposes:
☐ Has Not Changed During Preceding 12 Months
☐ Has Changed During Preceding 12 Months (Publisher must submit explanation of change with this statement)

13. Publication Title	14. Issue Date for Circulation Data Below
PHYSICAL MEDICINE AND REHABILITATION CLINICS OF NORTH AMERICA	MAY 2016

15. Extent and Nature of Circulation			Average No. Copies Each Issue During Preceding 12 Months	No. Copies of Single Issue Published Nearest to Filing Date
a. Total Number of Copies (Net press run)			280	321
b. Paid Circulation (By Mail and Outside the Mail)	(1)	Mailed Outside-County Paid Subscriptions Stated on PS Form 3541 (Include paid distribution above nominal rate, advertiser's proof copies, and exchange copies)	129	180
	(2)	Mailed In-County Paid Subscriptions Stated on PS Form 3541 (Include paid distribution above nominal rate, advertiser's proof copies, and exchange copies)	0	0
	(3)	Paid Distribution Outside the Mails Including Sales Through Dealers and Carriers, Street Vendors, Counter Sales, and Other Paid Distribution Outside USPS®	57	77
	(4)	Paid Distribution by Other Classes of Mail Through the USPS (e.g. First-Class Mail®)	0	0
c. Total Paid Distribution (Sum of 15b (1), (2), (3), and (4))		►	186	257
d. Free or Nominal Rate Distribution (By Mail and Outside the Mail)	(1)	Free or Nominal Rate Outside-County Copies included on PS Form 3541	11	24
	(2)	Free or Nominal Rate In-County Copies Included on PS Form 3541	0	0
	(3)	Free or Nominal Rate Copies Mailed at Other Classes Through the USPS (e.g. First-Class Mail)	0	0
	(4)	Free or Nominal Rate Distribution Outside the Mail (Carriers or other means)	0	0
e. Total Free or Nominal Rate Distribution (Sum of 15d (1), (2), (3) and (4))		►	11	24
f. Total Distribution (Sum of 15c and 15e)		►	197	281
g. Copies not Distributed (See Instructions to Publishers #4 (page #3))		►	83	40
h. Total (Sum of 15f and g)		►	280	321
i. Percent Paid (15c divided by 15f times 100)		►	94%	91%

* If you are claiming electronic copies, go to line 16 on page 3. If you are not claiming electronic copies, skip to line 17 on page 3.

16. Electronic Copy Circulation	Average No. Copies Each Issue During Preceding 12 Months	No. Copies of Single Issue Published Nearest to Filing Date
a. Paid Electronic Copies ►	0	0
b. Total Paid Print Copies (Line 15c) + Paid Electronic Copies (Line 16a) ►	186	257
c. Total Print Distribution (Line 15f) + Paid Electronic Copies (Line 16a) ►	197	281
d. Percent Paid (Both Print & Electronic Copies) (16b divided by 16c × 100) ►	94%	91%

☒ I certify that 50% of all my distributed copies (electronic and print) are paid above a nominal price.

17. Publication of Statement of Ownership

☒ If the publication is a general publication, publication of this statement is required. Will be printed
in the NOVEMBER 2016 issue of this publication. ☐ Publication not required.

18. Signature and Title of Editor, Publisher, Business Manager, or Owner

STEPHEN R. BUSHING - INVENTORY DISTRIBUTION CONTROL MANAGER

[signature] Stephen R. Bushing   Date 9/18/2016

I certify that all information furnished on this form is true and complete. I understand that anyone who furnishes false or misleading information on this form or who omits material or information requested on the form may be subject to criminal sanctions (including fines and imprisonment) and/or civil sanctions (including civil penalties).

Moving?

Make sure your subscription moves with you!

To notify us of your new address, find your **Clinics Account Number** (located on your mailing label above your name), and contact customer service at:

Email: **journalscustomerservice-usa@elsevier.com**

800-654-2452 (subscribers in the U.S. & Canada)
314-447-8871 (subscribers outside of the U.S. & Canada)

Fax number: **314-447-8029**

Elsevier Health Sciences Division
Subscription Customer Service
3251 Riverport Lane
Maryland Heights, MO 63043

*To ensure uninterrupted delivery of your subscription, please notify us at least 4 weeks in advance of move.

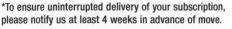